T0297224

Obstetrics: Evidence-Based Algorithms

COMPANION VOLUME:
Gynaecology: Evidence-Based Algorithms
Jyotsna Pundir and Arri Coomarasamy
(ISBN 9781107480698)

Obstetrics: Evidence-Based Algorithms

Jyotsna Pundir

Sub-Speciality Fellow in Reproductive Medicine and Surgery,
St Bartholomew's Hospital, London, UK

Arri Coomarasamy

Professor of Gynaecology, College of Medical and Dental Sciences,
University of Birmingham, and Birmingham Women's
Hospital Foundation Trust, Birmingham, UK

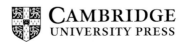

CAMBRIDGE
UNIVERSITY PRESS

University Printing House, Cambridge CB2 8BS, United Kingdom

One Liberty Plaza, 20th Floor, New York, NY 10006, USA

477 Williamstown Road, Port Melbourne, VIC 3207, Australia

4843/24, 2nd Floor, Ansari Road, Daryaganj, Delhi - 110002, India

79 Anson Road, #06-04/06, Singapore 079906

Cambridge University Press is part of the University of Cambridge.

It furthers the University's mission by disseminating knowledge in the pursuit of education, learning and research at the highest international levels of excellence.

www.cambridge.org
Information on this title: www.cambridge.org/9781107618930

First published 2016

A catalogue record for this publication is available from the British Library

Library of Congress Cataloging in Publication data
Pundir, Jyotsna, author.
Obstetrics : evidence-based algorithms / Jyotsna Pundir, Arri Coomarasamy.
  p. ; cm.
ISBN 978-1-107-61893-0 (Paperback)
I. Coomarasamy, Arri, author.   II. Title.
[DNLM: 1. Pregnancy Complications–diagnosis.   2. Pregnancy Complications–therapy.
3. Algorithms.   4. Decision Support Techniques. WQ 240]
RG563
618.2´075–dc23   2014035898

ISBN 978-1-107-61893-0 Paperback

"To my mother for everything I am today, to my husband and two lovely boys for their patience and endless support, to my brothers and in-laws for their faith and encouragement, and finally to my father for his wisdom." Jyotsna

"Dedicated to the memory of Poongo Aunty, who treaded the earth ever so gently." Arri

We would like to acknowledge Dr Justin Chu MBChB MRCOG, Academic Clinical Lecturer, Obstetrics and Gynaecology, College of Medical and Dental Sciences, University of Birmingham; and Helen Williams BSc (Hons), Research Associate, Institute of Metabolism and Systems Research, College of Medical & Dental Sciences, University of Birmingham for their help and time with editing the chapters.

TABLE OF CONTENTS

SECTION 5: Labour and Delivery

SECTION 6: Obstetric Emergencies

SECTION 7: Postnatal Care

SECTION 8: Miscellaneous

Evidence-based medicine is the conscientious, explicit, and judicious use of current best evidence in making decisions about the care of individual patients. With the evolution of evidence-based medicine, and the explosion of medical literature, there has been a continuous stream of guidelines published in obstetrics and gynaecology. These guidelines, designed to provide systematically developed recommendations, assist clinicians and patients in making decisions about appropriate treatment for specific conditions. They also provide crucial information for candidates preparing for the MRCOG examination.

Our attempt is to bring the essential information contained in these guidelines together in these comprehensive books. Where guidelines do not exist, we have relied on available evidence and accepted norms of practice. The information is presented in flowcharts, representing a step-by-step method of solving a clinical problem.

As our books are a revision guide for MRCOG candidates, we have focused primarily on RCOG and other UK national guidelines. However, many chapters contain a 'guideline comparator' box carrying information from other important international guidelines, thus providing an international perspective. Several chapters also contain a 'what not to do' box, which should act as a source of rich debate!

Our desire is that these books act as an essential tool for clinicians and exam candidates. However, they should not replace a close study of the guidelines themselves.

Jyotsna Pundir and Arri Coomarasamy

A1C – haemoglobin A1C
ABC – airway, breathing, circulation
AC – abdominal circumference
ACA – anticardiolipin antibodies
ACE – angiotensin-converting enzyme
ACOG – American Congress of
    Obstetricians and Gynecologists
ACS – acute chest syndrome
ADA – American Diabetes Association
AED – antiepileptic drug
AFC – antral follicle count
AFE – amniotic fluid embolism
AFI – amniotic fluid index
AFP – alpha fetoprotein
AFV – amniotic fluid volume
AIS – androgen insensitivity syndrome
ALP – alkaline phosphatase
ALT – alanine transaminase
AMH – anti-mullerian hormone
AMS – antenatal magnesium sulphate
ANC – antenatal care
ANCS – antenatal corticosteroids
ANP – atrial natriuretic peptide
anti-D Ig – anti-D immunoglobulin
antiHT – antihypertensive
APA – antiphospholipid antibodies
APC – activated protein C
APH – ante partum haemorrhage
APS – antiphospholipid antibody
    syndrome
APTT – activated partial
    thromboplastin time
ARBs – angiotensin II receptor blockers
ARDS – acute respiratory distress
    syndrome
AREDV – absent/reversed EDV
ARM – artificial rupture of membranes
ART – assisted reproductive techniques
ASAP – as soon as possible
ASRM – American Society for
    Reproductive Medicine
AST – aspartate aminotransferase
ATD – antithyroid drug
AV – atrioventricular
BASHH – British Association for Sexual
    Health and HIV
BG – blood glucose
BHIVA – British HIV Association
BMD – bone mass density
BMI – body mass index
BNF – British National Formulary
BNP – brain natriuretic peptide
BP – blood pressure

BPP – biophysical profile
BSO – bilateral salpingo-oopherectomy
BT – blood transfusion
BV – bacterial vaginosis
CAH – congenital adrenal hyperplasia
CC – clomiphene citrate
C-CBT – computerized CBT
C-CBT – computerized cognitive
    behaviour therapy
CEMACE – Centre for Maternal and
    Child Enquiries
CEMACH – Confidential Enquiry into
    Maternal and Child Health
CEMD – Confidential Enquiries into
    Maternal Death
CESDI – Confidential Enquiry into
    Stillbirths and Deaths in Infancy
CHC – combined hormonal contraception
CHD – congenital heart disease
ChT – chemotherapy
CI – cervical incompetence
CIN – cervical intraepithelial neoplasia
CKS – clinical knowledge summaries
CMP – cardiomyopathy
CMV – cytomegalovirus
COC – combined oral contraceptive pill
CRL – crown–rump length
CRP – C-reactive protein
CRS – congenital rubella syndrome
CS – caesarean section
CT – computerized tomography
CTG – cardiotocography
CTP – combined transdermal patch
CTPA – computed tomography
    pulmonary angiogram
Cu IUD – copper intrauterine device
CVP – central venous pressure
CVR – combined vaginal ring
CVS – chorionic villus sampling
DA – diamniotic
DAg – dopamine agonist
DAT – direct antiglobulin test
DBP – diastolic blood pressure
DC – dichorionic
DCDA – dichorionic diamniotic
DEET – di-ethyl 3-methyl benzamide
DHT – dihydrotestosterone
DIC – disseminated intravascular
    coagulation
DKA – diabetic ketoacidosis
DM – diabetes mellitus
DMPA – depot medroxyprogesterone
    acetate

DNA – deoxyribonucleic acid
DO – detruser overactivity
DOH – Department of Health
DR – detection rate
DS – Down syndrome
DSD – disorders of sex development
DtV – ductus venosus
DV – domestic violence
DVT – deep vein thrombosis
E2 – oestradiol
EAS – external anal sphincter
EBL – estimated blood loss
EBV – Epstein–Barr virus
EBW – estimated birth weight
EC – emergency contraception
ECV – external cephalic version
EDD – estimated date of delivery
EE – ethinyl oestradiol
EEG – electroencephalograph
EFM – electronic fetal monitoring
EFW – estimated fetal weight
eGFR – estimated glomerular filtration
    rate
EIN – endometrial intraepithelial
    neoplasia
ELCS – elective caesarean section
EMDR – eye movement desensitization
    and reprocessing
EPAU – early pregnancy assessment unit
EPS – extrapyramidal symptoms
ERCS – elective repeat caesarean section
ESBL – extended-spectrum beta-
    lactamases
ESHRE – European Society of Human
    Reproduction and Embryology
ET – endometrial thickness
EWS – early warning scoring
FAS – fetal alcohol syndrome
FASD – fetal alcohol spectrum disorder
FBC – full blood count
FBG – fasting blood glucose
FBS – fetal blood sampling
fFN – fetal fibronectin
FFP – fresh frozen plasma
FFTS – feto-fetal transfusion syndrome
FGR – fetal growth restriction
FHR – fetal heart rate
FIGO – The International Federation of
    Gynecology and Obstetrics
FISH – fluorescence in situ hybridization
FM – fetal movements
FMH – fetomaternal haemorrhage
FMU – fetal medicine unit

FNAC – fine needle aspiration cytology
FPG – fasting plasma glucose
FPR – false positive rate
Free T4 (fT4) and free T3 (fT3)
FSH – follicle stimulating hormone
FT3 – free T3
FT4 – free T4
FTC – first trimester combined
FTI – free thyroxine index
FTS – first trimester screening
FVS – fetal varicella syndrome
G6PD – glucose-6-phosphate dehydrogenase
GA – general anaesthesia
GAD – generalized anxiety disorder
GAS – group A *Streptococcus*
GBS – group B *Streptococcus*
GCT – glucose challenge test
GDM – gestational diabetes mellitus
GECS – graduated elastic compression stockings
GFR – glomerular filtration rate
GGT – gamma gluta-myltransferase
GIT – gastrointestinal tract
GnRH – gonadotropin-releasing hormone
GnRHa – GnRH agonist
GP – general practitioner
GTT – glucose tolerance test
GUM – genitourinary medicine
HAART – highly active antiretroviral therapy
Hb – haemoglobin
HBIG – hepatitis B specific immunoglobulin
HC – head circumference
hCG – human chorionic gonadotrophin
HCP – healthcare professional
HCV – hepatitis C virus
HDFN – hemolytic disease of the fetus and newborn
HDN – haemolytic disease of newborn
HELLP – haemolysis, elevated liver enzymes, and low platelet count
HER2 – human epidermal growth factor receptor 2
HF – hydrops fetalis
HFI – hormone-free intervals
HIE – hypoxic ischaemic encephalopathy
HIT – heparin-induced thrombocytopenia
HIV – human immunodeficiency virus
HMB – heavy menstrual bleeding
HNIG – human normal immunoglobulin
HNPCC – hereditary non-polyposis colonic cancer
HPA – Health Protection Agency UK
HR – heart rate
HRT – hormone replacement therapy
HSV – herpes simplex virus

HT – hypertension
HTA – Health Technology Assessment
HTAb – hydrothermablation
HVS – high vaginal swab
IADPSG – International Association of Diabetes and Pregnancy Study Groups
IAP – intrapartum antibiotic prophylaxis
IAS – internal anal sphincter
IBS – irritable bowel syndrome
ICS – International Continence Society
ICSI – intracytoplasmic sperm injection
ICU – intensive care unit
ID – iodine deficiency
IDDM – insulin-dependent DM
IFG – impaired fasting glycaemia
Ig – immunoglobulin
IgA – immunoglobulin A
IgG – immunoglobulin G
IgM – immunoglobulin M
IGT – impaired glucose tolerance
IHD – ischaemic heart disease
IM – intramascular
IMB – intermenstrual bleeding
INR – international normalized ratio
IOCS – intraoperative cell salvage
IOL – induction of labour
IPT – interpersonal psychotherapy
ITDM – insulin-treated diabetes
ITU/HDU – intensive therapy unit (ITU)/ high dependency unit (HDU)
IU – international unit
IUCD – intrauterine contraceptive device
IUD – intrauterine device
IUFD – intrauterine fetal death
IUGR – intrauterine growth restriction
IUI – intrauterine insemination
IUP – intrauterine pregnancy
IUS – intrauterine system
IUT – intrauterine transfusion
IV – intravenous
IVF – in vitro fertilization
IVH – intraventricular haemorrhage
IVIG – intravenous immunoglobulins
LAC – a lupus anticoagulant
LARC – long-acting reversible contraception
LB – live birth
LBR – live birth rate
LBW – low birth weight
LDH – lactate dehydrogenase
LFT – liver function test
LH – leutinizing hormone
LLETZ – large loop excision of the transformation zone
LLP – low-lying placenta
LMA – laryngeal mask airway
LMP – last menstrual period
LMWH – low molecular weight heparin
LN – lymph node
LND – lymph node dissection

LNG – levonorgestrel
LNG-IUS – levonorgestrel-releasing intrauterine system
LR – likelihood ratios:
LR– – negative test result
LR+ – positive test result
LSCS – lower segment caesarean section
LVSI – lymphovascular space involvement
MAP – mean arterial pressure
MAS – meconium aspiration syndrome
MBL – major blood loss
MC – monochorionic
MCA – middle cerebral artery
MCDA – monochorionic diamniotic
MCH – mean cell haemoglobin
MCHC – mean cell haemoglobin concentration
MCMA – monochorionic monoamniotic
MCMs – major congenital malformations
MCV – mean cell volume
MDT – multidisciplinary team
MEOWS – modified early obstetric warning system
MI – myocardial infarction
MIS – mullerian inhibitory substance
MLU – midwifery-led unit
MMI – methimazole
MOET – managing obstetric emergencies and trauma
MOH – massive obstetric haemorrhage
MoM – multiples of the median
MP – multiple pregnancy
MRI – magnetic resonance imaging
MRSA – methicillin-resistant *Staphylococcus aureus*
MSAFP – maternal serum alpha fetoprotein
MSL – meconium-stained liquor
MSU – midstream urine
MTHFR – methylene tetrahydrofolate reductase
MTX – methotrexate
MUI – mixed urinary incontinence
MVP – maximum vertical pocket
Mx – management
N – normal
NAATs – nucleic acid amplification tests
NEC – necrotizing enterocolitis
NET – norethisterone
NET-EN – norethisterone enantate
NGU – non-gonococcal urethritis
NICU – neonatal intensive care unit
NIFH – non-immune fetal hydrops
NND – neonatal deaths
NNT – number needed to treat
NPH – isophane
NPV – negative predictive value
NRT – nicotine replacement therapy

NSAID – non-steroidal anti–inflammatory
NSC – National Screening Committee
NT – nuchal translucency
NTDs – neural tube defects
OAB – overactive bladder
OC – obstetric cholestasis
OCD – obsessive–compulsive disorder
OCP – oral contraceptive pill
OGTT – oral glucose tolerance test
OH – overt hypothyroidism
OHSS – ovarian hyperstimulation syndrome
OligoH – oligohydramnios
ONTDs – open neural tube defects
OR – odds ratio
ORACLE – broad-spectrum antibiotics for preterm rupture of the fetal membranes: The ORACLE Randomized Trial
OVD – operative vaginal delivery
PAPP-A – pregnancy-associated plasma protein A
PCB – postcoital bleeding
PCOS – polycystic ovarian syndrome
PCP – *Pneumocystis carinii* pneumonia
PCR – polymerase chain reaction
PCS – planned CS
PCT – progesterone challenge test
PDS – polydiaxanone
PE – pulmonary embolism
PEA – pulseless electrical activity
PEDV – positive end-diastolic velocity
PEmTm – positron emission tomography
PET – pre-eclampsia
PFM – pelvic floor muscles
PFMT – pelvic floor muscle training
PGD – preimplantation genetic diagnosis
PGE2 – prostaglandin E2
PI – pulsatility index
PID – pelvic inflammatory disease
PIH – pregnancy-induced hypertension
PLN – pelvic lymph node
PMB – postmenopausal bleeding
PME – postmortem examination
PMHS – perinatal mental health services
PMS – premenstrual syndrome
PMW – postmenopausal women
PND – prenatal diagnosis
PNM – perinatal mortality
PNMR – perinatal mortality rate
POC – products of conception
POEC – progestogen-only emergency contraception
POF – premature ovarian failure
POICs – progestogen-only injectable contraceptives
POIM – progesterone only implant
POP – progestogen-only pill

POSDIs – progestogen-only subdermal implants
PP – postprandial
PPH – postpartum haemorrhage
PPROM – premature preterm rupture of membranes
PPT – postpartum thyroiditis
PPV – positive predictive value
PRECOG – pre-eclampsia community guideline
PRL – prolactin
PROM – premature rupture of membranes
PSV – peak systolic velocity
PTB – preterm birth
PTD – preterm delivery
PTL – preterm labour
PTSD – post-traumatic stress disorder
PTU – propylthiouracil
PUL – pregnancy of unknown location
PUPP – pruritic urticarial papules and plaques of pregnancy
PVL – periventricular leucomalacia
QF-PCR – quantitative fluorescent PCR
QOL – quality of life
RAADP – routine antenatal anti D prophylaxis
RAI – radioactive iodine
RBC – red blood cell
RBG – random blood glucose
RCOG – Royal College of Obstetricians and Gynaecologists
RCT – randomized controlled trial
RDS – respiratory distress syndrome
RFM – reduced fetal movements
RFT – renal function test
RhD – rhesus D
RI – resistance index
RPG – random plasma glucose
RR – relative risk
RT – radiotherapy
SA – semen analysis
SB – stillbirth
SBP – systolic blood pressure
SC – subcutaneous
SCBU – special care baby unit
SCC – sickle cell crisis
SCD – sickle cell disease
SCH – subclinical hypothyroidism
ScvO$_2$ – central venous oxygen saturation
SDP – single deepest pool
SDVP – single deepest vertical pocket
SFH – symphysis fundal height
SGA – small for gestational age
SHBG – sex hormone-binding globulin
SIDS – sudden infant death syndrome
SLE – systemic lupus erythematosus

SMM – surgical management of miscarriage
SOB – shortness of breath
SOGC – Society of Obstetricians and Gynaecologists of Canada
SPC – summary of product characteristics
SPD – symphysio-pubic dysfunction
SPTB – spontaneous preterm birth
SR – systematic review
SROM – spontaneous rupture of membranes
SSC – secondary sexual characteristic
SSPE – subacute sclerosing panencephalitis
SSRIs – selective serotonin reuptake inhibitors
STI – sexually transmitted infection
STL – second-trimester loss
SUI – stress urinary incontinence
T4 – thyroxine
TAH – total abdominal hysterectomy
TBG – T4-binding globulin
TC – trichorionic
TCAs – tricyclic antidepressants
TCRE – transcervical resection of the endometrium
TE – tracheoesophageal
TEDS – thromboembolic deterrent stockings
TENS – transcutaneous nerve stimulation
TFTs – thyroid function tests
TG – thyroglobulin
TIBC – total iron binding capacity
TNF – tumour necrosis factor
TOP – termination of pregnancy
TORCH – toxoplasmosis, rubella, cytomegalovirus, and herpes
TP – thromboprophylaxis
TPO – thyroid peroxidase
TRAbs – thyroid receptor antibodies
TRAP – twin reversed arterial perfusion
TRH – TSH-releasing hormone
TSAb – thyroid-stimulating antibodies
TSH – thyroid-stimulating hormone
TTN – transient tachypnoea of newborn
TTTS – twin–twin transfusion syndrome
TV – *Trichomonas vaginalis*
TV– transvaginal
TVS – transvaginal scan
U&E – urea and electrolytes
UAE – uterine artery embolization
UDCA – ursodeoxycholic acid
uE3 – unconjugated oestradiol
UI – urinary incontinence
UIC – urinary iodine concentration
UKOSS – United Kingdom Obstetric Surveillance System
UmAD – umbilical artery Doppler

UOP – urine output
UPA – ulipristal acetate
uPCR – urinary protein:creatinine ratio
UPSI – unprotected sexual intercourse
USCL – ultrasound cervical length
USS – ultrasound scan
UtAD – uterine artery Doppler
UTI – urinary tract infection
UUI – urge urinary incontinence

UV – umbilical vein
V/E – vaginal examination
V/Q – ventilation–perfusion lung scan
VA – valproic acid
VBAC – vaginal birth after caesarean
    section
VE – vaginal examination
VF – ventricular fibrillation
VSD – ventricular septal defect

VT – ventricular tachycardia
VTE – venous thromboembolism
VVC – vulvovaginal candidiasis
VZIG – varicella-zoster immunoglobulin
VZV – varicella-zoster virus
WHO – World Health Organization
WWE – woman with epilepsy
ZDV – zidovudine

CHAPTER 1 Prenatal screening for aneuploidy and neural tube defects

- Multiple marker screening uses a combination of maternal age and 2 or more biochemical tests, with or without an USS, to produce a single result for risk of Down syndrome, trisomy 18, and open neural tube defects (ONTDs).
- A screen is positive when the risk of one or more of the screened disorders falls above a designated risk cut-off.
- A risk cut-off – The risk of the condition being present in the fetus at term or at mid-trimester. The risk for the latter will be higher, because 23% of fetuses with Down syndrome are lost between mid-trimester and term (risk cut-off of 1:350 at term would be similar to 1:280 at mid-trimester).

- Detection rate (DR) or sensitivity: The proportion of affected individuals with positive screening results.
- False-positive rate (FPR): The proportion of unaffected individuals with positive screening results. It is the complement of the specificity.
- As screening performance improves, the FPR decreases and/or the DR increases.
- Multiples of the median (MoM): The absolute value of the assayed marker (serum or NT) divided by the gestation-specific median value of the serum marker in the measuring laboratory or by using standard or sonographer-specific curves for NT. This allows direct comparison of results between programmes.

Maternal age

- In the past screening was offered only to women ≥35 years at the EDD. This was considered to be the point at which the risk of a pregnancy loss was less than the chance of identifying a pregnancy with a significant chromosomal abnormality.
- The probability of conceiving a fetus with a trisomy increases with maternal age. However, maternal age screening is inferior to the use of multiple biochemical markers ± a first trimester USS NT assessment. The latter provides a greatly reduced FPR with a substantially improved DR across all age groups.
- Do not use maternal age alone for prenatal screening for aneuploidy.
- Do not offer amniocentesis to women ≥40 years without prior screening, because with a negative screening result, their risk of a chromosomal abnormality remains <1/200.

Factors potentially affecting screening performance

Gestational dating – USS improves the precision of gestational age estimation, and reduces the error for each screening marker. This effect is greater for markers whose concentrations change most with gestational age. For all marker combinations, the FPR is lower by about 2% when gestational age is estimated using a scan.

Insulin-dependent diabetes mellitus – Some second trimester serum markers tend to be lower in women with IDDM. After weight correction, AFP is ~10% lower and uE3 is ~5% lower in diabetic women. NT measurement, free β-hCG, and PAPP-A are not affected.

Ethnic origin – Adjusting for ethnic origin slightly increases the DR for a given FPR. Statistically significant differences in NT measurement have been found between ethnic groups. However, these differences may be too small to warrant correction.

Maternal weight – There is a negative association between the levels of maternal serum markers and maternal weight. With second trimester screening, maternal weight adjustment increases DR by about 1% for a given FPR.

- Weight adjustment is beneficial if there is a marginally elevated AFP when screening for ONTD. Weight adjustment does not appear to be necessary for NT risk adjustment, because it increases by only a clinically insignificant amount with increasing maternal weight.

Assisted reproduction – In the first trimester, a lower value of PAPP-A has been reported in IVF pregnancies, but data on NT and first trimester free β-hCG remain inconsistent.

Invasive prenatal diagnosis

- Offer to women who are at increased risk of fetal aneuploidy:
  * Non-invasive screen result above the risk cut-off.
  * Ultrasound findings.
  * A history of a previous child or fetus with a chromosomal abnormality.
  * Woman/her partner is a carrier of a chromosome rearrangement that increases the risk of having a fetus with a chromosomal abnormality.
- In these scenarios, the risk of a chromosomal abnormality not detected by screening is high enough to offer invasive testing without prior screening.

Screening options

Screen should provide – A DR for Down syndrome of 75% with <3% FPR in the first trimester (UK and SOGC) and a DR of 75% with <5% FPR in the second trimester (SOGC).

First trimester screening

Nuchal translucency (NT)

- NT – The subcutaneous layer of fluid behind the fetal neck and lower cranium visualized on ultrasound. It has a DR for Down syndrome ranging from 69 to 75%, with an FPR of 5–8%.
- Raised NT is also associated with numeric chromosome abnormalities, fetal anomalies such as cardiac defects, diaphragmatic hernia, and single gene disorders associated with decreased fetal movement.
- An NT >99th percentile has a sensitivity of 31% and specificity of 99% for major congenital heart defects when the fetal karyotype is normal. 1 in 33 fetuses with an NT >95th percentile and 1 in 16 with an NT >99th percentile have a major cardiac defect.
- Increased NT at 11–14 weeks with a normal fetal karyotype is an indication for a detailed USS at 18 to 20 weeks, to assess the fetal heart, including a 4-chamber view and view of the outflow tracts or a fetal echocardiogram.

First trimester combined (FTC)

- Maternal age + NT + hCG + PAPP-A
- 2 first trimester maternal serum biochemical markers: PAPP-A and hCG (total). PAPP-A is lower in Down syndrome pregnancies and hCG is higher.
- Combination of the maternal age-related risk, maternal serum PAPP-A, and free β-hCG provides a DR of 61% for Down syndrome, with a 5% FPR.
- Combination of the 2 first trimester biochemical markers with NT has a significant improvement over second trimester triple and quadruple screening.
- FTC detects 78% of cases with a 3% FPR using a term risk cut-off for Down syndrome of 1:300 (83% DR with a 5% FPR).
- FTC also screens for trisomies 13 and 18.

Nasal bone

- USS screening for delayed ossification of the fetal nasal bone in the first or second trimester.
- The first trimester USS, which determines the presence or absence of the nasal bone between 11 and 14 weeks of gestation, may be likely to be incorporated into other screening modalities. It detects 77% of Down syndrome cases.
- The difficulty in performing first trimester nasal bone sonography consistently in the general population might limit the usefulness of this screening technique.

Recommendations

- Given that timing is critical for serum analysis, accurate dating of the pregnancy is very important. Perform USS dating if menstrual or conception dating is unreliable. For any abnormal serum screen calculated on the basis of menstrual dating, perform an USS to confirm gestational age.
- Do not incorporate evaluation of the fetal nasal bone in the first trimester as a screening unless it is performed by sonographers trained and accredited for this service.
- For women who undertake first trimester screening, offer second trimester serum AFP screening and/or USS to screen for ONTDs.
- If local USS services are unable to provide a comprehensive screen for NTDs at 18 to 20 weeks' gestation, in patients undergoing first trimester screening for aneuploidy, offer MSAFP in the second trimester to screen for NTDs.

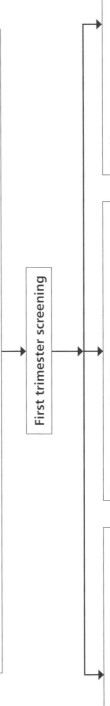

CHAPTER 1   Aneuploidy and neural tube defects

3

SECTION 1 Fetal Conditions

Combined first and second trimester

Integrated prenatal screening (IPS)

- PAPP-A and NT in the first trimester and the quad screen in the second trimester, with results released when all the testing completed.
- DR of 85–87% with an FPR of 0.8–1.5%.
- When Inhibin A is excluded from the IPS, the FPR increases to ~ 2.5%.
- The benefit of IPS over FTS is the achievement of a lower FPR and reduction of the number of invasive diagnostic procedures needed. However it requires two visits and delays results.
- IPS also screens for ONTDs and trisomy 18.

Serum integrated prenatal screening

- PAPP-A in the first trimester and triple or quad screening in the second trimester.
- This has an 83% DR for Down syndrome for a 4% FPR.
- Alternatively, PAPP-A and free β-hCG can be offered in the first trimester, followed by AFP and uE3 in the second with the same performance. The FPR is 4.2% if PAPP-A is measured at 10 completed weeks, and the FPR is doubled (8.5%) if it is measured at 13 completed weeks.
- Serum IPS is a practical option for areas where there is limited or no access to NT screening.

Second trimester screening

Triple marker testing

- Maternal age + MSAFP + unconjugated oestriol (uE3) + hCG measured between 15 and 20 weeks' gestation would detect 65% of fetuses with Down syndrome with a 5% FPR.
- Using a term risk cut-off of 1:385, the triple marker screening detects 72% of fetuses with Down syndrome with a 7% FPR.
- It also screens for ONTDs, other open fetal defects (e.g., gastroschisis, omphalocele), placental dysfunction, Smith–Lemli–Opitz syndrome, and trisomy.

Quadruple testing

- Maternal age + MSAFP + uE3 + hCG + **Inhibin A**
- Inhibin A will increase the DR of Down syndrome by 10%.
- With a risk cut-off of 1:230 at term, the DR is 75–80%, and the FPR is lowered to 3–5%.

Other screening options

Non-invasive prenatal testing (NIPT)

- Cell-free fetal DNA (cffDNA) comes from the placenta and can be detected from the first trimester of pregnancy onwards in maternal circulation. This technology is likely to become the primary screen for chromosomal abnormalities in pregnancy. This will enhance the information available to pregnant women while greatly reducing the loss of uncomplicated pregnancies as a result of miscarriage caused by unnecessary invasive procedures. NIPT is not considered diagnostic as yet. Results from an ongoing study will be used to assess the accuracy of NIPT in the lower-risk population, as the majority of previous studies have looked at high-risk women only. Further evaluation is being undertaken by the UK NSC before it considers whether to adopt NIPT in the NHS.

Contingent screening

- Majority of women receive their result after FTC. Women at high risk (risk >1/50) are offered invasive testing, and women at low risk (risk <1/1500) require no further testing. A proportion of women with a risk between the two cut-offs (1/50 and 1/1500) will go on to have second trimester screening and will receive a combined result.
- It is possible to select risk cut-offs that achieve performances similar to IPS, thus meeting the guideline recommendation, while achieving detection of a significant proportion of abnormal pregnancies by the end of the first trimester.
- It is suggested that contingent screening strategy had the best cost-effectiveness ratio, with fewer procedure-related euploid miscarriages and unnecessary terminations.
- However, the women in the intermediate risk group are likely to experience raised anxiety, and a proportion of them might wish to have an invasive test immediately.

UK National Screening Committee (UKNSC) recommendations for Down syndrome screening programme

- Offer all women screening test(s) with an FPR of <3% and a DR of >75%.
- Screen in the time window of 10 weeks + 0 days to 20 weeks + 0 days' gestation.
- Preferred strategy is to complete screening by 13 weeks + 6 days' gestation.
- Presently there is insufficient evidence for screening strategies for Down syndrome prior to 10 weeks of pregnancy.

First trimester combined (FTC)

- NT + hCG, PAPP-A (same time).
- Early diagnosis; screening is completed in one stage; gives a risk before 14 weeks of pregnancy allowing earlier decision making.
- Biochemistry or USS alone before 13 weeks will not meet the 2007 recommendation for DR.

Integrated testing (IT)

- NT + PAPP-A (1st trim.); hCG (all types), uE, and AFP (2nd trim.).
- Woman needs to attend twice for screening and has to wait until both samples have been processed for a final result.

Serum integrated testing (SIT)

- PAPP-A (1st trim.); hCG (all types), uE, and AFP (2nd trim.)
- Requires two visits but does not include USS NT.
- Women need to wait for a final result.

Quadruple testing (QT)

- hCG (all types), uE3, AFP, and Inhibin A.
- Tests in the second trimester for those women who book late (around 15% of the pregnant population).
- The second trimester screening test that just meets the 2007 recommendation for DR and FPR is the quadruple test.

The full screening window for:

- First trimester PAPP-A test – 10 weeks + 0 days to 13 weeks + 6 days.
- NT measurement – 11 weeks + 0 days to 13 weeks + 6 days.
- Second trimester serum testing – 15 weeks + 0 days to 20 weeks + 0 days.
- The optimal time for the PAPP-A measurement is 9–10 weeks' gestation with the performance of PAPP-A decreasing between 10 and 13 weeks. The proportion of pregnancies in which a satisfactory NT measurement can be obtained is the highest at 11 to 13 weeks' gestation. First trimester measurements are usually carried out between 11 and 14 weeks' gestation as a compromise to make the timing favourable for NT and PAPP-A.

- Offer the 'First trimester combined test' between 11 weeks 0 days and 13 weeks 6 days. For women who book later in pregnancy, offer the most clinically and cost-effective serum screening test (triple or quadruple test) between 15 weeks 0 days and 20 weeks 0 days. (NICE, CGN 62; 2008).
- **Threshold levels for risk measurements** – Categorize individual results as higher or lower risk based on a cut-off of 1 in 200 at term for second trimester screening strategies and 1 in 150 at term for first trimester screening strategies.
- Offer a confirmatory diagnostic test for all screen positive results – amniocentesis/CVS.
- Benchmark timeframe:
  A DR for Down's syndrome of >75% with a FPR of <3% (April 2007 to April 2010).
  A DR of >90% with a FPR of <2% (by April 2010).

This chapter is based on:
Prenatal Screening for Fetal Aneuploidy in Singleton Pregnancies; 2011; Joint SOGC–CCMG Clinical Practice Guidelines.
Screening for Down's syndrome: UK NSC Policy recommendations 2011–2014; Model of Best Practice; NHS Fetal Anomaly Screening Programme.
Antenatal Care – NICE Clinical Guideline 62; 2008.
Non-invasive prenatal testing for chromosomal abnormality using maternal plasma DNA. RCOG Scientific Impact – Paper No. 15; March 2014.
www. rapid.hhs.uk

CHAPTER 2 Routine fetal ultrasound screening

Use of first trimester USS

As part of prenatal screening, 11- to 14-week ultrasounds should be offered on a routine basis. (NICE CGN 62; 2008)

Indications/benefits

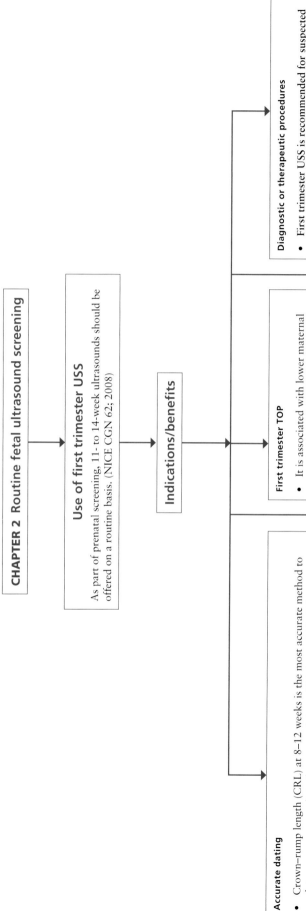

Accurate dating

- Crown–rump length (CRL) at 8–12 weeks is the most accurate method to date pregnancy; predicts the expected date of birth to within 5 days.
- It decreases the number of labour inductions for post-term pregnancy and helps to determine the timing of planned Css to prevent iatrogenic prematurity.
- It is important to assess fetal growth and interpret maternal serum screening.
- First trimester USS is indicated when LMP date is uncertain.

First trimester TOP

- It is associated with lower maternal morbidity than second trimester termination procedures. An inaccurate estimation of gestational age can be avoided by ultrasound examination prior to procedure selection.

Diagnostic or therapeutic procedures

- First trimester USS is recommended for suspected ectopic pregnancy, molar pregnancy, and suspected pelvic mass.
- First trimester USS is recommended during diagnostic or therapeutic procedures requiring visual guidance (e.g., CVS, amniocentesis) and prior to cervical cerclage placement.

Multiple gestation

- USS examination should include number of fetuses, viability, CRLs, chorionicity or amnionicity, and NT assessment.
- Maternal serum screening for aneuploidy is not effective and an NT assessment of risk for each fetus is recommended.
- The accurate diagnosis of a chorionicity in twin pregnancy is important because it selects a subgroup of twin pregnancies at higher risk for twin-to-twin transfusion syndrome, congenital anomalies, FGR, and perinatal mortality.
- First trimester USS is recommended for suspected multiple gestation to allow for reliable determination of chorionicity or amnionicity.

Early fetal anomaly review

- Awareness of variations in anatomical appearance at different gestational ages is essential to avoid false-positive diagnoses of anomalies. In an unselected, low-risk population, first-trimester sonography can detect 63% of structural abnormalities.
- Although routine screening for fetal development at 11 to 14 weeks is not recommended, offer such screening to women at increased risk of fetal structural and genetic abnormalities.
- Offer NT screening as part of a comprehensive prenatal screening and counselling programme. (NICE CGN 62; 2008)

Fetal anomaly screening by USS

The purpose of the anomaly scan

- The main aims are:
  - To identify lethal abnormalities.
  - To plan appropriate management of the pregnancy and delivery. For serious abnormalities there are 4 possible pathways: incompatibility with prolonged life; association with serious morbidity; amenability to postnatal treatment with relatively low morbidity; antenatal treatment.
  - To offer a choice about whether or not to continue with a pregnancy with an abnormal baby.
  - To identify abnormalities for which there may be intrauterine treatments.
  - To identify abnormalities amenable to immediate neonatal treatment.
- About 33 conditions could be looked for by an ultrasound anomaly scan.

- Offer all pregnant women an USS to detect abnormalities in the fetus – NICE CGN 62; 2008; UKNSC.
- Dating scanning is recommended so that the risk for trisomy 21 can be accurately assessed. To some degree the early dating scan is progressing towards being an early anomaly scan that can detect major structural anomalies such as anencephaly and can screen early for trisomy 18 and 13.
- Timing of the fetal anomaly scan – should be undertaken at 18+0 to 20+6 weeks. This allows sufficient time for reassessment and investigation of suspected problems, counselling, and then decision making, before 24 weeks of pregnancy, after which by UK laws TOP needs to be carefully considered.

Structures to be examined to constitute a minimum scan

- Head and neck – skull; neck skin fold (nuchal fold); brain; cavum septum pellucidum; ventricular atrium; cerebellum.
- Face – lips; chest – heart four-chamber view, outflow tracts, lungs.
- Abdomen – Stomach; short intrahepatic section of umbilical vein.
- Abdominal wall; bowel; renal pelvis; spine – vertebrae; skin covering.
- Limbs – femur length; hands; metacarpals (right and left) visible (not counted); feet metatarsals (right and left).
- Amniotic fluid volume; placenta.
- If these structures cannot be imaged sufficiently, refer to a diagnostic unit.
- Measure head circumference (HC), abdominal circumference (AC), and femur length (FL) to assess growth velocity in a pregnancy where the EDD has been assigned in line with nationally approved charts and tables. If the EDD has not been previously assigned then date the pregnancy by HC or FL.

Detection rate

- Although it is used as a screening tool, it is difficult to establish the sensitivity and specificity rates of many conditions because of the paucity of literature. Also prevalence changes with gestational age due to miscarriage or preterm birth.
- However, it is recommended that to screen for a condition, the minimum number needed to be detected by screening should be no lower than 50%.
- Conditions screened for as a minimum in the NHS in England

Condition	Detection rate	Condition	Detection rate
Anencephaly	98%	Gastroschisis	98%
Trisomy 18	95%	Trisomy 13	95%
Open spina bifida	90%	Bilateral renal agenesis	84%
Exomphalos	80%	Diaphragmatic hernia	60%
Cleft lip	75%	Lethal skeletal dysplasia	60%
Serious cardiac abnormalities	50%		

The potential harm

- The anxiety of a false-positive result and the possibility of the loss of a normal fetus following invasive investigation based on false-positive result.
- Offering screening to women who would never choose TOP is also vital as they have a chance to benefit from other options such as fetal therapy (pleural–amniotic shunting for chylothorax or transfusion for anaemia), preparation for postnatal management (changing the place of delivery for cardiac and surgically correctable abnormalities), and psychological preparation in the event that there are no therapeutic options.
- Ultrasound normal variants (soft markers), e.g., choroid plexus cysts, two-vessel cords, and echogenic foci in the heart, can generate distress. The NHS FASP statement (January 2010) – soft markers (normal variants) should not be used to assess the risk for a chromosomal condition or as a screening tool.

Service provision

- All women with a suspected or confirmed fetal anomaly should be seen by an obstetric ultrasound specialist within 3 working days or seen by a FMU within 5 working days of the referral being made.
- All women should be offered a single further scan at 23 weeks of pregnancy to complete the screening examination if the image quality of the first examination is compromised by: increased BMI; uterine fibroids; abdominal scarring; or suboptimal fetal position.
- Where the first examination is suboptimal and the sonographer is suspicious of a possible fetal abnormality, a second opinion should be sought ASAP.

The Use Of First Trimester Ultrasound. SOGC Clinical Practice Guidelines; No. 135, October 2003.

Ward P, Soothill P. Fetal anomaly ultrasound scanning: the development of a national programme for England. The Obstetrician & Gynaecologist 2011;13:211–217.

NHS Fetal Anomaly Screening Programme in collaboration with the Royal College of Obstetricians and Gynaecologists, British Maternal and Fetal Medicine Society and the Society and College of Radiographers. 18+0 to 20+6 Weeks Fetal Anomaly Scan National Standards and Guidance for England. Author Donna Kirwan and The NHS Fetal Anomaly Screening Programme (NHS FASP); 2010.

Antenatal Care. NICE, Clinical Guidance Number 62; 2008.

www.screening.nhs.uk

CHAPTER 2 Routine fetal ultrasound screening

7

CHAPTER 3 Amniocenteses and chorionic villus sampling

Approximately 5% of pregnant women (30 000 women/year in the UK) are offered invasive prenatal diagnostic tests (amniocentesis or CVS).

Amniocenteses – to obtain amniotic fluid

- Perform after 15+0 weeks of gestation.
- Additional risk of miscarriage following amniocentesis is around 1%.
- Blood stained amniotic fluid – 0.5% of cases.
- Systematic review – Post-amniocentesis pregnancy loss (background and procedure related) is 2%.
- 'Early amniocentesis' – Amniocentesis performed before 15 completed weeks of gestation. It has increased pregnancy loss compared with second-trimester amniocentesis and has a higher incidence of talipes when compared with CVS. Therefore, do not offer early amniocentesis.

CVS – aspiration or biopsy of placental villi

- Usually performed between 11+0 and 13+6 weeks of gestation.
- Systematic review – The additional risk of miscarriage following CVS may be slightly higher than that of amniocentesis carried out after 15 weeks of gestation.
- Transabdominal or transcervical – Several RCTs show almost identical miscarriage rates.
- Early CVS – The association between CVS, oromandibular limb hypoplasia, and isolated limb disruption defects is debated. CVS before 11+0 weeks can be technically difficult to perform, owing to a smaller uterus and thinner placenta. Therefore, do not offer CVS before 10+0 weeks of gestation.

Procedure

- Use maximum outer needle gauge size of 0.9 mm (20-gauge).
- With 'USS guidance' visualize the position of the placenta and the umbilical cord insertion prior to amniocentesis and note a suitable entry point on the mother's abdomen. The use of real-time ultrasound allows the insertion of the needle under 'continuous ultrasound control' and is the technique of choice. It reduces blood staining from 2.4% to 0.8%, has greater success in obtaining amniotic fluid, and reduces the risk of maternal bowel injury.
- Avoid transplacental passage of the amniocentesis needle unless it provides the only safe access to an adequate pool of liquor. Under these circumstances, place the needle through the thinnest available part of the placenta. Ensure that the placental cord insertion is avoided. Penetration of the placenta may not be associated with increased complications where continuous USS guidance is used.
- Local anesthetic does not reduce pain scores.

Risk of transmission of infection

- Blood borne viruses present a risk of maternal–fetal transmission. Do not perform invasive prenatal procedures without reviewing blood borne virus screening tests.

HIV –

- If no HIV test result is available, delay the test and perform a rapid HIV test.
- Review viral load and treatment regimens and consider delaying the procedure until there is no detectable viral load if the woman is already on treatment or consider antiretroviral therapy if women not yet on treatment for HIV.
- Testing earlier in pregnancy is safe provided that retroviral therapy is being used and the maternal viral load is low. There were no cases of transmission in women receiving HAART; however, there were significant rates of transmission where no treatment was in place (25%) and where mono or double therapy was used (6%). Whenever possible, delay procedures until treatment has optimized the maternal viral load.

Hepatitis B or C – Invasive prenatal testing in the first or second trimester can be carried out as there is currently no evidence that transmission is increased following amniocentesis. Severe sepsis, including maternal death, has been reported following invasive prenatal procedures. The risk of severe sepsis is likely to be <1/1000. Infection can be caused by inadvertent puncture of the bowel, skin contaminants, or organisms present on the ultrasound probe or gel.

Special circumstances

Multiple pregnancies

- CVS or amniocentesis needs to be performed by a specialist who has the expertise to subsequently perform a selective TOP if required. A high level of expertise in USS scanning is essential for operators because uterine contents have to be 'mapped' with great care. This is essential to ensure that separate samples are taken for each fetus.
- Most clinicians use two separate puncture sites.
- Miscarriage rate is likely to be higher than in singleton pregnancies (1.8%).
- The role of CVS in dichorionic placentas remains controversial because of a relatively high risk of cross-contamination of chorionic tissue, which may lead to false positive or false negative results. This risk may be minimized if two separate needles are used.

Third-trimester amniocentesis

- Most commonly indicated for late karyotyping and detection of suspected fetal infection in prelabour preterm rupture of the membranes.
- Does not appear to be associated with a significant risk of emergency delivery (0–0.7% for procedure-related delivery).
- Compared with mid-trimester procedures, complications including multiple attempts (over 5%) and blood-stained fluid (5–10%) are more common along with higher culture failure rates (9.7%). When carried out in the presence of PPROM, failure rates are higher.

- Check maternal RhD status in every case. Offer prophylaxis with anti-D immunoglobulin following each procedure in line with national recommendations.

Consent – amniocentesis

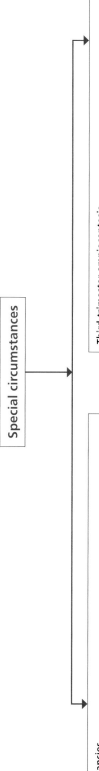

Discuss

- Explain the procedure – The procedure involves obtaining a sample of amniotic fluid from the pregnancy sac using a needle inserted through the woman's abdomen.
- Intended benefits – To provide information regarding the karyotype (chromosomal make-up) of fetus(es) and, less commonly, used to provide biochemical, metabolic or genetic information.
- Procedure – Involves the passage of a 20- or 22-gauge needle through the abdomen under direct ultrasound guidance into the amniotic sac followed by aspiration of 10–15 ml amniotic fluid.

Risks

Very common	1/1 to 1/10
Common	1/10 to 1/100
Uncommon	1/100 to 1/1000
Rare	1/1000 to 1/10000
Very rare	< 1/10000

- **Serious risks:**
  - * Failure to obtain a sample of amniotic fluid – 6%.
  - * Blood-stained samples – 0.8% with the use of continuous ultrasound guidance.
  - * Miscarriage rate – 1% over the norm.
  - * Fetal injury – rare.
  - * Maternal bowel injury – rare.
  - * Amniotic fluid leakage with the added risk of PTD.
  - * Chorioamnionitis – Severe sepsis, including maternal death, has been reported but the risk of severe sepsis is likely to be <1/1000.
  - * Failure of cell culture in the laboratory.
- **Frequent risks:**
  - * Mild discomfort at needle insertion site.

Amniocentesis and Chorionic Villus Sampling, RCOG Green-top Guideline No. 8; June 2010.
Amniocentesis. RCOG Consent Advice No. 6; 2006.

CHAPTER 4 Non-immune fetal hydrops

Hydrops fetalis (HF) is an excessive fluid accumulation within the fetal extravascular compartments and body cavities, characterized by a generalized skin thickness of >5 mm, placental enlargement, pericardial or pleural effusion, or ascites.

Immune – Rh alloimmunization
See Chapter 6 Fetal haemolytic disease

Non-immune fetal hydrops (NIFH) – 76–87% of cases of all fetal hydrops. Heterogeneous disorder, caused by a large number of underlying pathological processes.

Cardiovascular disorders

- Structural abnormalities and dysfunctioning (cardiac arrhythmias; myocardiopathies).
- High right atrial pressure or volume overload and right heart congestion, resulting in increased CVP and heart failure, or obstruction of venous or arterial blood flow which eventually leads to oedema.
- Inadequate diastolic ventricular filling occurring in rhythm disturbances or in cardiomyopathies leads to an increase in CVP.
- Hepatic venous congestion may complicate the clinical picture by decreasing hepatic function, thus leading to hypoalbuminaemia.

Chromosomal abnormalities

- Chromosomal causes are much higher in cases diagnosed prior to 20 weeks.
- Most common are trisomy 21 and Turner syndrome.

Hematological disorders

- Anaemia – resulting in cardiac failure
- Loss of oxygen-carrying capacity is the end stage. Rapidly generated anaemia usually causes immediate fetal death; hydrops occurs in the presence of slowly developing anaemia.
- Fetal anaemia can result from failure to manufacture normal haemoglobin (α-thalassaemia), fetal haemorrhage (intracranial bleeding), or haemolysis (glucose-6-phosphate dehydrogenase deficiency).

Lymphatic system

- Lymphatic drainage will be disturbed in lymph vessel dysplasias leading to liquid imbalance, thus producing hydrops.
- The central disturbance is a low output failure of the lymphatic system, that is, the overall lymphatic transport is reduced. This derangement occurs not only in lymphatic dysplasias but also in increased CVP, as this causes difficulties in draining the lymph into venous circulation.

Infectious agents

- The main targets of infection include fetal bone marrow, myocardium, and vascular endothelium.
- Intrauterine congestive heart failure, anaemia, and fetal sepsis leading to anoxia, endothelial cell damage, and increased capillary permeability are the mechanisms.
- Causative organisms include syphilis, cytomegalovirus, parvovirus B19, toxoplasmosis, herpes simplex, rubella, and coxsackievirus. **Parvovirus** – See Chapter 20 Parvovirus infection in pregnancy.
- Fetal parvovirus B19 infection results in an aplastic crisis, which leads to profound anaemia and hydrops, the outcome of which may be either fetal death or spontaneous resolution without long term morbidity.

Congenital malformations

- Congenital cystic adenomatoid malformations and congenital diaphragmatic hernia form intrathoracic masses which can compress the heart and limit its function, and may reduce venous return because of increased intrathoracic pressure.
- Fetal thoracic tumors, including cystic hygromas of the neck and chest, and arteriovenous malformations may also have an intrathoracic mass effect.

Others

- Twin-to-twin transfusion syndrome – Linked to volume disturbances and a subsequent increase in CVP.
- Maternal systemic lupus erythematosus in which anticardiolipin crossing the placenta causes fetal heart dysfunction.
- Inborn errors of metabolism – Anaemia or liver failure leading to hydrops.
- Structural fetal malformations include skeletal dysplasias, which may be associated with thoracic compression, impairment of venous return, and subsequent hydrops.
- The association of other structural malformations with NIFH, such as gastrointestinal, genitourinary, and neurological abnormalities, may represent chance occurrences.

Non-immune fetal hydrops (NIFH)

Background and definition

- Definition – Presence of fetal subcutaneous oedema and abnormal fluid accumulations in one or more fetal compartments, with absence of antibodies against red-cell antigens in the mother.
- It represents an end-stage condition of different disease processes.
- The most common causes are cardiovascular pathology, chromosomal abnormalities, haematological disorders, and infections.
- An SR of the aetiology for NIFH has reported the causes of NIFH as: cardiovascular (21.7%), chromosomal (13.4%), haematological (10.4%), infections (6.7%), thoracic (6.0%), lymphatic dysplasia (5.7%), FFTS-placental (5.6%), syndromic (4.4%), urinary tract malformations (2.3%), inborn errors of metabolism (1.1%), extrathoracic tumors (0.7%), gastrointestinal (0.5%), miscellaneous (3.7%), and idiopathic (17.8%).

Prevalence and incidence

- Affects 1:1500 to 1:3750 pregnancies.
- PNM ranges from 55 to 98%.
- In a series of pre-screened populations:
  * The survival rate was up to 48% with PNM up to 40%.
  * Prenatal identification of cause was possible in up to 56% of cases.
  * Unexplained in 18% even after postnatal investigations.
- 61% of those that survive have no long-term morbidity.
- Parvovirus infection is associated with good prognosis.

DDx

Diagnosis – USS

- Detection of abnormal or increased fluid accumulation in fetal body cavities (pericardial effusion, pleural effusion, ascites), subcutaneous oedema, cystic hygroma, polyhydramnios, and placental thickening.
- Skin thickness of at least 5 mm is required to diagnose subcutaneous oedema, and a placental thickness of at least 6 cm is required to diagnose placentomegaly.

Exclude immune causes – Screen for antibodies associated with blood group incompatibility.

Referral to FMU

- MDT – Obstetricians, neonatologists, clinical geneticists, and other paediatric subspecialists.

Maternal history

- Age, parity, gestation, ethnicity.
- Previous scan findings in the current pregnancy.
- Past medical and obstetric history.
- Family history of any genetic disorders (e.g., metabolic disorders).
- Recent infections or contacts.

Maternal investigations

- Full blood count, blood group, and antibodies.
- Haemoglobin electrophoresis (α-thalassaemia carrier).
- Kleihauer–Betke stain (feto-maternal haemorrhage).
- Glucose-6-phosphate dehydrogenase deficiency screen.
- Infectious screen:
  * TORCH (toxoplasmosis, rubella, cytomegalovirus, and herpes simplex) titres.
  * Rapid plasma reagent test.
  * Parvovirus B19 IgG and IgM titres.
- Auto-antibody screen (SLE, anti Ro, and La).
- Oral GTT.

Fetal investigations

Non-invasive

- Detailed fetal sonographic anatomy survey – for possible structural malformations.
- Fetal echocardiography – with particular attention to fetal rhythm disturbances.
- FHR monitoring for 12 to 24 hours – to rule out underlying fetal arrhythmia.
- M-mode study of heart – cardiac biometry; heart rate and rhythm.
- Doppler studies of umbilical artery and MCA. MCA peak systolic velocity to identify fetal anaemia.
- Placental morphology; amniotic fluid index (AFI).

Invasive

- CVS/Amniocentesis –
  * Fetal karyotype – FISH or PCR for a rapid diagnosis of the common aneuploidies.
  * PCR testing for infectious agents.
  * Metabolic testing.
- Cordocentesis – FBC, blood group and Coombs test, thalassaemia screen, karyotype, G6PD in male fetus; viral screen – TORCH, parvovirus.
- Gross fluid collection in the fetus – Drained under USS guidance and sent to lab for lymphocyte count and protein content evaluation.

Management

Non-infectious NIFH

- Presence of hydrops together with a structural malformation, such as cardiac abnormality, is associated with a very poor prognosis.
- Counsel regarding the possibility of elective TOP, depending on the gestational age at presentation.

Fetal therapy

- Pleuro-amniotic shunt; thoracoamniotic shunt; peritoneoamniotic shunt – for thoracic masses or persistent pleural/peritoneal effusions.
- Digoxin and other antiarrhythmic agents in cardiac dysrhythmias.
- Consider maternal steroids in cases of complete heart block in association with the presence of maternal auto-antibodies to Anti Ro and Anti La.
- Open fetal surgical resection of thoracic masses, such as congenital cystic adenomatoid malformation and bronchopulmonary sequestration; resection of fetal sacrococcygeal teratoma.

Infectious NIFH – Anaemia

- Fetal surveillance – With serial USS for signs of fetal hydrops. Scans weekly for at least 8 weeks from the time of exposure.
- Mild hydrops – Conservative management, since spontaneous resolution can occur.
- Worsening of hydrops – cordocentesis and IUT – To assess fetal haematocrit along with the facilities for immediate IUT. IUT if fetal haematocrit <30%; with Group O, irradiated, packed red cells that are CMV negative, Rh(D) negative, Kell negative, and cross-matched compatible with maternal serum. The unit of red cells should be packed with a haematocrit of at least 80%. The volume of packed red cells to be transfused depends on the starting haematocrit, haematocrit of transfused blood, target haematocrit, and a correction factor for the volume of blood in the placental circulation.
- For many fetuses with anaemia secondary to parvovirus B19 infection, one transfusion may be sufficient to maintain a normal fetal haematocrit, as the initial insult to the fetal marrow is generally self-limiting.
- Combined intravascular and intraperitoneal transfusion – With the intravascular aliquot of blood designed to provide an acute increase in fetal haematocrit and the intraperitoneal aliquot designed to provide a slower sustained increase in haematocrit.
- It is not advisable to transfuse a hydropic fetus to a final haematocrit that is 4 times the initial haematocrit as it is associated with fluid overload and sudden intrauterine fetal death.

Fetal surveillance

- Repeat sonographic fetal anatomy surveys should be performed at least every 2 weeks to confirm appropriate fetal growth and to improve the chances of detecting an underlying structural fetal malformation.

Time and mode of delivery

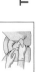

- Timing of delivery is uncertain.
- Depending on the gestational age, premature delivery may be indicated if fetal testing becomes non-reassuring.
- Otherwise, continue expectant management until 37 weeks of gestation.
- Maternal complications :
  * Pre-eclampsia in up to 50% of cases; may necessitate preterm delivery.
  * Polyhydramnios – may precipitate PTL; periodic reduction amniocenteses may be required to relieve maternal discomfort from severe polyhydramnios.

- The optimal mode of delivery – uncertain, as the overall prognosis is poor regardless of the form of delivery.
- Because of the risk of soft-tissue dystocia associated with hydrops, it is generally advisable to deliver all potentially viable fetuses with NIFH by CS. This should minimize the chances of maternal and fetal trauma.
- In cases in which the fetus is not expected to survive, the option of therapeutic thoracocentesis or paracentesis to optimize a vaginal delivery is also reasonable.
- The optimal location of delivery is a tertiary care centre with the immediate availability of skilled neonatologists and other appropriate paediatric subspecialists.

Neonatal care

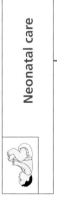

- Immediate availability of a multidisciplinary neonatal resuscitation team.
- Immediate neonatal endotracheal intubation is commonly needed.
- A high frequency ventilator and high airway-pressure settings – to achieve adequate gas exchange.
- Paracentesis and thoracocentesis, with placement of bilateral chest tubes – to allow adequate ventilation.
- Umbilical artery and umbilical vein lines may be needed.
- Blood products, albumin, and diuretics – to maintain adequate intravascular volume without significant fluid overload.
- Transport to a NICU.
- To confirm absence of significant structural malformation – a thorough physical examination, radiological investigations, and echocardiography.
- Specific therapy to the individual abnormalities, if any detected.

Bellini C, Hennekam RCM, Fulcheri E, Rutigliani M, Morcaldi G, Boccardo F, Bonioli E. Etiology of nonimmune hydrops fetalis: A systematic review. Am J Med Genet Part A 2009;149A:844–851.

Santo S, Mansour S, Thilaganathan B, Homfray T, Papageorghiou A, Calvert S, Bhide A. Prenatal diagnosis of non-immune hydrops fetalis: what do we tell the parents? Prenat Diagn 2011;31(2):186–195.

14

CHAPTER 5   Late intrauterine fetal death and stillbirth

Background and prevalence

- Stillbirth (SB) – baby delivered with no signs of life after 24 completed weeks of pregnancy.
- Intrauterine fetal death (IUFD) – babies with no signs of life in utero.
- Late intrauterine fetal death (after 24 completed weeks of pregnancy).
- The SB rate has remained constant since 2000 in the UK. Rising obesity rates and average maternal age might be associated with the lack of improvement (risk factors for SB).
- Stillbirth incidence in the UK – 1 in 200 babies.
- Sudden infant death – 1 per 10000 live births.
- 4037 stillbirths in the UK (2007) at a rate of 5.2/1000 total births.
- Over one third of SB are SGA fetuses with half of them unexplained.
- 8th Annual CESDI report - suboptimal care was evident in half of these pregnancies.

History

- History of no FMs may be present. After the diagnosis of late IUFD, mothers sometimes continue to experience (passive) FMs.
- If the mother reports passive FMs after a diagnosis of IUFD, offer a repeat scan.
- A detailed history of events during pregnancy.

Examination

- Auscultation of the fetal heart is inaccurate for diagnosis. It can give false reassurance as maternal pelvic blood flow can result in an apparently normal FHR pattern.
- Do not use auscultation and CTG to investigate suspected IUFD.
- Clinical examination for PET, chorioamnionitis, and placental abruption.

Investigations

- Real-time USS is essential for the accurate diagnosis. It allows direct visualization of the fetal heart. Ideally, real-time ultrasonography should be available at all times.
- Imaging can be technically difficult, in the presence of maternal obesity, abdominal scars, and oligohydramnios.
- Other secondary features on USS – collapse of the fetal skull with overlapping bones, hydrops, or maceration resulting in unrecognizable fetal mass, intrafetal gas within the heart, blood vessels, and joints.
- Although evidence of occult placental abruption might be identified, the sensitivity can be as low as 15%. Even large abruptions can be missed.
- Get a second opinion whenever practically possible.

Risks or complications

- Profound emotional, psychological, and social effects on parents.
- Moderate risk of maternal disseminated intravascular coagulation (DIC): 10% within 4 weeks after late IUFD, rising to 30% thereafter.

Causes of late IUFD

- Antepartum conditions – congenital malformation, congenital fetal infection, APH, PET, and maternal disease such as diabetes mellitus.
- Intrapartum conditions – placental abruption, maternal and fetal infection, cord prolapse, idiopathic hypoxia–acidosis, and uterine rupture.
- Transplacental infections – CMV, syphilis, parvovirus B19, listeria, rubella, toxoplasmosis, herpes simplex, coxsackievirus, leptospira, Q fever, Lyme disease, malaria parasitaemia, etc.
- Ascending infection with or without membrane rupture, with *E. coli, Klebsiella,* GBS, *Enterococcus,* mycoplasma/ureaplasma, *Haemophilus influenza,* and *Chlamydia.*

To determine the cause of death, the chance of recurrence, and possible means of avoiding further pregnancy complications:
- No specific cause is found in almost half of stillbirths.
- When a cause is found it can crucially influence care in a future pregnancy.
- An abnormal test result is not necessarily related to the IUFD; seek correlation between blood tests and postmortem examination (PME). Further tests might be indicated following the results of the PME.
- The proportion of unclassified late IUFDs can be significantly reduced with the use of customised weight-for-gestational-age charts.

To assess maternal wellbeing (including coagulopathy) and ensure prompt management of any potentially life-threatening maternal disease – undertake comprehensive investigations even if one cause is particularly suspected.

Maternal investigations

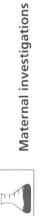

- Haematology, LFT, RFT, CRP, and bile salt.
- Platelet count for occult DIC.
- Maternal coagulation times and plasma fibrinogen for DIC.
- Repeat above investigations twice weekly in women who choose expectant management.
- Kleihauer for lethal FMH and to decide dose of anti-D gammaglobulin for all women, not simply those who are RhD-negative. Undertake before birth as red cells might clear quickly from maternal circulation.
- In RhD-negative women, perform a second Kleihauer test to determine whether sufficient anti-RhD has been given.
- Maternal bacteriology – blood cultures; MSU; vaginal and cervical swabs for suspected maternal infection including *Listeria* and *Chlamydia*. Abnormal bacteriology is of doubtful significance in the absence of clinical or histological evidence of chorioamnionitis.
- Maternal serology: viral screen; syphilis; tropical infections for occult maternal–fetal infection (if history of travel to endemic areas); parvovirus B19, rubella (if non-immune at booking); CMV, herpes simplex, and *Toxoplasma gondii*.
- Stored serum from booking tests can provide baseline serology.
- Hydrops may not necessarily be a feature of parvovirus-related late IUFD.

- Maternal random blood glucose – for occult maternal diabetes mellitus (DM). Rarely a woman will have type 1 DM, usually with severe ketosis.
- Maternal thyroid function (TSH, FT4, and FT3) – for occult maternal thyroid disease.
- Maternal thrombophilia screen – if evidence of FGR or placental disease. The association between inherited thrombophilias and IUFD is weak, and management in future pregnancy is uncertain. Repeat antiphospholipid screen if abnormal.
- Anti-red cell antibody serology – immune haemolytic disease; indicated if fetal hydrops is evident clinically or on PME.
- Maternal anti-Ro and anti-La antibodies – occult maternal autoimmune disease; indicated if evidence of hydrops, endomyocardial fibroelastosis, or AV node calcification at PME.
- Maternal alloimmune antiplatelet antibodies – alloimmune thrombocytopenia; indicated if fetal intracranial haemorrhage found on PME.
- Parental bloods for karyotype – parental balanced translocation, parental mosaicism. It is indicated if: fetal unbalanced translocation; other fetal aneuploidy, e.g., 45X; fetal genetic testing fails and history suggestive of aneuploidy (fetal abnormality on PME, previous unexplained IUFD, recurrent miscarriage).
- Maternal urine for cocaine metabolites for occult drug use – with consent, if history and/or presentation are suggestive.

Fetal investigations

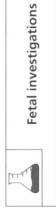

- Fetal and placental microbiology: fetal blood (cord or cardiac blood), fetal swabs, placental swabs for fetal infections. More informative than maternal serology for viral infections.
- Sexing the baby – if potential difficulty in sexing, two experienced HCPs should inspect the baby when examining the external genitalia of extremely preterm, severely macerated, or grossly hydropic infants. If there is any doubt, request a rapid karyotyping using quantitative fluorescent PCR (QF-PCR) or FISH. QF-PCR with additional Y chromosome markers can provide accurate result within 2 days in >99.9% of samples. If these fail, sex can be determined on cell culture or at postmortem. Stillborn babies can be registered as indeterminate sex.
- Cytogenetic analysis of the baby – 6% of SB babies have a chromosomal abnormality; some are recurrent and can be tested for in future pregnancies.
- Fetal and placental tissues for karyotype (and possible single-gene testing): for aneuploidy and single gene disorders. Cell culture provides the greatest range of genetic information. Use samples from multiple tissues to increase the chance of culture – skin, cartilage, and placenta. Skin specimens are associated with a higher rate of culture failure (~60%). Placenta has the advantages of more rapid cell culture, but has the disadvantages of maternal contamination and placental pseudomosaicism.
- If cultures fail, QF-PCR is a reliable (<0.01% failure rate), efficient, and cheap technique for detecting common aneuploidies.
- Microdeletions need to be requested specifically.

Postmortem examination (PME)

- Full PME helps to explain the cause of an IUFD. PME provides more information than other tests and can be crucial to the management of future pregnancy.
- Avoid attempts to persuade parents to choose PME. Respect individual, cultural, and religious beliefs. Obtain written consent. Provide information leaflet.
- Parents who decline full PME – offer a limited examination (sparing certain organs). Offer less invasive methods such as needle biopsies, but these are much less informative and reliable than conventional PME.
- Do not offer USS and MRI as a substitute for conventional PME. MRI can be a useful adjunct to conventional PME.
- PME includes external examination with birth weight and length, microscopy, histology of relevant tissues, and skeletal X-rays.
- Pathological examination of the cord, membranes, and placenta whether or not PME is requested.
- Autopsy alone can provide a classification of death in 46% of cases. When combined with other diagnostic tests, it offers information on recurrence risk in 40% of cases and/or management of next pregnancy in 51%.

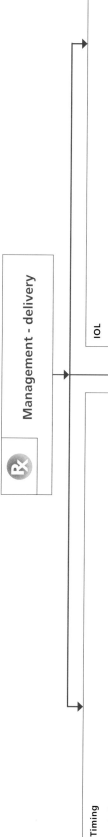

Management - delivery

Timing

- Take into account the mother's preferences, her medical condition, and previous intrapartum history.
- Commence immediate delivery if there is sepsis, PET, placental abruption or membrane rupture, but take a more flexible approach if these factors are not present.
- Well women with intact membranes and no laboratory evidence of DIC are unlikely to come to physical harm if labour is delayed for a short period (for 48 hours), but they may develop severe medical complications and suffer greater anxiety with prolonged intervals.
- Test women who delay labour for periods >48 hours for DIC twice weekly.
- Advise women contemplating prolonged expectant management that the appearance of the baby may deteriorate and the value of PME may be reduced.

Mode of delivery

- Vaginal birth for most women. Vaginal birth can be achieved within 24 hours of IOL for IUFD in about 90% of women. It has the advantages of immediate recovery and quicker return to home.
- CS might occasionally be clinically indicated by virtue of maternal condition.

IOL

- A combination of mifepristone and a prostaglandin preparation is the first-line intervention for IOL.
- Mifepristone can be used alone to increase the chance of labour significantly within 72 hours (avoiding the use of prostaglandin).
- Misoprostol can be used in preference to prostaglandin E2 because of equivalent safety and efficacy with lower cost but at doses not currently marketed in the UK.
- Vaginal misoprostol is as effective as oral therapy but associated with fewer adverse effects.
- Previous CS:
  * Discuss the safety and benefits of IOL. Monitor closely for features of scar rupture.
  * Women with a single lower segment scar – IOL with prostaglandin is safe but not without risk; misoprostol can be safely used but not yet marketed in the UK.
  * Women with 2 previous LSCS – the absolute risk of IOL with prostaglandin is only a little higher than for women with a single previous LSCS.
  * Women with >2 LSCS deliveries or atypical scars – the safety of IOL is unknown.
- Oxytocin augmentation can be used but the decision should be made by a consultant obstetrician.
- Use mechanical methods for IOL only in the context of a clinical trial.

Intrapartum care

Suitable facilities for labour

- Labour in an environment that provides appropriate facilities for emergency care.
- Care in labour by an experienced midwife.
- Maternity units should have a special labour ward room for women with an otherwise uncomplicated IUFD that pays special heed to emotional and practical needs without compromising safety.

Intrapartum antimicrobial therapy

- Treat women with sepsis with IV broad-spectrum antibiotics (including antichlamydial agents).
- Do not use routine antibiotic prophylaxis.
- Do not give intrapartum antibiotic prophylaxis to women with uncomplicated GBS colonization.
- It is suggested that artificial rupture of membranes may facilitate ascending infection.

Pain relief in labour

- All options including regional anaesthesia and patient-controlled anaesthesia.
- Use diamorphine in preference to pethidine. Diamorphine and morphine have greater analgesic qualities and longer duration of action than pethidine.
- Assess for DIC and sepsis before giving regional anaesthesia. DIC increases the chance of subdural and epidural haematomata with regional anaesthesia.

Postpartum care

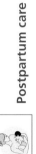

Thromboprophylaxis

- Assess for thromboprophylaxis, but IUFD in itself is not a risk factor.
- Given the association of late IUFD with obesity, advanced maternal age, infection, and maternal diseases it is likely that many women with an IUFD fall into the moderate or high-risk categories.
- Discuss heparin thromboprophylaxis with a haematologist if the woman has DIC.

Suppression of lactation

- Almost one third of women who choose non-pharmacological measures are troubled by excessive discomfort.
- Bromocriptine inhibits lactation in >90% of women with few side effects and is significantly more effective than breast binders.
- Cabergoline is superior to bromocriptine. Both have very similar effectiveness, but cabergoline is simpler to use and has significantly lower rates of rebound breast activity and adverse events.
- Dopamine agonists can increase BP and have been associated with intracerebral haemorrhage. Therefore avoid in women with HT or PET.
- Do not use oestrogens to suppress lactation.

Psychological and social care

Psychological problems

- Mother, partner, and children are all at risk of prolonged severe psychological reactions including post-traumatic stress disorder but their reactions might be very different.
- Increased rates of admission owing to postnatal depression; unresolved normal grief responses can evolve into post-traumatic stress disorder.
- Women with poor social support are particularly vulnerable.

Interventions that might aid psychological recovery

- Be aware of possible variations in individual and cultural approaches to death.
- Offer counselling to all women and their partners. Consider other family members, especially existing children and grandparents, for counselling.
- Advise about support groups.
- Appoint bereavement officers to coordinate services.
- Debriefing services must not care for women with symptoms of psychiatric disease in isolation.

Seeing, holding, naming, and mementos

- Avoid persuading parents to have contact with their stillborn baby, but support such desires when expressed.
- After registration a name cannot be entered at a later date, nor can it be changed.
- If parents do decide to name their baby, use the name, including at follow-up meetings.
- Offer but do not persuade parents to retain artefacts of remembrance. If the parents do not wish to have mementos, offer to store them securely in the maternal case record for future access.

Spiritual guidance, burial, cremation, and remembrance

- Maternity units should have arrangements with all common faiths and non-religious spiritual organizations as a source of guidance and support for parents. The legal responsibility for the child's body rests with the parents but can be delegated to hospital services.
- A leaflet about the options should be available.

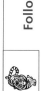

Follow-up

Timing of follow-up meetings

- Consider the wishes of the woman and her partner.
- Ensure that all available results are readily to hand.
- 6–8 weeks is common practice for the timing of the appointment, when the placental and the postmortem histology results usually become available, but a flexible approach is appropriate according to the needs of the parents and the range of tests performed.

Content of the follow-up appointment

- Discuss the cause of late IUFD, chance of recurrence, and any specific means of preventing further loss.
- Advise to avoid weight gain if they are already overweight or to consider weight loss.
- Discuss the potential benefit of delaying conception until severe psychological issues have been resolved.
- Provide general prepregnancy advice.
- While mothers tend to experience greater anxiety when conception occurs soon after a fetal loss, partners are more likely to suffer anxiety if conception is delayed.
- Document the discussion at the meeting and an agreed plan for future pregnancy.

Fertility

- Inform about fertility and contraception.
- The absolute chance of adverse events with a pregnancy interval less than 6 months remains low and is unlikely to be significantly increased compared with conceiving later.

Pregnancy following unexplained stillbirth

- Clearly mark the history of SB in the case record.
- Recommend:
  * Obstetric consultant-led care.
  * Screening for GDM, since these women have a rate of GDM four times higher than expected.
  * For women in whom a normally formed SB baby had shown evidence of being SGA – arrange serial assessment of growth by USS biometry.
- Women with a history of SB (but otherwise low-risk) compared with pregnancies after live birth have a:
  * 12-fold increased risk of intrapartum SB.
  * Placental abruption (OR 9.4).
  * Fetal distress (OR 2.8).
  * Extreme PTD (OR 4.2).
  * An increased risk of PET (OR 3.1).
  * Ischaemic placental disease (OR 1.6).
  * Chorioamnionitis (OR 2.3).
  * Early neonatal mortality (OR 8.3).

Management of future delivery

- Recommend birth at a specialist maternity unit.
- Take into account the gestational age of the previous IUFD, previous intrapartum history, and the safety of IOL.
- A retrospective study – history of SB conferred a greater risk of subsequent early IUFDs between 20 and 28 weeks (HR 10) than of late IUFDs (over 29 weeks) (HR 2.5).
- There have been no studies that adequately tested fetal benefit from routine IOL.
- Be vigilant for postpartum depression in women with a previous IUFD.

Late Intrauterine Fetal Death and Stillbirth. RCOG Green-top Guideline No. 55, October 2010.

CHAPTER 6 Fetal haemolytic disease

Incidence

- UK – deaths attributed to RhD alloimmunization fell from 46/100 000 births before 1969 to 1.6/100 000 in 1990.
- New immunizations continue to occur: around 500 per year in England and Wales. The incidence of RhD alloimmunization post introduction of anti-D prophylaxis is 1–2 per 1000 RhD-negative pregnancies.
- Clinically significant antibodies are seen in 0.09–0.24%.
- Race – incompatibility involving Rh antigens (anti-D or anti-c) occurs in about 10% of all pregnancies among Whites and Blacks; in contrast, it is very rare in Asian women.
- Fetal sex – 13-fold increase is observed in fetal hydrops in RhD-positive male fetuses compared with female fetuses in similarly sensitized pregnancies.
- Red cell antibodies during pregnancy may be the result of alloimmunization during the pregnancy or antibodies that predate conception.

Do not routinely screen for red cell antibodies pre-pregnancy.

Prevention – previous blood transfusion is an important cause for alloimmunization with antibodies other than anti-D. Prevention is possible by routine screening and matching donor blood for c and Kell type for women before or during childbearing age.

Women with red cell antibodies – provide pre-pregnancy counselling particularly if there is a risk of fetal anaemia or if there is a significant risk of blood being required during the pregnancy where compatible blood (i.e. red cells) is rare and difficult to obtain.

All pregnant women

Routine antenatal screening – red blood cell antibody screen at booking and at 28 weeks.

Booking history:

- A history of hydropic birth increases the risk of fetal hydrops in the next pregnancy to 90%; the fetal hydrops occurs at about the same time or earlier in gestation in the subsequent pregnancy.
- Any history of blood transfusion in the past.

Risks

Fetal – haemolytic disease of the fetus and newborn (HDFN) – transplacental passage of maternal IgG antibodies results in immune haemolysis of fetal/neonatal red cells.

- Nearly 50% of the affected newborns do not require treatment, have mild anaemia and hyperbilirubinemia at birth, survive, and develop normally.
- Approximately 25% are born near term but become extremely jaundiced without treatment and either die (90%) or become severely affected by kernicterus (10%).
- Remaining 25% of affected newborns are severely affected in utero and become hydropic; about half are affected before 34 weeks, and the other half between 34 weeks and term.
- Fetuses requiring intrauterine transfusion (IUT) – perinatal mortality is around 10–15%.
- Overall rate of neurodevelopmental impairment is 10%.
- Hearing loss is increased 5- to 10-fold over the general population in infants who require IUT, probably because of their prolonged exposure to elevated levels of bilirubin and its toxic effect on the developing eighth cranial nerve.

Maternal – maternal red cell antibody can cause difficulty in timely provision of blood and blood components because of difficulty in obtaining antigen-negative blood and/or cross matching issues.

Causes

- Almost 50 different red cell surface antigens have been found to be responsible for HDFN.
- Clinically significant HDN can be caused by: anti-RhD, anti-Rhc, and anti-Kell and Fya.
- Other antibodies that potentially cause fetal anaemia include anti-E, -Jka, -C, and -Ce.
- The most important cause of anti-D antibodies is immunization during pregnancy, when no overt sensitizing event has occurred. Late immunization during a first pregnancy is responsible for 18–27% of cases. Immunization during a second or subsequent pregnancy accounts for a similar proportion of cases.
- Alloimmunization due to Kell antigen accounts for 10% of severely affected fetuses.
- Anti-K causes anaemia secondary to erythroid suppression but hyperbilirubinemia is not a prominent feature. Severe fetal anaemia can occur even at relatively low antibody titres.
- ABO incompatibility occurs during the first pregnancy and is present in approximately 12% of pregnancies, with evidence of fetal sensitization in 3% of live births. Less than 1% of births are associated with significant haemolysis. In particular, naturally occurring anti-A and anti-B antibodies of the IgG subclass in a group O mother can cross the placenta and cause haemolysis of fetal erythrocytes.
- Spontaneous FMH occurs with increasing frequency and volume with advancing gestational age. There is a reported presence of 0.01 ml of fetal cells in 3%, 12%, and 46% of women in each of the three successive trimesters.

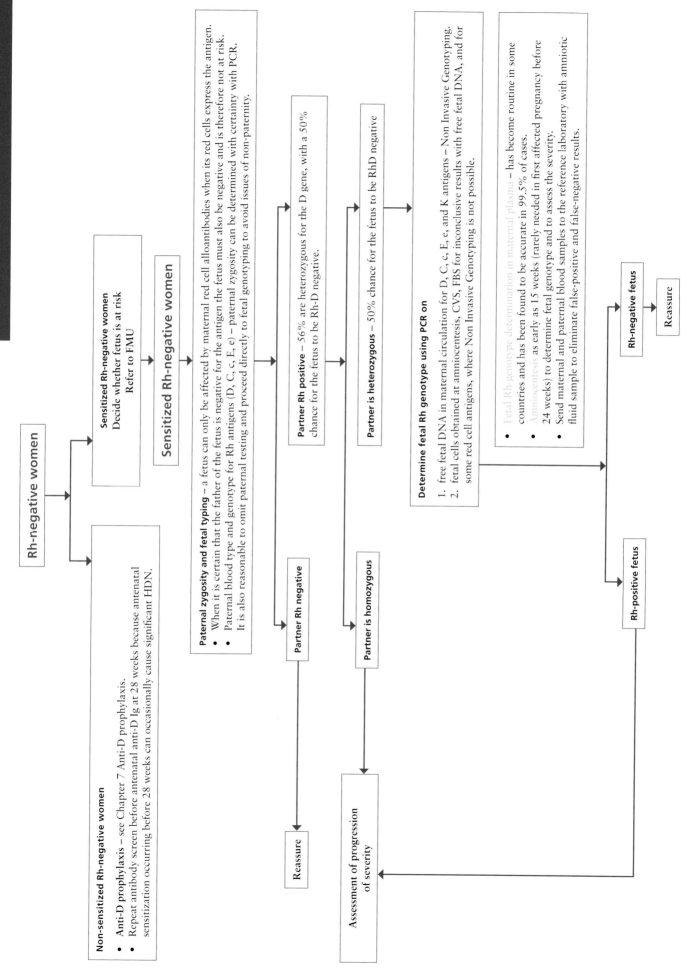

Rh-negative women

Non-sensitized Rh-negative women
- Anti-D prophylaxis – see Chapter 7 Anti-D prophylaxis.
- Repeat antibody screen before antenatal anti-D Ig at 28 weeks because antenatal sensitization occurring before 28 weeks can occasionally cause significant HDN.

Sensitized Rh-negative women
Decide whether fetus is at risk
Refer to FMU

Sensitized Rh-negative women

Paternal zygosity and fetal typing – a fetus can only be affected by maternal red cell alloantibodies when its red cells express the antigen.
- When it is certain that the father of the fetus is negative for the antigen the fetus must also be negative and is therefore not at risk.
- Paternal blood type and genotype for Rh antigens (D, C, c, E, e) – paternal zygosity can be determined with certainty with PCR. It is also reasonable to omit paternal testing and proceed directly to fetal genotyping to avoid issues of non-paternity.

Partner Rh negative

Reassure

Partner Rh positive – 56% are heterozygous for the D gene, with a 50% chance for the fetus to be Rh-D negative.

Partner is homozygous

Assessment of progression of severity

Partner is heterozygous – 50% chance for the fetus to be RhD negative

Determine fetal Rh genotype using PCR on

1. free fetal DNA in maternal circulation for D, C, c, E, e, and K antigens – Non Invasive Genotyping.
2. fetal cells obtained at amniocentesis, CVS, FBS for inconclusive results with free fetal DNA, and for some red cell antigens, where Non Invasive Genotyping is not possible.

- Fetal Rh-genotype determination in maternal plasma – has become routine in some countries and has been found to be accurate in 99.5% of cases.
- Amniocentesis as early as 15 weeks (rarely needed in first affected pregnancy before 24 weeks) to determine fetal genotype and to assess the severity.
- Send maternal and paternal blood samples to the reference laboratory with amniotic fluid sample to eliminate false-positive and false-negative results.

Rh-negative fetus

Reassure

Rh-positive fetus

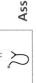

Assessment and fetal monitoring

Serial maternal serological monitoring

- At regular intervals after 18 weeks until the critical titre for the laboratory is exceeded.
- Critical titres – The cut-off level used to select patients for serial diagnostic tests for signs of anaemia and fetal hydrops. Severe fetal disease may occur when the titre is 1:16 or above. Other data suggest that significant fetal anaemia is not expected when the anti-D titre remains below 1:64.
- The utility of antibody titres above the threshold in predicting fetal risk is greatest during the first sensitized pregnancy. In subsequent pregnancies once the threshold is crossed, titre and history are inadequate measures to direct management.
- In the UK, RhD immunization is followed by serial quantification using an autoanalyzer. Severe fetal disease is not expected with anti-D levels <4 IU/ml and is rare <10–15 IU/ml.
- Measure anti-D, anti-c, and anti-K levels every 4 weeks to 28 weeks then every 2 weeks until delivery or referral to FMU. If anti-D titres >4 IU/ml – monitor every 2 weeks.

USS monitoring

- **Serial USS monitoring can detect moderate anaemia and early signs of hydrops.** Other signs of fetal anaemia include polyhydramnios, skin oedema, and cardiomegaly.
- Fetal middle cerebral artery (MCA) peak systolic velocity (MCA PSV) is a reliable screening tool to detect fetal anaemia. The sensitivity for detection of moderate and severe fetal anaemia is up to 100%, with a false-positive rate of 10%. It performs better in cases of clinically significant fetal anaemia.
- For anti-D, anti-c, and anti-K antibodies – weekly USS MCA PSV.
- For other less common antibodies – 1–2-weekly USS MCA PSV is reasonable.
- MCA Doppler studies can be started as early as 18 weeks but use it with caution after 36 weeks as its sensitivity for the detection of fetal anaemia decreases. It can be used to time the subsequent IUT.

Referral to FMU – depend on the type of antibody and its levels or titres:
- Rising antibody levels/titres or once above a titre of 32 or
- Ultrasound features suggestive of fetal anaemia.
- History of unexplained severe neonatal jaundice, neonatal anaemia requiring transfusion or exchange transfusion.

Thresholds for the various antibodies to trigger referral:
- **anti-D** – refer if anti-D levels are >4 IU/ml. Level of
  >4 IU/ml but <15 IU/ml correlates with a moderate risk of HDFN.
  >15 IU/ml can cause severe HDFN.
- **anti-c** – refer if anti-c levels are >7.5 IU/ml. Level of
  >7.5 IU/ml but <20 IU/ml correlates with a moderate risk of HDFN
  >20 IU/ml correlates with a high risk of HDFN.
- **anti-K** or anti-Fy – refer once detected, as severe fetal anaemia can occur even with low titres as there is a poor correlation between antibody levels and severity of disease.
- For other antibodies – a history of previous significant HDFN, or once above a titre of 32 or further rising antibody titres, or a 4-fold increase in any antibody titre.
- The presence of anti-E potentiates the severity of fetal anaemia due to anti-c antibodies, therefore referral at lower titres is indicated.

Invasive treatment (FBS and IUT) if the MCA PSV rises above the gestational threshold or if there are other signs (e.g., hydrops) of fetal anaemia.

Invasive monitoring

With experience in performing MCA Doppler study, serial amniocentesis for detecting fetal anaemia has been used to a lesser extent.

Amniocentesis

- Historically, the spectral analysis of amniotic fluid at 450 nm (ΔOD450) has been used to measure the level of bilirubin, an indirect indicator of the degree of fetal haemolysis. The original Liley curve was divided into three zones and remains useful after 27 weeks' gestation.
- Serial procedures are undertaken at 10-day to 2-week intervals and continued until delivery.
- A rising or plateauing trend of ΔOD450 values that reaches the 80th percentile of zone two or zone 3 on the Liley curve necessitates investigation by fetal blood sampling (FBS).
- Extrapolating Liley curves to earlier gestational ages underestimates the level of fetal disease and should not be used.
- Risks – fetal loss and FMH further increasing the risk of alloimmunization

Fetal blood sampling (FBS)

- USS-directed FBS (cordocentesis) allows direct access to the fetal circulation to obtain haematocrit, direct Coombs, fetal blood type, reticulocyte count, and total bilirubin.
- Site – either the placental cord insertion site or the intrahepatic vein. Intrahepatic approach is less likely to cause fetal distress but is technically more difficult.
- Indicated in patients with elevated ΔOD450 values or elevated peak MCA PSV.
- Blood should be available for intravascular IUT if fetal anaemia is detected (haematocrit <30% or < two standard deviations for gestational age).
- Risks of cordocentesis:
  - * Bradycardia, haemorrhage, cord haematoma and tamponade, and fetal death.
  - * 1–3% fetal loss rate in low-risk patients; as high as 20% if the fetus is hydropic.
  - * A significant risk of FMH thereby boosting maternal antibody levels.

Treatment – intrauterine transfusion (IUT)

- The total amount of red cells to transfuse will depend on the initial fetal haematocrit, gestational age, and haematocrit of the donor unit.
- A final target haematocrit of 40–50% is used; a decline of approximately 1% per day can be anticipated between transfusions.
- In the extremely anaemic fetus, the initial haematocrit should not be increased by more than four-fold to allow the fetal cardiovascular system to compensate for the acute change in viscosity. A repeat procedure is undertaken 48 hours later to normalize the fetal haematocrit.
- Hydropic features usually reverse rapidly after one or two IUTs.
- If the fetus is not severely anaemic at the first IUT, subsequent procedures are scheduled at 14-day intervals until suppression of fetal erythropoiesis is noted on Kleihauer–Betke stains. This usually occurs by the third IUT. The interval for repeat procedures can be determined based on the decline in haematocrit for the individual fetus, usually a 3- to 4-week interval.
- Procedure-related loss rates are around 2–4%. The loss rate depends on the gestation, site of sampling, and underlying pathology.

Sites:

- 1. Historically intraperitoneal transfusion.
- 2. Cordocentesis – by puncturing the umbilical cord at its placental insertion under USS guidance; has replaced intraperitoneal transfusion. Compared with intraperitoneal transfusion, intravascular transfusion is advantageous to the hydropic fetus where absorption of cells from the peritoneal cavity is compromised.
- 3. The intrahepatic portion of the umbilical vein may be slightly safer.
- Combining the procedure with an additional intraperitoneal transfusion has been advocated, to lengthen the interval between transfusions.
- The blood – ABO compatible with the fetus and mother (to avoid ABO HDFN from the woman's anti-A or -B antibodies); RhD negative; K negative; negative for the antigens(s) corresponding to maternal red cell antibodies; CMV-negative. Cells are packed to a haematocrit of 75–85% to prevent volume overload. It is processed to order as it only has 24 hours' shelf life after processing.
- K-negative blood is recommended to reduce additional maternal alloimmunization risks. In exceptional cases, for example HDFN because of anti-c alloimmunization, it may be necessary to give O RhD-positive, c-negative blood.

Delivery

- Timing of delivery depends on the antibody levels/titres, rate of rise, and if any fetal intervention has been required.
- In the past, delivery after 32–34 weeks was considered safer than continuing transfusions until near term.
- Most authorities now perform the final IUT up to 35 weeks, with delivery at 37–38 weeks. It allows maturation of both the pulmonary and hepatic enzyme systems, eliminating the need for neonatal exchange transfusions.
- In patients with relatively easy access to the fetal circulation, IUTs up to 36 weeks may be performed, with an aim for near-term and usually vaginal delivery.
- Prior IUT is not an indication for elective CS.
- Continuous electronic fetal heart monitoring is advised during labour.

Neonatal care

- Cord samples for a direct antiglobulin test (DAT), haemoglobin and bilirubin levels.
- Monitor neonate's neurobehavioural state, development of jaundice and/or anaemia, and bilirubin and haemoglobin levels.
- Encourage mother to feed the baby regularly to ensure that the baby does not become dehydrated as dehydration can increase the severity of jaundice.
- **If bilirubin levels rise rapidly or above the interventional threshold, phototherapy and/or exchange transfusion may be required.**
  * In milder cases phototherapy may be sufficient.
  * Early severe anaemia particularly in the presence of heart failure and severe hyperbilirubinaemia is treated with exchange transfusions. The aim is to remove both the antibody-coated red cells and the excess bilirubin. Exchanging the estimated volume of the baby's blood in a 'single volume exchange' will remove 75% of red cells, while a double-volume exchange removes 90% of the initial red cells. A double-volume exchange can remove 50% of available intravascular bilirubin.
- **When 3 or more IUTs are given:**
  * Blood of the fetus consists of almost 100% adult donor RhD-negative red cells. These neonates may hardly show signs of haemolytic disease.
  * Passively acquired maternal antibodies may remain in the neonatal circulation for weeks causing continuing haemolysis resulting in persisting anaemia for a few weeks following birth.
  * Suppression of erythropoiesis (hyporegenerative) may occur resulting in late anaemia. This results in a 1- to 3-month period in which the infant may need several top-up red cell transfusions. Assess weekly haematocrit and reticulocyte counts.
  * For late anaemia, occurring 2–6 weeks postpartum, especially in neonates who received IUTs, treatment with recombinant erythropoietin may reduce the need for top-up transfusions.
- Whether or not IV gammaglobulin is useful in the management of neonatal haemolytic disease is still unclear.
- Overall survival is 84%. Survival of non-hydropic fetuses (92%) is better than those with hydrops (70%).
- Long-term developmental outcome of children who where transfused in utero seems excellent and no different from normal controls.
- Sensorineural hearing loss is more common in infants affected by haemolytic disease of the newborn because of the toxic effect of prolonged exposure of bilirubin on the developing eighth cranial nerve. Newborns should have their hearing frequently tested.

Future pregnancies

- Refer all women with a history of an infant with HDFN to FMU for early assessment in all further pregnancies.
- Risk of recurrence depends on the type of antibody, the paternal genotype (heterozygous or homozygous), as well as the severity and gestational onset of the fetal anaemia.

The management of women with red cell antibodies during pregnancy. RCOG Green-top Guideline No. 65; May 2014.

Maternal issues

- Do not offer antenatal or postnatal anti-D Ig prophylaxis in women who are already sensitized with positive immune anti-D detected.
- Give Anti-D Ig to D negative women with non-anti-D antibodies for routine antenatal prophylaxis, for potential antenatal sensitizing events, and postnatal prophylaxis.
- For antibodies other than anti-D, anti-c, anti-C, anti-E, or anti-K, liaise with the transfusion laboratory to assess and plan for any possible transfusion requirements, as obtaining the relevant blood may take longer.
- Pregnant women who are assessed as at high risk of requiring a blood transfusion (placenta previa) should have a cross-match sample taken every week. Blood samples for cross-matching red cells during pregnancy should be no more than 7 days old and ideally should be fresh, as new antibodies may form; particularly in the last trimester.
- If maternal transfusion is required – use same ABO/O group and RhD type, K negative and CMV negative blood.
- When blood is required for women with multiple or rare antibodies, planning is required as rare blood donors may need to be called up to donate, or frozen blood may need to be obtained from the National Frozen Blood Bank in Liverpool.
- Local blood transport time and time for cross-match should be taken into account when the decision for transfusion is made.
- Emergency transfusion – ABO, RhD, and K compatible blood that is not matched for other antibodies has the risks of a haemolytic transfusion reaction with associated complications, including renal failure versus severe haemorrhage; balance these with the benefit. Give this for resuscitation if necessary with IV methylprednisolone 1 g cover and monitor closely. If a severe transfusion reaction develops, IV immunoglobulin may be required. The presence of maternal red cell antibodies has no implications for other blood components such as platelets, fresh frozen plasma, cryoprecipitate, or fractionated products.

Early onset/severe HDN

- Early transfusions, before 18–20 weeks, carry a higher fetal loss risk. Patients with a previously affected fetus at or before 20 weeks of gestation pose a great challenge.
- Plasmapheresis, IV immunoglobulins, and 'prophylactic' intraperitoneal transfusions can be considered, but the optimal approach is unknown.
- Stem cell therapy may be an option in the future.
- Maternal IV immunoglobulin has shown some benefit in severe cases of HDN. The extreme expense of this therapy warrants its use only in cases of early perinatal loss when technical limitations of IUT make success unlikely.
- IV immunoglobulin does not eliminate the need for IUT but can prolong the interval before the first procedure is necessary.

CHAPTER 6 Fetal haemolytic disease

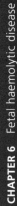

23

CHAPTER 7 Anti-D immunoglobulin for rhesus D prophylaxis

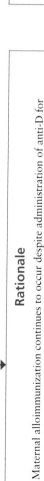

Background and prevalence

- Development of anti-D antibodies usually occurs as a result of fetomaternal haemorrhage (FMH) in a rhesus D (RhD)-negative woman with an RhD-positive fetus.
- Postdelivery immunoprophylaxis with anti-D immunoglobulin (anti-D Ig) began in the UK in 1969. Deaths attributed to RhD alloimmunization fell from 46/100 000 births before 1969 to 1.6/100 000 in 1990.
- The most important cause of allo-immunization now is during pregnancy where there has been no overt sensitizing event. Late immunization, during the third trimester of a first pregnancy, is responsible for 18–27% of cases.
- Anti-D Ig is a blood product extracted from the plasma of donors who have high circulating levels of anti-D, from deliberate immunization of Rh-negative donors.
- **Risks** – Concerns of viral and prion transmission. Donors undergo specific virology testing and the end product is subject to a viral inactivation process. Very low rate of adverse events (<1/85 000 doses) with only a minority of these classified as serious.

Anti-D Ig preparations, dose, and administration

- **Dose** – 500 IU of anti-D Ig IM will neutralize an FMH of up to 4 ml. For each ml of FMH in excess of 4 ml, a further 125 IU of anti-D Ig is necessary.
- Minimum recommended doses:
  * <20+0 weeks of gestation – 250 IU.
  * ≥20+0 weeks of gestation – 500 IU.
- Request a test for the size of FMH when anti-D Ig is given ≥20+0 weeks.
- Give it ASAP after the potentially sensitizing event but always within 72 hours. If it is not given before 72 hours, still give anti-D Ig within 10 days as it may provide some protection.
- Give anti-D Ig via the SC or IV route for women with a bleeding disorder.
- Do not give anti-D Ig to women who are already sensitized to RhD.
- IM anti-D Ig is best given into the deltoid muscle as injections into the gluteal region often only reach the subcutaneous tissues and absorption may be delayed.
- Women who have a weak expression of the RhD blood group (Du) do not form anti-D and therefore do not require prophylaxis.

Routine antenatal anti-D prophylaxis (RAADP)

Rationale

- Maternal alloimmunization continues to occur despite administration of anti-D for recognized sensitizing events. In a significant number of cases (55–80%) there is no recognized sensitizing event with 'silent' sensitization secondary to occult FMH. This occurs with increasing frequency as gestation advances. Less than 10% of cases of silent FMH occur before 28 weeks of gestation. The rationale for RAADP is to protect against these unpredictable sensitizations and to prevent potential morbidity in subsequent pregnancies.
- In the absence of RAADP, approximately 1% of RhD-negative women who deliver an RhD-positive baby will become sensitized. RAADP reduces the incidence of rhesus alloimmunization in these women.
- Meta-analysis – the rate of sensitization in a subsequent pregnancy is reduced from 0.95% to 0.35% (OR 0.37). On the basis of this risk reduction, the number of Rh-negative women needed to treat to prevent one case of sensitization is 166. The overall number needed to treat is 278 as only 60% of RhD-negative women will be carrying an RhD-positive baby.
- There is evidence that RAADP given in a first pregnancy continues to confer benefit in subsequent pregnancies, although the mechanism for this remains unexplained.

Recommendations

- Offer RAADP to all non-sensitized RhD-negative women.
- RAADP is not required in women who are RhD sensitized.
- Take the routine 28-week antibody screening sample before giving the first dose of anti-D.
- Give RAADP irrespective of whether anti-D Ig has been given at an earlier gestation.
- Cover any sensitizing events that occur after administration of RAADP with an additional dose of anti-D Ig.

Regimens for RAADP

- Two regimens:
  * Two doses of 500 IU anti-D Ig at 28 and 34 weeks of gestation.
  * A single dose of 1500 IU at 28 weeks of gestation.
- There are no studies comparing the efficacy of the single-dose and two-dose regimen. Two-dose regimen results in a slightly higher residual anti-D level at term.
- A small proportion of women will have undetectable levels of anti-D 12 weeks after a single injection of 1500 IU of anti-D Ig. Therefore, if anti-D Ig is given at 28 weeks of gestation, there is a risk that some women will be unprotected if their pregnancy progresses beyond 40 weeks of gestation. However, if anti-D Ig is administered later than 28 weeks of gestation, the proportion of occult FMH that will not be covered will increase.

Anti-D Ig prophylaxis – other events in pregnancy

To all non-sensitized RhD-negative women

Miscarriage

- Provide prophylaxis:
  * Spontaneous complete or incomplete miscarriage at or after 12+0 weeks.
  * Surgical evacuation of the uterus, regardless of gestation.
  * Medical evacuation of the uterus, regardless of gestation. Medically induced evacuation of the uterus with prostaglandins is likely to result in increased uterine contractions and bleeding compared with spontaneous miscarriage. There is a lack of evidence but it seems reasonable to consider anti-D administration in this situation.
- Do not provide for spontaneous miscarriage before 12+0 weeks, provided there is no instrumentation of the uterus. There is evidence that significant FMH occurs only after curettage to remove pregnancy tissue but does not occur after complete spontaneous miscarriages.

Threatened miscarriage

- Provide prophylaxis:
  * Threatened miscarriage after 12+0 weeks.
  * Provide at 6-weekly intervals if bleeding continues intermittently after 12+0 weeks.
  * Consider if there is heavy or repeated bleeding or associated abdominal pain as gestation approaches 12+0 weeks.
- Do not provide routine anti-D Ig prophylaxis in the event of threatened miscarriage before 12 weeks, as the evidence that these women get sensitized is scant.

Termination of pregnancy

- Provide prophylaxis – for TOP by surgical or medical methods, regardless of gestational age.

Ectopic pregnancy

- Provide prophylaxis for ectopic pregnancy – regardless of management option. There is a paucity of evidence regarding the risk of alloimmunization associated with medical and conservative management of ectopic pregnancy. However, given the potential for sensitization, it is reasonable to offer anti-D Ig.

Antenatal sensitizing events

- Antenatal events which require anti-D Ig, in include:
  * Invasive prenatal diagnosis (amniocentesis, CVS, cordocentesis, intrauterine transfusion).
  * Other intrauterine procedures (e.g., insertion of shunts, embryo reduction, laser).
  * Antepartum haemorrhage.
  * Fetal death.
  * External cephalic version (including attempted).
  * Abdominal trauma (direct/indirect, sharp/blunt, open/closed).

- Dose – Give a minimum dose of 250 IU for sensitizing events up to 19+6 weeks and 500 IU for events at or after 20+0 weeks along with a test to identify FMH >4 ml (give additional anti-D Ig as required).
- Recurrent vaginal bleeding after 20+0 weeks – give anti-D Ig at a minimum of 6-weekly intervals. If there is concern about the frequency of recurrent bleeding, perform an estimation of FMH at 2-weekly intervals; if positive, give an additional dose of anti-D Ig (500 IU or greater, depending on the size of the FMH).

Test for the size of FMH

- 99% of women have an FMH of <4 ml at delivery.
- Of the cases where the FMH is >4 ml, 50% will have occurred during normal delivery.
- Clinical circumstances likely to be associated with a large FMH are:
  * Traumatic deliveries including CS.
  * Stillbirths and fetal deaths.
  * Twin pregnancies (at delivery).
  * Manual removal of the placenta.
  * Abdominal trauma in third trimester.
  * Unexplained hydrops fetalis.
- **Always test to quantify the size of FMH with a Kleihauer screening test performed within 2 hours of delivery.** Where there is no facility to perform the Kleihauer test at delivery, it is reasonable to administer a standard postnatal dose of 1500 IU anti-D Ig.
- Up to 0.3% of women have an FMH >15 ml, which would not be covered if routine 1500 IU of anti-D Ig is given (>200 women each year in the UK).
- Flow cytometry – results are more accurate and more reproducible than those from the Kleihauer test and it detects RhD-positive cells, making it particularly helpful in women with high fetal haemoglobin levels. Flow cytometry is most effectively employed in those cases where a Kleihauer test indicates a large FMH which requires accurate quantitation and follow-up.

Inadvertent transfusion

RhD-positive blood

- Calculate dose on the basis that 500 IU of anti-D Ig will suppress immunization by 4 ml of RhD-positive red blood cells.
- When < 15 ml of RhD-positive blood has been transfused – give appropriate dose of anti-D Ig.
- When > 15 ml has been transfused – use larger anti-D Ig IM preparation (2500 IU or 5000 IU).
- When > 2 units of RhD-positive blood have been transfused – consider an exchange transfusion. Immediate exchange transfusion will reduce the load of RhD-positive red cells (a single-blood-volume exchange will achieve a 65–70% reduction in RhD-positive cells, and a two-volume exchange 85–90%).
- Following exchange transfusion, estimate the residual volume of RhD-positive red cells using flow cytometry or rosetting. IV anti-D Ig is the preparation of choice, achieving adequate plasma levels immediately and being twice as effective as IM anti-D Ig at clearing red cells. Undertake follow-up tests for RhD-positive red cells every 48 hours and give further anti-D Ig until all RhD-positive red cells have been cleared from the circulation.

RhD-positive platelets

- RhD-negative platelets can be provided for women of childbearing age who need a platelet transfusion. If an appropriate product is not available, it may be necessary to use RhD-positive platelets – give prophylaxis against possible Rh alloimmunization by red cells contaminating the platelet products.
- Each unit of platelets prepared from one whole blood donation contains < 1 × 10⁹ L (< 0.1 ml) red cells. Give 250 IU (50 µg) anti-D Ig following every 3 adult doses (i.e. derived from up to 18 routine donations) of platelets.
- Give anti-D Ig SC to avoid the possibility of a haematoma following IM injection in women with thrombocytopenia.

Postnatal prophylaxis

- Give at least 500 IU of anti-D Ig to every non-sensitized RhD-negative woman within 72 hours following the delivery of an RhD-positive infant. This includes women with alloantibodies other than anti-D.
- Undertake a test to detect FMH >4 ml so that additional anti-D Ig can be given as appropriate.
- If the pregnancy is non-viable and no sample can be obtained from the baby, give anti-D Ig to a non-sensitized RhD-negative woman.

What not to do

- Anti-D prophylaxis in women with a weak expression of the RhD blood group (Du).
- Anti-D for spontaneous miscarriage before 12+0 weeks, provided there is no instrumentation of the uterus.
- Routine administration of anti-D Ig in threatened miscarriage in first 12 weeks of pregnancy.
- RAADP in women who are already RhD sensitized.

The use of anti-D immunoglobulin for rhesus D prophylaxis. RCOG Green-top Guideline No. 22; March 2011.

Background and incidence

- SGA – neonate with an estimated fetal weight (EFW) or abdominal circumference (AC) less than the 10th centile.
- Severe SGA is a neonate with EFW or AC less than the 3rd centile.
- 50–70% of SGA fetuses are constitutionally small, with fetal growth appropriate for maternal size and ethnicity.
- Fetal growth restriction (FGR) – fetus with a pathological restriction of the genetic growth potential. There may be evidence of fetal compromise (abnormal umbilical Doppler studies, reduced liquor volume).
- A fetus with growth restriction may not be SGA.
- The likelihood of FGR is higher in severe SGA infants.
- Low birth weight (LBW) – an infant with a birth weight < 2500 g.
- SGA –
  1. Normal (constitutionally) small.
  2. Non-placenta-mediated growth restriction (structural or chromosomal anomaly, inborn errors of metabolism, and fetal infection).
  3. Placenta-mediated growth restriction.
- The use of centiles customized for maternal characteristics (maternal height, weight, parity, and ethnic group), as well as gestational age at delivery and infant sex, identifies small babies at higher risk of morbidity and mortality than those identified by population centiles.

Risks or complications

- Structurally normal SGA fetuses are at increased risk of perinatal mortality and morbidity but most adverse outcomes are concentrated in the growth-restricted group.
- Greater risk of stillbirth, birth hypoxia, neonatal complications.
- Impaired neurodevelopment.
- Type 2 (non-insulin-dependent) diabetes and hypertension in adult life.

Prevention

- Interventions to promote smoking cessation may prevent SGA birth. Offer it to all women who are pregnant and smoke. Women who are able to stop smoking by 15 weeks of gestation can reduce the risk back to that of non-smokers.
- Antiplatelet agents may be effective in women at high risk of PET. In women at high risk of PET, commence antiplatelet agents at or before 16 weeks of pregnancy.
- Antithrombotic therapy appears to be promising for preventing SGA in high-risk women. However, do not offer in view of limited data and potentially serious side effects.
- No consistent evidence that dietary modification prevents SGA.

Screening

1st and 2nd trimester – medical and obstetric history; examination; maternal serum screening and uterine artery Doppler.
2nd and 3rd trimester – abdominal palpation and measurement of symphysis fundal height (SFH).

1. **History** – At booking assess for risk factors for a SGA fetus.
- **Risk factors with OR ≥ 2.0:**
  * Maternal age > 40 years, smoker ≥ 11 cigarettes per day, cocaine, daily vigorous exercise.
  * Previous SGA baby, previous stillbirth, previous preterm unexplained stillbirth.
  * Maternal SGA, chronic hypertension, diabetes with vascular disease, moderate and severe renal impairment (especially when associated with HT), antiphospholipid syndrome, paternal SGA.
- SLE and certain types of congenital heart disease (particular cyanotic congenital heart disease) are associated with increased likelihood of a SGA neonate but there are no papers reporting ORs. Assess the risk on an individual basis.
- **Minor risk factors with OR > 1 to < 2.0:**
  * Maternal age ≥ 35 years, nulliparity, BMI < 20, BMI > 25, smoker 1–10 cigarettes per day, moderate alcohol intake, maternal caffeine consumption ≥ 300 mg per day in the 3rd trimester, IVF singleton pregnancy, low fruit intake pre-pregnancy.
  * African American or Indian/Asian ethnicity, social deprivation, unmarried status, domestic violence.
  * Pre-eclampsia, pregnancy interval < 6 months, pregnancy interval ≥ 60 months, heavy bleeding in 1st trimester.
- Asthma, thyroid disease, IBS, and depression – if uncomplicated and adequately treated, these are not risk factors.
- Evidence regarding recurrent miscarriage is conflicting.
- Low maternal weight gain is associated with an SGA infant in a preterm population but it is no longer recommended that women are routinely weighed during pregnancy.

- Women who have a major risk factor (OR > 2.0) – serial USS of fetal size and UmAD from 26 to 28 weeks onwards.
- Women who have ≥ 3 minor risk factors – uterine artery Doppler at 20–24 weeks.

2. Clinical examination

- Abdominal palpation has limited accuracy for the prediction of a SGA neonate. Physical examination of the abdomen by inspection and palpation detects as few as 30% SGA fetuses.
- SFH – perform serial measurement of SFH at each antenatal appointment from 24 weeks of pregnancy as this improves prediction of a SGA neonate.
- SFH – measure from the fundus (variable point) to the symphysis pubis (fixed point) with the cm values hidden from the examiner.
- Maternal obesity, abnormal fetal lie, large fibroids, hydramnios, and fetal head engagement limit the predictive accuracy of SFH measurement.
- SFH is associated with significant intra- and interobserver variation and serial measurement may improve accuracy.
- Plot SFH on customized chart rather than a population-based chart as this may improve prediction of an SGA neonate. A customized SFH chart is adjusted for maternal characteristics (maternal height, weight, parity, and ethnic group). Use of customized charts is also associated with fewer referrals for investigation and fewer admissions.
- The impact on perinatal outcome of measuring SFH is uncertain.

3. Biochemical markers used for Down syndrome (DS) screening

- A low level (< 0.4 MoM) of the 1st trimester marker PAPP–A – **major risk factor.**
- 2nd trimester DS markers (AFP; elevated hCG; and inhibin A; low unconjugated estriol and the combined triple test) have limited predictive accuracy.

4. Uterine artery Doppler (UtAD)

- Low-risk population – do not offer UtAD, as it has limited accuracy to predict a SGA neonate and it has shown no benefit to mother or baby.
- Women with major risk factor for a SGA neonate – UtAD has insufficient predictive value as a screening test to negate the risk associated with a major risk factor and therefore does not change care. Arrange serial USS of fetal size and UmAD from 26 to 28 weeks onwards.
- Women with multiple minor risk factors – consider UtAD screening at 20–24 weeks –
  * Women with an **abnormal UtAD** (defined as a pulsatility index [PI] > 95th centile) and/or notching – serial USS of fetal size and UmAD from 26 to 28 weeks onwards. In these women subsequent normalization of flow velocity indices is still associated with an increased risk of a SGA neonate. Do not repeat UtAD as it has limited value.
  * Women with a **normal UtAD** do not require any further referral unless they develop specific pregnancy complications, for example APH or HT. However, offer them a scan for fetal size and UmAD during the 3rd trimester.

5. Fetal echogenic bowel

- Fetal echogenic bowel is associated with a SGA neonate (OR 2.1) and fetal demise (OR 9.6) – major risk factor.

6. Re-assess the risk 20–24 weeks

- Additional screening information and pregnancy complications may develop.
- Major risk factor (OR ≥ 2.0) –
  * PAPP–A < 0.4 MoM, echogenic bowel.
  * Low maternal weight gain, unexplained APH, severe PIH, PET, heavy bleeding.
- Minor risk factor (OR > 1 to < 2.0) –
  * Mild PIH; placental abruption; caffeine ≥ 300 mg/day in third trimester.

- Single SFH which plots < 10th centile or serial measurements show slow or static growth by crossing centiles – USS of fetal size
- Women in whom measurement of SFH is inaccurate (BMI > 35, large fibroids, hydramnios) – serial USS of fetal size and UmAD from 26 to 28 weeks onwards.

One major risk factor – serial USS of fetal size and UmAD from 26 to 28 weeks. **≥ 3 minor risk factors** – UtAD screening at 20–24 weeks.

Abnormal UtAD – serial USS of fetal size and UmAD from 26 to 28 weeks. **Normal UtAD** – one scan for fetal size and UmAD during the 3rd trimester

DDx | Diagnosis

- Designed to predict size but predict fetal wellbeing. The diagnosis of SGA would rely on biometric tests.

Ultrasound biometry

- Use < 10th centile threshold for AC and EFW to diagnose SGA.
- Customized ultrasound EFW charts (adjusted for variables, such as maternal weight, maternal height, ethnic group, and parity) may improve prediction of a SGA neonate and normal/adverse perinatal outcome.
- Routine measurement of fetal AC or EFW in the 3rd trimester in low-risk pregnancy does not improve perinatal outcome. Do not offer routine fetal biometry.
- Serial measurements of AC and EFW (growth velocity) are superior to single estimates in the prediction of FGR and predicting poor perinatal outcome.
- When using 2 measurements of AC or EFW to estimate growth velocity, they should be at least 3 weeks apart to minimize false-positive rates. More frequent measurements may be appropriate where birth weight prediction is relevant outside of the context of diagnosing SGA/FGR.
- Mean growth rates for AC and EFW after 30 weeks of gestation are 10 mm/14 days and 200 g/14 days although greater variation exists in the lower limits. However a change in AC of < 5mm over 14 days is suggestive of FGR.
- There is no evidence to recommend one specific method of measuring AC nor which growth chart to use.
- Ratio measures, such as HC/AC and FL/AC ratios, are poorer than AC or EFW alone in predicting SGA.
- **Where the fetal AC or EFW is < 10th centile or there is evidence of reduced growth velocity – offer serial assessment of fetal size and UmAD.**

Biophysical tests

- Not designed to predict size but predict fetal wellbeing. The presence of fetal wellbeing implies the absence of fetal acidaemia.
- Abnormal biophysical tests are more indicative of FGR than SGA.
- All biophysical tests, including amniotic fluid volume (AFV), umbilical Doppler, CTG, and biophysical scoring, are poor at diagnosing a SGA fetus.
- Amniotic fluid volume (AFV) – has minimal value in diagnosing FGR. Serial measurements of AFI also have disappointing results.
- Uterine artery Doppler (UtAD) – has limited use in predicting FGR.
- Although various Doppler studies of fetal circulation such as aortic to middle cerebral artery pulsatility index ratio are used to predict FGR fetuses, their use needs to be evaluated further.

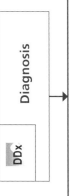

Investigations for severe SGA fetus – refer to FMU

- Detailed fetal anatomical survey and UtAD if identified at 18–20 weeks scan.
- Karyotype in fetuses with structural anomalies and in those detected before 23 weeks of gestation, especially if UtAD is normal.
- In severe SGA, the incidence of chromosomal abnormalities is up to 19%. The most common chromosomal defect is triploidy in fetuses before 26 weeks and trisomy 18 in those after 26 weeks. The risk of aneuploidy is higher in fetuses with a structural abnormality, a normal amniotic fluid volume, a higher head circumference/AC ratio or a normal UtAD.
- Fetal infections – responsible for up to 5% of SGA fetuses. Screen for CMV and toxoplasmosis infection. Test for syphilis and malaria in high-risk populations.
- UtAD has limited accuracy to predict adverse outcome in SGA fetuses diagnosed during the 3rd trimester.

Surveillance

The purpose is to predict fetal acidaemia thereby allowing timely delivery prior to irreversible end-organ damage and in utero death.

Umbilical artery Doppler (UmAD)

- Do not offer screening to the low-risk population by UmAD, as it does not reduce perinatal mortality or morbidity.
- UmAD measurements reduce perinatal morbidity and mortality in high-risk population (SGA).
- Normal UmAD indices – repeat surveillance every 14 days. More frequent Doppler surveillance may be appropriate in a severely SGA fetus.
- However, compared to normally grown fetuses, SGA fetuses with a normal umbilical artery Doppler are still at increased risk of neonatal morbidity and adverse neurodevelopmental outcome.
- Indices of UmAD – PI, RI, systolic/diastolic ratio, and diastolic average ratio. RI has the best discriminatory ability to predict a range of adverse perinatal outcomes.
- For abnormal UmAD indices (pulsatility (PI) or resistance index (RI) > +2 SDs above mean for gestational age) where delivery is not indicated, the optimal frequency of surveillance is unclear. **Repeat surveillance twice weekly in fetuses with positive end-diastolic velocity (PEDV) and daily in fetuses with absent/reversed EDV (AREDV).**

Amniotic fluid volume (AFV) –

- Do not use AFV as the only form of surveillance.
- Use single deepest vertical pocket (SDVP) to interpret AFV.
- Both AFI and single-pocket measurements poorly correlate with actual AFV.
- AFV assessment – See Chapter 11 Amniotic fluid abnormalities.

CTG –

- Do not use CTG as the only form of surveillance.
- No evidence that antenatal CTG in high-risk pregnancies improves perinatal outcome.
- Interpret CTG based on short-term fetal heart rate variation from computerized analysis.
- Computerized CTG (cCTG) is objective and consistent, unlike conventional CTG, which has high intra- and interobserver variability. FHR variation – a short-term variation ≤ 3 ms (within 24 hours of delivery) is associated with a higher rate of metabolic acidaemia and early neonatal death.

Biophysical profile (BPP) –

- BPP as a surveillance tool in high-risk pregnancies does not improve perinatal outcomes and it is associated with an increased risk of CS.

Middle cerebral artery (MCA) Doppler

- Cerebral vasodilatation secondary to increase in diastolic flow is a sign of the 'brain-sparing effect' of chronic hypoxia, and results in decreases in Doppler indices of the MCA. Reduced MCA PI is therefore an early sign of fetal hypoxia in SGA fetuses.
- In the preterm SGA fetus, MCA Doppler has limited accuracy to predict acidaemia and adverse outcome, therefore do not use it to time delivery.
- **In the term SGA fetus with normal UmAD, an abnormal MCA Doppler (PI < 5th centile) has moderate predictive value for acidosis at birth, therefore use it to time delivery.**

Ductus venosus (DtV) and umbilical vein (UV) Doppler

- The DtV Doppler flow velocity pattern reflects atrial pressure–volume changes during the cardiac cycle. As FGR worsens velocity reduces in the DtV a-wave owing to increased afterload and preload, as well as increased end-diastolic pressure, resulting from the directs effects of hypoxia/acidaemia and increased adrenergic drive. A retrograde a-wave and pulsatile flow in the umbilical vein (UV) signifies the onset of overt fetal cardiac compromise.
- DtV Doppler has moderate predictive value for acidaemia and adverse outcome. **In preterm SGA fetus with abnormal UmAD, use DtV Doppler for surveillance and to time delivery.**

Serial USS of fetal size and UmAD from 26 to 28 weeks onwards.

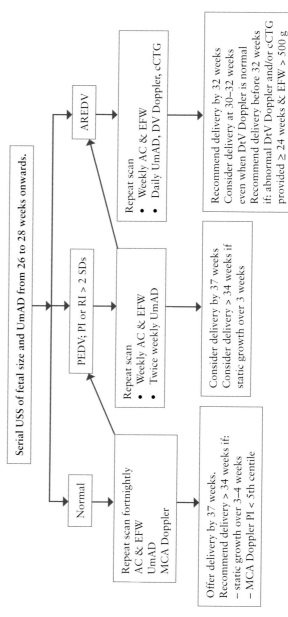

Normal

Repeat scan fortnightly
AC & EFW
UmAD
MCA Doppler

Offer delivery by 37 weeks.
Recommend delivery > 34 weeks if:
– static growth over 3–4 weeks
– MCA Doppler PI < 5th centile

PEDV; PI or RI > 2 SDs

Repeat scan
- Weekly AC & EFW
- Twice weekly UmAD

Consider delivery by 37 weeks
Consider delivery > 34 weeks if static growth over 3 weeks

AREDV

Repeat scan
- Weekly AC & EFW
- Daily UmAD, DV Doppler, cCTG

Recommend delivery by 32 weeks
Consider delivery at 30–32 weeks even when DtV Doppler is normal
Recommend delivery before 32 weeks if: abnormal DtV Doppler and/or cCTG provided ≥ 24 weeks & EFW > 500 g

Mode of delivery

↓

- Term and near term SGA fetuses are at increased risk of FHR decelerations in labour, emergency CS for suspected fetal compromise, and metabolic acidaemia at delivery.
- SGA fetus with umbilical artery AREDV – deliver by CS.
- SGA fetus with normal UmAD or with abnormal umbilical artery PI but PEDV – IOL can be offered but rates of emergency CS are increased. Monitor with continuous EFM from the onset of uterine contractions.
- Admit early women in spontaneous labour with a SGA fetus in order to commence continuous EFM.
- Deliver in a unit where optimal neonatal expertise and facilities are available.
- A neonatologist should be present if gestation is extremely preterm or growth restriction is severe.

What not to do

- Second trimester DS markers or abdominal palpation to predict an SGA neonate.
- Use of UtAD in a low-risk population to predict an SGA neonate.
- Repeat UtAD in women with an abnormal UtAD at 20–24 weeks of pregnancy.
- Routine fetal biometry in the 3rd trimester in low-risk population.
- Use of UtAD to predict adverse outcome in SGA fetuses diagnosed during the 3rd trimester.
- Use of dietary modification, progesterone or calcium to prevent SGA.
- Antithrombotic therapy for preventing SGA in high-risk women.
- CTG and ultrasound assessment of AFV as the only form of surveillance in SGA fetuses.
- Biophysical profile for fetal surveillance in preterm SGA fetuses.
- Use of MCA Doppler in the preterm SGA fetus to time delivery.

The Investigation and Management of the Small-for-Gestational-Age Fetus. RCOG Guideline No. 31; 2nd Edition; February 2013.

When do obstetricians recommend delivery for a high-risk preterm growth-retarded fetus? The GRIT Study Group. Growth Restriction Intervention Trial. Eur J Obstet Gynecol Reprod Biol. 1996 Aug;67(2):121–126.

CHAPTER 9 Reduced fetal movements (RFM)

Background and definition

- A significant reduction or sudden alteration in FM may be a warning sign of impending fetal death. Studies have shown an association between RFM and poor perinatal outcome.
- About 55% of women experiencing a SB perceived a reduction in FMs prior to diagnosis.
- There is no universally agreed definition of RFM, due to the paucity of studies on fetal activity patterns and maternal perception of fetal activity in normal pregnancies.
- There is an association of RFM with FGR, SGA fetus, placental insufficiency, and congenital malformations.

Normal fetal movements (FM) during pregnancy

- Perceived FMs – defined as the maternal sensation of any discrete kick, flutter, swish or roll. Such fetal activity provides an indication of the integrity of the central nervous and musculoskeletal systems. Changes in the number and nature of FMs as the fetus matures are a reflection of normal neurological development of the fetus.
- FMs show diurnal changes, the afternoon and evening periods being periods of peak activity. FMs are usually absent during fetal 'sleep' cycles, which occur regularly throughout the day and night and usually last for 20–40 minutes. These sleep cycles rarely exceed 90 minutes in the normal, healthy fetus.
- By term, the average number of generalized movements/hour is 31, with the longest period between them ranging from 50 to 75 minutes.
- Most women are aware of FMs by 20 weeks and up to and including the onset of labour.
- Some multiparous women may perceive FMs as early as 16 weeks of gestation and some primiparous women may perceive movement much later than 20 weeks of gestation.
- The frequency of FMs tends to increase until the 32nd week and plateaus until the onset of labour. Although FMs tend to plateau at 32 weeks, there is no reduction in their frequency in the late third trimester.

Assessment of FMs

Subjective maternal perception

- Studies on the correlation between maternal perception and concurrent detection of FM on USS show wide variation. Large FMs lasting more than 7 seconds are most likely to be felt.
- The greatest number of FMs are noted when the mother is lying down, and the number appears to be greatest in the evening.
- The difference in mean time to perceive 10 movements varies between 21 minutes for focused counting to 162 minutes with unfocused perception of FMs.
- Objective assessments – Doppler or real-time USS. Studies report slightly increased sensitivity for FMs recorded by USS.

Role of routine FM counting in a formal manner

- Formal FM counting relies on a woman counting FMs and, if she perceives fewer movements than a specified alarm limit, contacting her care provider. Problems with this strategy:
  * There is a wide range of 'normal' FMs, leading to wide variability among mothers.
  * The most frequently used alarm limit was developed in high-risk patients who counted FMs while as inpatients; therefore, these observations may not be applicable to a general population.
- Ideally, an alarm limit would be developed using the whole obstetric population and then be proved to reduce SB rates in a prospective study. There is insufficient evidence to recommend formal FM counting using specified alarm limits.
- Advise women to be aware of their baby's individual pattern of FMs.
- Instructing women to monitor FMs is associated with increased maternal anxiety. Any study on the utility of FMs as a screening test must take into account the potentially deleterious effects on maternal stress and anxiety.

Factors which influence perception of FMs

- There is some evidence that women perceive most FMs when lying down, fewer when sitting, and fewest while standing. When attention is paid in a quiet room and careful recordings are made, FMs that were not previously perceived are often recognized clearly.
- Fetal presentation has no effect on perception of FMs. Fetal position might influence maternal perception: 80% of fetal spines lay anteriorly in women who were unable to perceive FMs despite being able to visualize them on USS.
- There may be an increase in FMs following the elevation of glucose concentration in maternal blood.

Factors associated with reduced FMs

- Sedating drugs which cross the placenta such as alcohol, benzodiazepines, methadone, and other opioids can have a transient effect on FMs.
- From 30 weeks of gestation onwards, the level of carbon dioxide in maternal blood influences fetal respiratory movements, and cigarette smoking may be associated with a decrease in fetal activity.
- Corticosteroids has been reported to decrease FMs and fetal heart rate variability on CTG over the 2 days following administration.
- Fetuses with major malformations. A lack of vigorous motion may relate to abnormalities of the central nervous system, muscular dysfunction or skeletal abnormalities.

Women presting with RFM

Aim – To exclude fetal death; to exclude fetal compromise, and to identify pregnancies at risk of adverse pregnancy outcome while avoiding unnecessary interventions.

History

- Duration of RFM, whether there has been absence of FMs, and whether this is the first occasion the woman has perceived RFM.
- Evaluate SB risk for the presence of factors such as multiple consultations for RFM, known FGR, HT, DM, extremes of maternal age, primiparity, smoking, placental insufficiency, congenital malformation, obesity, racial/ethnic factors, poor past obstetric history, genetic factors, and issues with access to care.

Examination

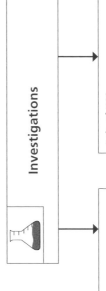

- **Confirm fetal viability.** Auscultate fetal heart using a handheld Doppler device to exclude fetal death. If the presence of a fetal heart beat is not confirmed, refer immediately for USS assessment of fetal cardiac activity.
- Clinically assess fetal size to detect SGA fetuses – abdominal palpation and measurement of SFH. Consider USS for fetal biometry in women in whom clinical assessment is likely to be less accurate, for example, those with a raised BMI.
- BP and urine for proteinuria as PET is associated with placental dysfunction.

Investigations

Role of CTG

- CTG for at least 20 minutes to exclude fetal compromise if the pregnancy is > 28+0 weeks. The presence of a normal FHR pattern is indicative of a healthy fetus with a properly functioning autonomic nervous system.
- If the term fetus does not experience a FHR acceleration for > 80 minutes, fetal compromise is likely to be present.
- **Routine CTG monitoring of 'at risk' pregnancies** – a systematic review did not confirm or refute any benefits.
- In an observational study of women presenting with RFM who had an initial CTG and an USS, 21% had an abnormality detected that required action and 4.4% were admitted for immediate delivery.

Role of USS

- There are no RCTs of USS versus no USS in women with RFM.
- A study from Norway investigated a protocol of CTG and USS within 2 hours if women reported no FMs, and within 12 hours if they reported RFM to assess AFV, fetal size, and fetal anatomy. There was a significant reduction in all SBs from 3.0 to 2.0 per 1000, and from 4.2% to 2.4% of women presenting with RFM. There was more than a doubling in the number of USS (OR 2.64) but this seemed to be compensated by a reduction in additional follow-up consultations and admissions for IOL. The addition of Doppler studies did not show any additional benefit.
- Perform USS assessment in a woman presenting with RFM after 28+0 weeks if RFM persists despite a normal CTG or if there are any additional risk factors for FGR/SB. Perform it within 24 hours and include assessment of AC and/or EFW to detect the SGA fetus, AFV, and fetal morphology if this has not previously been performed.
- There may be a role for the selective use of biophysical profile (BPP). A systematic review – evidence from RCTs does not support the use of BPP as a test of fetal wellbeing in high-risk pregnancies. However, there is evidence from observational studies that BPP in high-risk women has good NPV, i.e. fetal death is rare in women in the presence of a normal BPP.
- The basis of the BPP is the observed association between hypoxia and alterations of measures of central nervous system performance such as FHR patterns, FM, and fetal tone.

Management of RFM

Before 24+0 weeks of gestation

- Confirm fetal heartbeat by auscultation with a Doppler handheld device. While placental insufficiency rarely presents before the first trimester, it is done to exclude fetal demise.
- Women who present with no FMs at all may have a fetus with an underlying neuromuscular condition.
- If FMs have never been felt by 24 weeks of gestation, refer to a specialist FMU to look for any fetal neuromuscular conditions.

Between 24+0 and 28+0 weeks of gestation

- Confirm fetal heartbeat by auscultation with a Doppler handheld device.
- Undertake a comprehensive SB risk evaluation.
- Placental insufficiency may present at this gestation. If there is clinical suspicion of FGR, consider USS.
- **There is no evidence to recommend the routine use of CTG surveillance in this group.**

After 28+0 weeks of gestation

- Advise women to contact their maternity unit, and not to wait until the next day for assessment of fetal wellbeing.
- If women are unsure whether FMs are reduced, advise them to lie on their left side and focus on FMs for 2 hours. If they do not feel 10 or more discrete movements in 2 hours, advise them to contact their midwife or maternity unit.
- Undertake a history and examination as above.
- Confirm fetal heartbeat by auscultation with a Doppler handheld device.

- Reassure – if woman does not have RFM any longer, there are no other risk factors for SB and FHR is present on auscultation.'
- However, if the woman still has concerns, advise her to attend her maternity unit.

- Women noticing a sudden change in fetal activity or in whom other risk factors for SB are identified.

Refer to maternity unit for further investigation.

CTG to exclude fetal compromise.

Normal investigations:

- Reassure that 70% of pregnancies with a single episode of RFM are uncomplicated.
- There are no data to support formal FM counting (kick charts) in these women.
- There are no studies of the follow-up of women who have normal investigations.
- Advise women to contact their maternity unit if they have another episode of RFM.

USS – if

- The perception of RFM persists despite a normal CTG.
- Recurrent RFMs.
- Any additional risk factors for FGR/SB.

Recurrent episode of RFM

- Review to exclude predisposing causes.
- Women who present on two or more occasions with RFM are at increased risk of a poor perinatal outcome (SB, FGR or PTD) compared with those who attend on only one occasion (OR 1.9).
- There are no studies to determine whether intervention (e.g., delivery or further investigation) alters perinatal morbidity or mortality. Therefore, the decision whether or not to induce labour at term in these women when the growth, liquor volume, and CTG appear normal must be made after careful consultant-led counselling on an individualized basis.

What not to do

- The addition of Doppler studies to fetal size and AFV on USS.
- Routine use of CTG surveillance between 24+0 and 28+0 weeks of gestation.
- Formal FM counting (kick charts) in these women.

Reduced Fetal Movements. RCOG Green-top Guideline 57; February 2011.

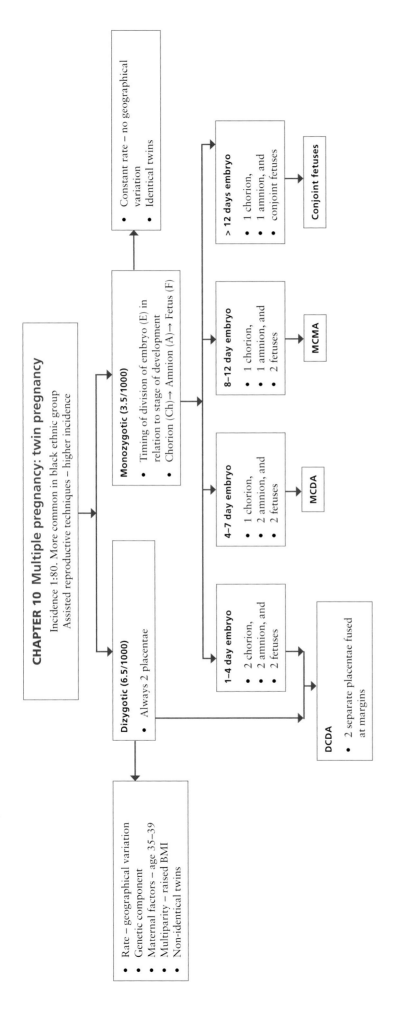

CHAPTER 10 Multiple pregnancy: twin pregnancy

Incidence 1:80. More common in black ethnic group
Assisted reproductive techniques – higher incidence

Dizygotic (6.5/1000)
- Always 2 placentae

- Rate – geographical variation
- Genetic component
- Maternal factors – age 35–39
- Multiparity – raised BMI
- Non-identical twins

Monozygotic (3.5/1000)
- Timing of division of embryo (E) in relation to stage of development
- Chorion (Ch) → Amnion (A) → Fetus (F)

- Constant rate – no geographical variation
- Identical twins

1–4 day embryo
- 2 chorion,
- 2 amnion, and
- 2 fetuses

DCDA
- 2 separate placentae fused at margins

4–7 day embryo
- 1 chorion,
- 2 amnion, and
- 2 fetuses

MCDA

8–12 day embryo
- 1 chorion,
- 1 amnion, and
- 2 fetuses

MCMA

> 12 days embryo
- 1 chorion,
- 1 amnion, and
- conjoint fetuses

Conjoint fetuses

Background

- Chorionicity: the number of chorionic (outer) membranes that surround babies in a multiple pregnancy, indicating whether babies share a placenta. In monochorionic (MC) pregnancies babies share one placenta; in dichorionic pregnancies (DC) there are two placentas; in trichorionic triplet pregnancies each baby has a separate placenta.
- Amnionicity: the number of amnions (inner membranes) surrounding babies in a multiple pregnancy. Pregnancies with one amnion (so that all babies share an amniotic sac) are monoamniotic (MA); with two amnions are diamniotic (DA); and with three amnions are triamniotic.
- Zygosity: pregnancies are either monozygous (arising from one fertilized egg) or dizygous (arising from two separate fertilized eggs). Monozygous twins are identical; dizygous twins are non-identical.

History and examination

- History – hyperemesis, assisted conception
- Examination – large for dates

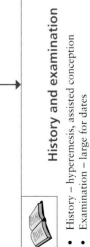

Risks or complications

- **Maternal risks:**
Hyperemesis, anaemia, PTL, PET/PIH, placenta praevia, APH, PPH, hydramnios
- **Fetal risk:**
Miscarriage, congenital abnormalities, loss of one twin, IUGR, TTTS, TRAP
  - PNM 3 times higher in MC compared to DC

Service provision - MDT

- Core team – specialist obstetricians, specialist midwives, ultrasonographers.
- Enhanced team for referrals – perinatal mental health professional; physiotherapist; infant feeding specialist; dietician.
- Coordinate clinical care to: minimize the number of hospital visits; provide care as close to the woman's home as possible; provide continuity of care within and between hospitals and the community.

Investigations

- First trimester USS when CRL measures 45 mm to 84 mm (at 11 weeks 0 days to 13 weeks 6 days) to estimate gestational age, determine chorionicity, and screen for Down syndrome. Use the largest baby to measure gestational age.
- Assign nomenclature to babies in twin and triplet pregnancies and document this in the notes to ensure consistency throughout pregnancy.

Chorionicity – Determine chorionicity using the number of placental masses, the lambda or T-sign, and membrane thickness.

- Lamda sign is formed by a tongue of placental tissue within the base of dichorionic membranes.
- For women presenting after 14 weeks 0 days, use all of the above features and discordant fetal sex.
- Do not use 3D USS to determine chorionicity.

Problems determining chorionicity:

- Poor transabdominal views because of a retroverted uterus or high BMI – use TVS.
- If it is not possible to determine chorionicity seek a second opinion or refer to a HCP competent in determining chorionicity by USS, ASAP.
- If it is still difficult after referral, manage as MC until proved otherwise.

Indications for referral – FMU

- MCMA twin/triplet pregnancies.
- MCDA/DCDA triplet pregnancies.

Maternal care

- Book at 10 weeks.
- Higher incidence of anaemia – Perform a FBC at 20–24 weeks to identify a need for early supplementation with iron or folic acid, and repeat at 28 weeks.
- **Hypertension** – Measure BP and test urine for proteinuria at each appointment.
- 75 mg of aspirin daily from 12 weeks until the birth of the babies if they have one or more of the following risk factors for hypertension: * First pregnancy. * ≥age 40 years or older. * Pregnancy interval of more than 10 years. * BMI of 35 or more at first visit. * Family history of PET.

Preterm birth (PTB)

- **Predict the risk of PTB**
  - * Higher risk if history of a spontaneous PTB in a previous singleton pregnancy.
  - * Do not use cervical length (with or without fetal fibronectin) routinely to predict the risk of PTB.
  - * Do not use the following to predict the risk of PTB: fetal fibronectin testing alone; home uterine activity monitoring.
- **Preventing PTB** – do not use the following routinely to prevent spontaneous PTB: bed rest at home or in hospital; IM or vaginal progesterone; cervical cerclage; oral tocolytics.
- **Untargeted corticosteroids** – do not use single or multiple untargeted (routine) courses of corticosteroids.

Antenatal care - plan care according to chorionicity

Screening for Down syndrome

- Inform women:
  - * Greater likelihood of Down syndrome in MPs. * Different options for screening.
  - * Higher false positive rate of screening tests. * Greater likelihood of being offered invasive testing and of complications from this testing. * Physical and psychological risks related to selective fetal reduction.
  - * Calculate risk per pregnancy in MC pregnancies and for each baby in DC and TC pregnancies.
- Twin pregnancies
  - * Use the 'combined test'.
  - * Consider second trimester serum screening if woman books too late. Explain the potential problems (increased likelihood of pregnancy loss associated with double invasive testing because the risk cannot be calculated separately for each baby).
- Triplet pregnancies
  - * Use NT and maternal age. * Do not use second trimester serum screening.
- Refer to FMU – Women whose risk of Down's syndrome exceeds 1:150.

Fetal anomaly and growth scans

- Structural abnormalities (anomaly scan at 18+0 to 20+6 weeks) – Consider scheduling scans slightly later.
- Serial growth scans:
  - * MC – Clinic appointment and scan FFTS starting at 16/40 – every 2 weeks up to 24 weeks; 28 weeks, 32 weeks, 34 weeks, and 36 weeks.
  - * DC – Scan starting at 20 weeks – every 4 weeks. Clinic appointment at 16 and 34 weeks.
- Monitor for IUGR:
  - * EFW discordance using 2 or more biometric parameters at each USS from 20 weeks.
  - * Aim to undertake scans at intervals of < 28 days.
  - * Consider a 25% or greater difference in size between twins or triplets as a clinically important indicator of IUGR and refer to FMU.
- Fetal Growth: USS – 4 weekly for DC; 2 weekly for MC.
- Do not use: abdominal palpation or SFH measurements to predict IUGR; umbilical artery Doppler ultrasound to monitor for IUGR or birth weight differences.

For monochorionic pregnancies (MC twins; DC and MC triplets)

Feto-fetal transfusion syndrome (FFTS)

- Do not monitor for FFTS in the first trimester.
- Monitor with USS for FFTS (including identification of membrane folding) from 16 weeks.
- Repeat fortnightly until 24 weeks.
- If membrane folding or other possible signs (pregnancies with inter twin membrane infolding and amniotic fluid discordance) are found, monitor weekly to allow time to intervene if needed.

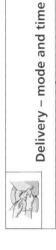

Delivery – mode and time

Uncomplicated twin pregnancies

- About 60% of twin pregnancies result in spontaneous birth before 37 weeks.
- Continuing twin pregnancies beyond 38 weeks increases the risk of fetal death.
- Offer elective birth at:
  * 36 weeks for MC twin pregnancies, after a course of corticosteroids.
  * 37 weeks for DC twin pregnancies.

Uncomplicated triplet pregnancies

- About 75% of triplet pregnancies result in spontaneous birth before 35 weeks.
- Continuing triplet pregnancies beyond 36 weeks increases the risk of fetal death.
- Offer elective birth from 35 weeks, after a course of corticosteroids.

If elective birth is declined, offer weekly appointments with an USS, fortnightly fetal growth scans, and weekly biophysical profile.

Mode of delivery

Vaginal delivery
- Cephalic/cephalic, cephalic/breech presentations.

Indications for CS:
- MCMA pregnancies – risk of cord entanglement – best delivered at 32/40 by CS, after corticosteroids.
- Breech/breech, breech/cephalic presentations.
- Any complications – PET, IUGR.

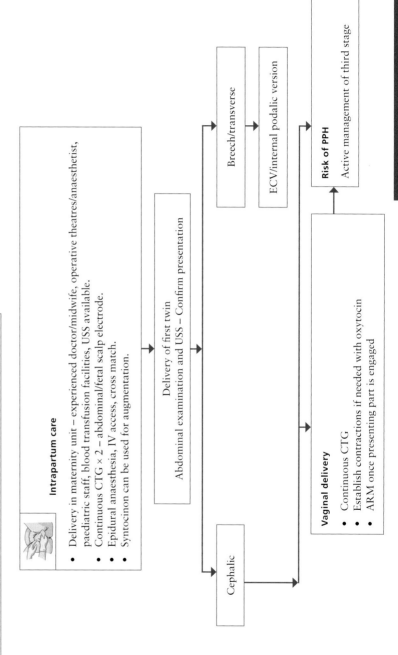

Intrapartum care

- Delivery in maternity unit – experienced doctor/midwife, operative theatres/anaesthetist, paediatric staff, blood transfusion facilities, USS available.
- Continuous CTG × 2 – abdominal/fetal scalp electrode.
- Epidural anaesthesia, IV access, cross match.
- Syntocinon can be used for augmentation.

Delivery of first twin
Abdominal examination and USS – Confirm presentation

Cephalic

Breech/transverse

ECV/internal podalic version

Vaginal delivery
- Continuous CTG
- Establish contractions if needed with oxytocin
- ARM once presenting part is engaged

Risk of PPH
Active management of third stage

Monochorionic twin pregnancies

Around one-third of twin pregnancies in the UK

USS monitoring

- 10–13 weeks – assess viability, major congenital malformation, NT, and chorionicity. Overall, the correct diagnosis can be made in 96%.
- NT and CRL discordance may be useful in identifying MC twin pregnancies at risk of FFTS.
- Uncomplicated MC pregnancies – USS monitoring from 16/40 every 2 weeks.
- USS at 16 to 24/40 – focus on detection of FFTS. After 24/40, when first presentation of FFTS is uncommon, the main purpose is to detect IUGR.
- Umbilical artery waveforms may show cyclical absent or reversed EDF. More common in discordant growth restriction (45%) than uncomplicated (5%) or severe FFTS (2%). The significance of Doppler findings, in terms of timing intervention, is not clear.

Fetal risks

- MC pregnancies have higher fetal loss rates than DC:
  * Main risk of fetal death < 24 weeks.
  * Remain at higher risk of PNM > 24/40 (3.3%).
  * Higher neurodevelopmental morbidity.
- For uncomplicated MCDA pregnancy there may be a higher risk of unexplained fetal demise despite intensive fetal surveillance.
- Significant intrauterine size discordance occurs in MC twins in the absence of FFTS in 10% of cases. It may be differentiated from FFTS by the absence of polyhydramnios in one of the amniotic sacs, although the small twin may have oligohydramnios owing to placental insufficiency.
- Consequences to the co-twin of fetal death.
- Discordant malformations.
- MCMA pregnancy (1% of twin pregnancies) – cord entanglement.
- FFTS.

Fetal death of the co-twin in MC pregnancy

Management – FMU

- Rapid delivery is usually unwise.
- Evidence of fetal compromise (abnormal CTG) could represent continuing damage to the brain and other organs, as well as already existing damage.
- A conservative policy is often appropriate, with brain imaging by 4 weeks to establish whether serious cerebral morbidity has occurred.
- The appearances of such manifestations on USS of the fetal CNS are variable and may take up to 4 weeks to occur.
- Fetal MRI provides earlier & more detailed information.
- Fetal anaemia may be assessed in the surviving twin by measurement of the fetal MCA peak systolic velocity using Doppler.
- There are a few reports of IUT of anaemic surviving co-twins but the value of this intervention is not established, in terms of preventing perinatal and long-term neurological morbidity.
- TOP would be an option.
- The gestational age at the time of diagnosis will have an important influence on management options.

Risks to survivor twin

- The odds of death and neurological damage – 6 and 4 times greater in MC than in DC.
- Death – 12% in MC and 4% in DC.
- Neurological abnormality – 18% MC and 1% DC.
- Preterm birth – 68% MC and 57% in DC.
- Serious compromise in the surviving fetus may be anticipated, including a significant risk of long-term morbidity.
- Damage to MC twins after the death of a co-twin is due to the acute haemodynamic changes around the time of death, with the survivor essentially haemorrhaging part of its circulating volume into the circulation of the dying twin.
- This may cause transient or persistent hypotension and low perfusion, leading to the risk of ischaemic organ damage, notably but not exclusively to the brain.

FFTS

Diagnosis

- Symptoms – sudden increases in abdominal size or breathlessness.
- Based on USS criteria:
  * Presence of a single placental mass.
  * Concordant gender.
  * Oligohydramnios with maximum vertical pocket (MVP) < 2 cm in one sac and polyhydramnios in other sac (MVP ≥ 8 cm).
  * Discordant bladder appearances – severe TTTS.
  * Haemodynamic and cardiac compromise – severe FFTS.

Quintero system of staging

I. Discrepancy in AFV with oligohydramnios – MVP ≤ 2 cm in one sac and polyhydramnios in other sac (MVP ≥ 8 cm). The bladder of the donor twin is visible and Doppler studies are normal.

II. Bladder of the donor twin is not visible but Doppler studies are not critically abnormal.

III. Doppler studies are critically abnormal in either twin and are characterized as abnormal or reversed EDF in the umbilical artery, reverse flow in the ductus venosus or pulsatile umbilical venous flow.

IV. Ascites, pericardial or pleural effusion, scalp oedema or overt hydrops.

V. One or both babies are dead.

- Some prognostic value but the course of the condition is unpredictable.
- There is a relationship between Quintero stage at diagnosis and mean gestational age at delivery and perinatal survival.
- Disease progression is often unpredictable, with 28% of pregnancies improving, 35% worsening, and 37% remaining in the same grade.
- Pregnancies may progress from stage I to stage III without passing through stage II.

Surveillance/investigations – FMU

- Detailed USS with extended views of the fetal heart.
- Fetal echocardiographic assessment in severe FFTS. 11% of fetuses have secondary, structural heart disease, predominantly pulmonary stenosis.

Management of severe FFTS

Termination/selective termination

- Some women may request TOP.
- Selective TOP using bipolar diathermy of one of the umbilical cords. This may be appropriate if there is severe hydrops fetalis in the recipient or evidence of cerebral damage in either twin.
- Treat severe FFTS presenting < 26/40 by laser ablation rather than by amnioreduction or septostomy.
- Laser ablation versus amnioreduction – more babies survive without neurological abnormality at 6 months of age after laser ablation.
- Anastomoses may be missed at laser ablation and FFTS can recur later in up to 14%.

Optimal timing and mode of delivery

- Uncomplicated MC pregnancies – aim for vaginal birth unless there are specific indications for CS.
- Some units deliver all MCDA twins by CS due to 10% risk of acute transfusion in labour, although the evidence base for this is unclear.
- Acute transfusion can occur during labour, therefore continuous EFM in labour.

What not to do

- 3D USS to determine chorionicity.
- Second trimester serum screening.
- Abdominal palpation or SFH measurements to predict IUGR; umbilical artery Doppler ultrasound to monitor for IUGR or birth weight differences.
- Monitor for FFTS in the first trimester.
- Routine use of cervical length to predict the risk of PTB.
- Use fetal fibronectin test alone; home uterine activity monitoring to predict the risk of PTB.
- Routine use of bed rest at home or in hospital; IM or vaginal progesterone; cervical cerclage; oral tocolytics to prevent PTB.
- Single or multiple untargeted (routine) courses of corticosteroids.

Multiple Pregnancy: the Management of Twin and Triplet Pregnancies in the Antenatal Period; NICE CGN 129, September 2011.
Management of Monochorionic Twin Pregnancy. RCOG Green-top Guideline No. 51; December 2008.

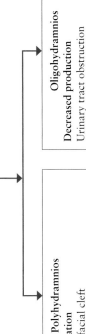

Amniotic fluid dynamics

- Early transudation across skin and placental surfaces becomes negligible by skin maturation at about 22 weeks. Amniotic fluid is formed primarily from lung fluid (about 100 ml/day) and fetal urine (7–10 ml/kg/hour) and is eliminated primarily by fetal swallowing, up to 1 l/day. Near term, urine concentration increases and volume of production falls. Other normal fetal functions also contribute – regurgitation, diuresis (e.g., caffeine or hyperglycaemia from maternal diabetes), and efficiency of fetal swallowing.
- Impact of anomalies – these dynamics are markedly altered by fetal abnormalities. Abnormal swallowing (obstruction or neurological) means many fetuses with anomalies, including aneuploidy, have polyhydramnios; urinary tract anomalies are related to oligohydramnios.

Polyhydramnios

Decreased elimination
Choanal atresia, facial cleft
TE fistula, oesophageal atresia
Imperforate anus, reduced swallowing, drug induced
Polyuria – abnormal kidneys, brain injury, diabetes

Oligohydramnios

Decreased production
Urinary tract obstruction
Renal failure (bad kidneys)
Oliguria
Placental failure
Renal agenesis
Absent lung fluid (e.g., tracheal atresia)

Amniotic fluid volume measurement

- Invasive studies, using amniocentesis to instill dye, and remeasuring after mixing reported – neither single deepest vertical pool nor the four-quadrant amniotic fluid index (AFI) produced very accurate evaluation.
- Review (11 studies) – no significant difference in sensitivity, while specificity for oligohydramnios was superior for single deepest vertical pool set at 2 cm to the AFI threshold of 5 cm.
- Categorization of polyhydramnios by single deepest vertical pool is more closely associated with clinical outcome, but neither method is very accurate.
- In management comparisons (especially for oligohydramnios), single deepest vertical pool gives better performance, the same predictive accuracy, fewer false alarms, and better correlation with biophysical and Doppler variables.
- Meta-analysis – the use of AFI led to more diagnoses of oligohydramnios, more IOL, and CS for fetal distress without improving perinatal outcome. The single deepest vertical pool measurement appears to be the more appropriate method for assessing AFV during fetal surveillance.

CHAPTER 11 Amniotic fluid abnormalities

Background and definition

- Amniotic fluid regulation represents a complex interaction of many systems – fetal respiratory, cardiovascular, fluid balance, urinary tract, gastrointestinal, skin, neurological, placenta and membranes, and maternal factors.
- Amniotic fluid functions can be categorized as physical (preventing fetal injury, increasing placental surface, regulating temperature), functional (mobility for practice breathing movement, swallowing exercises the digestive tract, skeletal muscle movement of every kind), and homeostasis (maintaining amnion integrity, fighting infection, discouraging contractions, maintaining cervical length and consistency).

Risks or complications

- Perinatal mortality and morbidity: fetal abnormalities (renal agenesis with oligohydramnios, duodenal atresia, gross neurological anomalies with polyhydramnios); birth weight (IUGR with oligohydramnios, diabetic macrosomia with polyhydramnios).
- The more severe the hydramnios the greater likelihood of a congenital anomaly.
- AFV and perinatal outcome: controversial studies – this does not eliminate the value of amniotic fluid monitoring in an obstetric population. It might be fairer to say that obstetric decisions should not be made based on AFV alone.

Amniotic fluid volume measurement

- The dye-dilution test is considered the 'gold standard.' This, however, necessitates amniocentesis; therefore it is seldom used clinically.
- USS – amniotic fluid index (AFI), single deepest vertical pool, and the subjective assessment of the AFV.
- TVS – no significant difference was noted between the mean measurement of forewaters of patients with oligohydramnios and that of control subjects.
- Concurrent use of colour Doppler imaging with AFI may lead to over diagnosis of oligohydramnios.
- Difficulties with current ultrasonographic methods of amniotic fluid assessment:
  * The 2D nature of real-time ultrasound representation of the true 3D amniotic fluid pockets that are dispersed unequally throughout the amniotic cavity.
  * The presence of a constantly active fetus and loops of umbilical cord in the amniotic fluid cavity, with resulting differences in fluid dispersion throughout the amniotic cavity.
  * The description of a number of cut-off threshold points in the diagnosis of abnormally low amniotic fluid levels.

Polyhydramnios (PH)

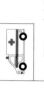

Prevalence and background

- Prevalence is approximately 1–2% depending on the method for diagnosis. In 50%–60% of cases, it is idiopathic.

Degree of polyhydramnios

- AFI – defines polyhydramnios as an AFI of >24 cm or >25 cm, which is >95 or >97.5 percentile in normal singleton pregnancies.
- The AFI has been subdivided into categories – mild as an AFI >25–30 cm, moderate >30.1–35 cm, and severe as an AFI >35.1.
- The definition of polyhydramnios with the SDP is > 8 cm.

Degree	SDP	AFI	Frequency	PNM	Anomalies
Mild	>8	>24	68%	50	6% or less
Moderate	>11	>32	19%	190	Up to 45%
Severe	>15	>44	13%	540	Up to 65%

Risks or complications

- PTL and delivery, malpresentation, abruption from sudden uterine decompression; a 4-fold increase in CS, and a 6-fold increase in PPH.
- Idiopathic PH is associated with increased risk of: PNM 2- to 5-fold, macrosomia 2- to 3-fold, malpresentation, CS, PTD, meconium, NICU admission.
- Only in pregnancies complicated by congenital anomalies and diabetes, the severity of PH correlates with the risk of PTD. In pregnancies with idiopathic PH, the overall rate of PTD is not influenced by its severity and is not higher than the overall rate of PTD.
- The combination of PH and SGA was found to be an independent risk factor for PNM (OR 20.6), neonatal morbidity (OR 2.7), and neonatal mortality (OR 29.7).

Causes of polyhydramnios

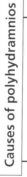

Maternal diabetes

- Fetuses with incompletely controlled diabetes account for about 25%. It is thought that fetal hyperglycaemia produces fetal polyuria due to its osmotic effect.
- Macrosomic diabetic infants also have increased cardiac output and increased blood volume, which increase fetal GFR and urine production.
- Most PH in this group are also in the mild category.

Fetal anomalies

- Abnormalities causing gastrointestinal obstruction – tracheoesophageal (TE) fistula and oesophageal atresia may generate PH of severe proportion for which antenatal imaging is often inconclusive.
- Underlying neurological disorders and PH due to absent or reduced swallowing. This is often associated with reduced activity, symmetrical IUGR, and non-gastrointestinal anomalies (e.g., cardiac anomalies, spina bifida, akinesia).
- Fetuses with borderline cardiac failure or diuresis due to elevated atrial natriuretic peptide (ANP) or brain natriuretic peptide (BNP) are associated with mild to moderate PH.
- In most, the fetal condition precedes PH, but in some (e.g., intermittent severe supraventricular tachycardia), elevated AFV may exist for several weeks before the underlying cause is determined.

Fetal infections – CMV, syphilis, toxoplasmosis, parvovirus.

Twins:

- Twins account for about 7% of PH, two thirds due to recipient status of TTF syndrome, which may reach severe proportions.
- In this case, pure hypervolaemia and corresponding maladaptive responses cause virtually continuous fetal diuresis.

Other causes :

- Isoimmunization, FMH.
- Placental tumours, chorioangioma.

Idiopathic

- The majority fall into the mild group and are idiopathic (55%).
- No long-term sequelae are attributed to this and there are many documented cases of women with serial pregnancies affected by PH, so maternal factors may be influential.

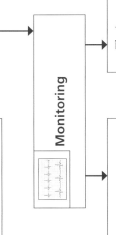

Investigations – rule out possible causes.

- High-level USS; fetal MRI.
- Testing for karyotype and metabolic disorders.
- Use of amniocentesis for the detection of chromosomal abnormalities is controversial.
- Additional tests based on the maternal history of exposure and acute titre suggestive of a recent infection with parvovirus, toxoplasmosis, or CMV.

- Severe PH – **refer to a FMU** (MDT care) for:
  * Close monitoring of contractions, cervical status, and potential interventions to prolong the pregnancy.
  * Counselling regarding possible long-term neurological sequelae.

Monitoring

- Several studies support an association between PH and adverse pregnancy outcome. Thus antepartum fetal surveillance is often employed, but the optimal test (if any) for this surveillance has not been established by rigorous study, nor has the optimal timing for delivery.
- Uterine artery Doppler velocimetry in pregnancies complicated by PH, but without fetal congenital anomalies or diabetes, was not significantly different from controls with normal AFV.
- MCA Doppler velocimetry – the rate of an abnormal MCA pulsatility index was significantly higher in the pregnancies with PH compared to the control group.

- The inverse relationship between amniotic fluid pressure (which correlates with AFV) and umbilical cord pH suggest that conventional antenatal testing (BPP, CTG) may have a role in the antenatal assessment of these pregnancies.
- However, the exact role of either Doppler velocimetry or of the CTG or BPP has not been determined by high quality investigation.
- Periodic assessments of AFV seems reasonable.
- Depending on the gestational age and the presence of other comorbidities, antenatal testing is often performed (CTG or BPP). If these are reassuring, in most cases delivery need not occur before term.

Management

- In pregnancies with an AFV that continues to increase – management depends on the gestational age of the fetus and the presence of maternal complications (e.g., respiratory compromise).
- In the presence of dramatically increasing or symptomatic PH – deliver at or beyond 37 weeks.
- If preterm – consider serial amnioreductions or judicious indomethacin therapy.
- Amnioreduction and the use of indomethacin – neither have been studied in RCTs.

Amnioreduction

- Comparisons of rapid versus slow drainage, large volume versus repeated small volumes, and the use of tocolysis during amnioreduction have not shown significant differences.
- Complications – relate to initial severity, gestational age at presentation, and PTL.
- Serial amniodrainage has been successfully conducted in a number of cases, reducing the impact of prematurity. This benefit must be weighed against the potential risk to mother and fetus should PTL or placental abruption follow the procedure.

Indomethacin

- Renovascular effect reduces fetal urine production – AFV falls, especially in those with normal amniotic fluid (e.g., cases of cervical incompetence), non-obstructive causes (maternal anaemia or maternal renal failure), and after 26 weeks' gestation (fetal renovascular responsiveness earlier is limited).
- The lack of RCT data suggests cautious application.
- The tocolytic effect of indomethacin in prolonging such pregnancies should not be overlooked – reduced amniotic fluid may simply be a side effect.

Oligohydramnios (OH)

Isolated oligohydramnios – The presence of an appropriate-for-gestational-age, non-compromised fetus in the absence of maternal disease.

Risks or complications

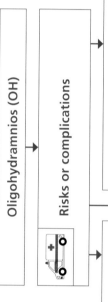

Early OH:

- Even when the fetus is initially normal, chronic OH from PROM (iatrogenic from CVS/amniocentesis, or spontaneous) may cause pulmonary hypoplasia, abnormal chest wall compliance, contractures, and lethal infection.
- Onset, duration, and severity of amniotic fluid loss are important cofactors, but the gestational age at delivery remains the main issue.
- USS visualization is more difficult due to lack of contrast and lack of fetal mobility.
- If anomalies due to aneuploidy are suspected, amniocentesis may be very difficult.
- Severe OH with fetal distress at early gestation means intervention (often classical CS) without a certainty about a normal outcome. In such dilemmas, amnioinfusion may be helpful.

Late OH – OH later in the third trimester:

- Adverse perinatal outcome – results from an increase in umbilical cord compression, potential uteroplacental insufficiency, and an increased incidence of meconium-stained amniotic fluid (and its inherent risks of meconium aspiration syndrome).
- Fetal – stillbirth and neonatal death, fetal distress in labour, low Apgar score, and neonatal complications.
- Maternal – severe PET, reduced success with ECV, IOL or VBAC, poor pain control in labour, and postpartum sepsis.

Investigations

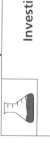

- USS – to determine if kidneys are present, do they work, and will normal renal function be maintained? Any information to suggest inadequate prerenal volume (e.g., severe IUGR with markedly abnormal placental Dopplers, donor status in TTT syndrome).
- It appears logical to infer that in the presence of fetal urine production (as evident by a distended fetal bladder), fetal renal perfusion is unimpaired.
- Decreased AFV in a structurally normal fetus is considered to reflect impaired uteroplacental flow. Redistribution of oxygenated fetal blood towards essential organs resulting in decreased peripheral and renal perfusion would explain decreased urine output and associated oligohydramnios. Normal umbilical artery Doppler velocimetry indices will rule out placental insufficiency as an underlying cause of the OH.
- If all of these observations appear to be normal, there may be a uterine or maternal reason, e.g., occult PROM.

- A meta-analysis – either direct or dye measurement suggested a cut-off of 318 ml for OH.
- Various cut-off criteria have been suggested for the diagnosis of volume OH according to different sonographic volume assessment modalities:
1. Single deepest vertical pool – definitions are in the range <0.5 cm, <1.0 cm, <2 cm, and <3 cm.
2. Two-diameter pocket; vertical × horizontal <15 cm.
3. AFI – definitions of oligohydramnios include <5 cm (which represents <first centile), <5th centile for gestational age (AFI 9.7–7.1 cm), <5 cm, <7 cm, and <8 cm.
- USS is at best imprecise in the detection of OH.
- Using multiple assessments (AFI and deepest pocket) does not add to estimation accuracy.
- Meta-analysis – use of the AFI led to more diagnoses of oligohydramnios, more inductions of labor, and CS for fetal distress without improving perinatal outcome. The single deepest vertical pool measurement appears to be the more appropriate method for assessing AFV during fetal surveillance.

- In patients at <41 weeks' gestation with normal AFI values, a repeated AFI assessment is not necessary for 7 days.
- Post term – because of concerns about uteroplacental insufficiency and the rapid decrease of AFV that may occur, twice-weekly AFV assessments are uniformly practised.
- Doppler velocimetry – pregnancies with OH and normal umbilical artery Doppler velocimetry were significantly less likely to have an abnormal perinatal outcome than those with abnormal Doppler velocimetry. These data suggest that avoiding intervention in pregnancies with OH and normal umbilical artery Doppler velocimetry may decrease iatrogenic morbidity related to prematurity by as much as 26%.

Management

- Amnioinfusion for the restoration of AFV in the mid-trimester and early third trimester has not been fully studied. There is probably no significant maternal danger and fetal outcomes have not been proven to be worse, so it may be considered in individual cases.
- Amnioinfusion lacks benefit antenatally but has specific intrapartum application. Prophylactic transabdominal or transcervical amnioinfusion immediately before or in early labour at term eliminate FHR decelerations from cord compression.
- For isolated OH when other fetal testing is reassuring, amnioinfusion may allow safe vaginal delivery.
- It may reduce meconium aspiration syndrome.

- Studies on maternal hydration (increased water intake, oral or intravenous with oral follow-up) for borderline OH. There was no increase in fluid defined by single deepest vertical pool, no increase in normal AFI, and increased AFI was not sustained >48 hours.
- The severity of this problem has generated attempts to patch iatrogenic holes in the membrane, glue the cervix shut, or chronically replace the fluid.

Time and mode of delivery

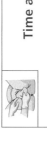

- The reported increased incidence of adverse perinatal outcome in association with OH has led to recommendation for delivery, at least at >37 weeks' gestation.
- However, the original reports of this association included fetuses with structural anomalies, SGA, growth-restricted fetuses, postmaturity, and mothers with various underlying medical conditions that may affect AFV. Furthermore, OH may be a transient finding.
- AFI <5 cm as a trigger for delivery is associated with increased fetal distress, more CSs, and significant maternal morbidity. Many of those women would labour on their own before the MVP trigger of only 2 cm is reached, with significant improvement in obstetric parameters.
- Although IOL in post-term patients with oligohydramnios (AFI <5 cm or no vertical pocket >2 cm) is considered the standard of care, adherence to this practice results in subsequent increases in labour complications and the incidence of operative delivery without significantly improving outcome.

- The finding of OH in the clinical settings of FGR, postdates pregnancy, or pregnancies complicated by maternal disease may indicate increased risk for intrauterine fetal demise or neonatal morbidity and may be an indication for delivery.
- When oligohydramnios accompanies abnormal Doppler ultrasound indicating placental insufficiency, or abnormal BPP or FHR testing indicating increased risk of asphyxia, delivery is the principal treatment.
- Before term, oligohydramnios is probably not reliable as a sole factor indicating delivery.

- Women who underwent IOL for isolated OH between 37 and 42 weeks' gestation were matched to women presenting in spontaneous labour with normal AFI – neonatal outcome measures did not differ. Significantly higher CS rates were observed among women in whom labour was induced than controls.
- Isolated OH may not be a marker for fetal compromise and IOL may not be warranted in most cases.
- In a study in which women with isolated OH diagnosed by AFI values <5 cm were randomly allocated to expectant management versus IOL – the majority of patients managed expectantly entered spontaneous labour within 3 days of ultrasonographic diagnosis.
- In the presence of an appropriate-for-gestational-age fetus, with reassuring fetal wellbeing and the absence of maternal disease, OH is not associated with an increased incidence of adverse perinatal outcome.
- Given the poor current ultrasonographic capability to diagnose correctly decreased AFV (other than overt OH), the reported transient nature of OH, and evidence that AFV may be increased with maternal hydration, it appears that IOL at term for decreased AFV should be reconsidered.

Harman CR. Amniotic fluid abnormalities. Semin Perinatol. 2008 Aug;32(4):288–294.

Magann EF, Chauhan SP, Doherty DA, Lutgendorf MA, Magann MI, Morrison JC. A review of idiopathic hydramnios and pregnancy outcomes. Obstet Gynecol Surv. 2007 Dec;62(12):795–802.

Dashe JS, McIntire DD, Ramus RM, Santos-Ramos R, Twickler DM. Hydramnios: anomaly prevalence and sonographic detection. Obstet Gynecol. 2002 Jul;100(1):134–139.

Nabhan AF, Abdelmoula YA. Amniotic fluid index versus single deepest vertical pocket: a meta-analysis of randomized controlled trials. Int J Gynaecol Obstet. 2009 Mar;104(3):184–188. Epub 2008 Nov 30.

Hofmeyr GJ, Essilfie-Appiah G, Lawrie TA. Amnioinfusion for preterm premature rupture of membranes. Cochrane Database Syst Rev. 2011 Dec 7;(12):CD000942.

Hofmeyr GJ, Xu H. Amnioinfusion for meconium-stained liquor in labour. Cochrane Database Syst Rev. 2010 Jan 20;(1):CD000014.

Sherer DM, Langer O. Oligohydramnios: use and misuse in clinical management. Ultrasound Obstet Gynecol. 2001 Nov;18(5):411–419.

CHAPTER 12 Human immunodeficiency virus

Background and prevalence

- A retrovirus, which preferentially targets CD4 lymphocytes, causing progressive immunosuppression. When CD4 lymphocytes fall below a critical level, infected individuals become more susceptible to opportunistic infections and malignancies.
- Transmission is through sexual intercourse, intravenous drug use, transfusion of blood or blood products, and from mother to child during pregnancy and breastfeeding.
- Prevalence – HIV infection in women giving birth in the UK in 2008 was 1/486 (0.2%); highest in London (0.37%).
- Proportion of exposed infants (born to both diagnosed and undiagnosed HIV-infected women) who became infected has decreased from 12% in 1999 to approximately 2% in 2007.

Effect on pregnancy and HIV

- Pregnancy does not adversely affect HIV progression or survival, although long-term data are lacking.
- Women using HAART in pregnancy may be at increased risk of GDM, PET, and PTD.
- In the pre-HAART era, HIV infection was associated with PET. There are conflicting data on the risk of PET in women taking HAART.

Preconception management

Serodiscordant couples

- The risk of transmission for each act of sexual intercourse is 0.001% – 0.03%. This risk is significantly reduced, if the male partner has a viral load of <50 copies/ml and is taking HAART. The risk can be further reduced by limiting exposure to the fertile period of the cycle and ensuring that all genital infections have been treated.
- Couples who are serodiscordant choosing to have intercourse should use condoms as it is associated with an 80% reduction in transmission. They should practice self-insemination during the fertile time of the cycle using quills, syringes, and sterile containers.
- Couples who are serodiscordant where the female partner is HIV negative – assisted conception with either donor insemination or sperm washing is significantly safer than timed unprotected intercourse.
- Sperm washing is simple and is significantly safer than timed unprotected intercourse, with no case of seroconversion in either female partner or child born in over 3000 cycles of sperm washing combined with IUI, IVF or ICSI reported in the literature.

HIV positive mother

- To optimize health of mother and baby – advise to delay conception until:
  * HAART regimen is optimised and is effectively suppressing viraemia.
  * Prophylaxis against PCP is no longer required.
  * Any opportunistic infections are treated.
- Folate supplementation – higher dose folate (5 mg) for women taking cotrimoxazole.
- Yearly cervical cytology because of the association of HIV, immunosuppression, and cervical neoplasia.

Risks of mother-to-child transmission

Untreated women – transmission rate is 15–20% in non-breastfeeding women in Europe and 25–40% in breastfeeding African populations.

- In non-breastfeeding women, over 80% of transmissions occur perinatally, around the time of labour and delivery.
- There is a linear correlation between maternal viral load and the risk of transmission.
- Obstetric factors associated with transmission are:
  * Mode of delivery.
  * Duration of membrane rupture.
  * Delivery before 32 weeks of gestation.
  * Presence of other STIs.
  * Chorioamnionitis.
- Breastfeeding doubles the risk from 14 to 28%.

Treated women (HAART, appropriate management of delivery and avoidance of breastfeeding) – transmission rates are reduced to <2% from 25–30% (<1% in UK).

- For non-breastfeeding women taking HAART, where viral load is <50 copies/ml at delivery, mother-to-child transmission rate is <1%, irrespective of mode of delivery. (In the UK/Irish cohort – 0.1%.)
- Principal risk factors for transmission:
  * High plasma viraemia at delivery.
  * Short duration of HAART.
  * Delivery at <32 weeks of gestation.
- In contrast to women who are untreated, the few transmissions that occur in women receiving HAART are likely to be as a result of in utero transmission occurring before treatment.

Antenatal HIV screening

- Screen all pregnant women for HIV, syphilis, hepatitis B, and rubella at their booking antenatal visit. HIV positive women can take up interventions that can prevent mother-to-child transmission and can significantly improve their own health by reducing their risk of disease progression and death.
- consider repeat HIV test in women who are HIV negative at booking but are at continued high risk of acquiring HIV.
- If a woman declines an HIV test, document her reasons and explore them sensitively. Offer screening again at around 28 weeks.
- Fourth-generation laboratory assays test for both HIV antibody and p24 antigen and reduce the diagnostic window to 1 month, as p24 antigen is detectable during seroconversion.
- At least 20% of the infants born to undiagnosed women had a negative antenatal HIV test. The timing of maternal seroconversion in these cases is unknown.
- Where a woman books for antenatal care at 26 weeks of gestation or later, request the test urgently and issue the results within 24 hours.
- Rapid HIV tests (results within 20 minutes; test for antibody only) for women who present in labour. Act immediately on reactive results.

HIV positive pregnant women

- Refer for assessment and management within an MDT – an HIV physician, obstetrician, specialist midwife, health advisor, and paediatrician.
- Maintain confidentiality. Encourage women to disclose their HIV status to their partner.
- Advise about safer-sex practices and the use of condoms to prevent transmission of HIV and other STIs to an uninfected partner.
- Manage difficult disclosure cases with a MDT approach, with a low threshold for legal advice.
- Women with existing children of unknown HIV status should have them tested for HIV.
- If the mother continues to refuse any intervention package, then seek legal permission at birth to treat the infant for 4 weeks with antiretroviral therapy and to prevent breastfeeding.

Interventions

- Interventions to prevent disease progression in the mother to prevent mother-to-child transmission:
  * Antiretroviral therapy.
  * Appropriate management of delivery.
  * Avoidance of breastfeeding.

Antiretroviral therapy

- BHIVA guidelines recommend initiation of HAART for those with symptomatic HIV infection and/or a falling or low CD4 lymphocyte count (<350 × 10⁶/l). Delaying treatment until the CD4 lymphocyte count has fallen <200 × 10⁶/l is associated with a substantially greater risk of disease progression and death.
- Those with CD4 lymphocyte counts <200 × 10⁶/l are at risk of opportunistic infections; provide prophylaxis against *Pneumocystis carinii* pneumonia (PCP) – cotrimoxazole is the first-line agent.
- In pregnancy, the criteria for initiating HAART for maternal health reasons and for PCP prophylaxis are the same. However, it may be possible to delay treatment until after the first trimester.
- Advise all pregnant HIV-positive women to take antiretroviral therapy:
  * For women who require HIV treatment for their own health – prescribe their HAART regimen throughout pregnancy and postpartum.
  * For women who do not require HIV treatment for their own health – initiate HAART between 20 and 28 weeks and discontinue at delivery.
  * For women who do not require HIV treatment for their own health, have a viral load <10000 copies/ml, and are prepared to be delivered by elective CS – an acceptable alternative to HAART is zidovudine monotherapy initiated between 20 and 28 weeks, given orally twice daily, IV at delivery, and discontinued immediately thereafter.

- HAART safety data are reassuring; the rate of major and minor congenital abnormality is 2.8%, with no significant difference according to timing of exposure or class of anti-retroviral.
- There is no increased risk of abnormalities in infants exposed to efavirenz or didanosine in the first trimester.
- Cotrimoxazole, a folate antagonist, raises the possibility of neural tube defects.

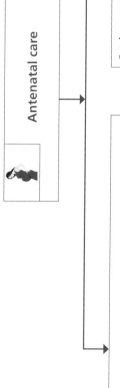

Antenatal care

Fetal

- Aneuploidy screening as per the general population.
- Counsel women who are considering invasive diagnostic test in a FMU and seek advice from the HIV physicians about reducing the risk of transmission.
  * Observational studies in the pre-HAART era suggested an increased risk of HIV transmission with amniocentesis and other invasive procedures. More recent studies found no transmission among the mothers receiving HAART.
  * For women who have started HAART but whose viral load is >50 copies/ml, it may be advisable to delay the amniocentesis until the maternal viral load is <50 copies/ml.
  * For women not already taking HAART, administration of antiretrovirals to cover the procedure is advised.
  * When performing amniocentesis, the placental route is contraindicated.
- Dating and anomaly scans as per the general population.

Maternal

- At booking – test for hepatitis B, C, varicella zoster, measles, toxoplasma, syphilis, and rubella.
- Screen for genital infections at booking and again at 28 weeks. Treat any infection detected, even if asymptomatic.
- Women on HAART at the time of booking – even though the evidence for the association of HAART with GDM is conflicting, screen these women for GDM at the time of booking.
- Hepatitis B and pneumococcal vaccination can be administered in pregnancy.
- Influenza vaccination can be safely administered in pregnancy. The decision to immunize depends on the time of year.
- Varicella zoster and MMR vaccines are contraindicated in pregnancy. Consider immunization in postpartum period for non-immune women depending on their CD4 count.

Management of maternal HIV

- Maternal plasma viral load is the most important predictor of transmission. Measure viral load every trimester, at 36 weeks and at delivery.
- Monitor for drug toxicities – FBC, urea and electrolytes and liver function tests regularly.
- Complications of HIV – for women who become acutely unwell, liaise with HIV physicians. Consider HIV-related complications in pregnant women whose HIV status is unknown, particularly those who are not booked.
- Pregnant women with advanced HIV are at increased risk of opportunistic infections, particularly PCP. Symptoms of PCP include fever, dry cough, and shortness of breath and patients are typically hypoxic.
- Adverse effects of HAART – gastrointestinal disturbances, skin rashes, and hepatotoxicity. Lactic acidosis (including two fatal cases) has been reported with stavudine and didanosine. Symptoms of lactic acidosis are often non-specific – gastrointestinal disturbances, fever, and breathlessness.
- Presentation with symptoms suggestive of PET, cholestasis or other signs of liver dysfunction may indicate drug toxicity therefore seek early liaison with HIV physicians.

Antenatal complications

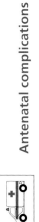

1. Preterm labour and PPROM

- Screen for genital infection and treat any infections, even if asymptomatic.
- The usual indications for steroids apply.

Preterm labour (PTL)

- PTD rate is higher in women taking HAART (14%) than in women on mono or dual therapy (10%). The association of HAART and prematurity is even stronger for deliveries before 32 weeks; 3.6% compared with 1.4%.
- It is unclear whether the increased risk of PTD is due to spontaneous labour, PROM or obstetric intervention in response to antenatal complications.
- Women presenting with threatened PTL:
  - * Assess in accordance with general guidelines.
  - * Initiate tocolysis as appropriate.
  - * Seek urgent MDT advice for a detailed plan of care about the choice of antiretroviral therapy.
- In women taking HAART, delivery <32 weeks is a risk factor for perinatal transmission, particularly if the duration of HAART is short.
- Infants born <32 weeks are at increased risk of HIV but may be unable to tolerate oral medication, so administering antiretroviral therapy to the mother just before and during delivery will provide prophylaxis to the neonate.

PPROM <34 weeks of gestation

- Oral erythromycin in accordance with national guidelines.
- Consider broad-spectrum IV antibiotics.
- Chorioamnionitis and fetal distress are indications for delivery.
- Decide whether to expedite delivery after MDT consultation on the adequacy of maternal HAART, plasma viraemia, and the presence of any other pregnancy or HIV-related comorbidities.
- Timing of delivery – take into consideration the risk of complications associated with prematurity, the availability of neonatal facilities, and the risk of perinatal HIV transmission.

PPROM > 34 weeks of gestation

- Expedite delivery. At this gestation, the small risk of neonatal morbidity and mortality associated with prematurity is outweighed by the risk to mother and neonate of chorioamnionitis and the risk of perinatal HIV transmission.
- Consider augmentation if the viral load is <50 copies/ml and there are no obstetric contraindications.
- Consider broad-spectrum IV antibiotics.

Prelabour rupture of the membranes at term

- Expedite delivery.
- Consider broad-spectrum IV antibiotics if there is evidence of genital infection or chorioamnionitis.
- Before the use of HAART – rupture of membranes for >4 hours was associated with a doubling of the risk of HIV transmission; a 2% incremental increase in transmission risk for every hour of ruptured membranes up to 24 hours.
- For women on HAART whose viral loads are low, data regarding transmission risk are reassuring. The studies provide some data to support immediate augmentation rather than CS where plasma viral load is <50 copies/ml, provided that there is no evidence of any genital infection or chorioamnionitis and no obstetric contraindications.

Antenatal complications contd.

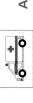

2. Prolonged pregnancy

- For women on HAART with a plasma viral load of <50 copies/ml – consider IOL, particularly if cervix is favourable.
- There is no contraindication to membrane sweep or to the use of prostaglandins.
- Otherwise, an elective CS is an option.

3. Vaginal birth after CS

- Consider VBAC for women taking HAART whose plasma viral load is <50 copies/ml.
- It is unknown whether scar rupture in HIV infected women is associated with an increased risk of transmission from prolonged fetal exposure to maternal blood. However, in women taking HAART with a plasma viral load of <50 copies/ml, this risk is likely to be very low.

4. Women diagnosed in late pregnancy but before the onset of labour

- MDT assessment and commence HAART ASAP.
- A woman diagnosed HIV positive beyond 32 weeks may still have her pregnancy managed with a view to planned vaginal delivery if HAART is commenced and a viral load of <50 copies/ml is achieved by 36 weeks.
- If the viral load is >50 copies/ml at 36 weeks, deliver by elective CS at 38 weeks; continue her HAART regimen and give IV ZDV at delivery.

Management of delivery

- **Make a plan of care for antiretroviral therapy and mode of delivery at 36 weeks.**
- Before the introduction of HAART – there was a significant reduction in transmission of HIV with elective CS at 38 weeks compared with planned vaginal birth (RR 0.17). A systematic review showed a 50% reduction in the transmission rate in women who underwent elective CS.
  - However, current data for women with plasma viral loads of <50 copies/ml who are taking HAART support the option of a planned vaginal delivery.

Caesarean section

- Delivery by elective CS at 38 weeks to prevent labour and/or ruptured membranes is recommended (earlier delivery is justified because the risk of perinatal HIV transmission associated with labour and/or ruptured membranes may outweigh the risk of transient tachypnoea of the newborn):
  - * In women taking HAART who have a plasma viral load >50 copies/ml.
  - * In women taking ZDV monotherapy as an alternative to HAART.
  - * In women with HIV and hepatitis C virus co-infection.
- Delay delivery by elective CS for obstetric indications or maternal request until after 39 weeks in women with plasma viral loads of <50 copies/ml, to reduce the risk of TTN.
- For women co-infected with HCV and HIV but not receiving antiretroviral therapy – there is a reported 3-fold increased risk of HCV transmission and an increased risk of HIV transmission. Whether CS is protective in women co-infected with HIV and HCV is uncertain; currently elective CS is recommended.

- Clamp the cord as early as possible after delivery.
- Keep surgical field as haemostatic as possible and take care to avoid rupturing the membranes until the head is delivered through the surgical incision.
- Peripartum antibiotics in accordance with national guidelines.
- Some studies have suggested that the complications of CS are higher in women with HIV. The most frequent reported complication is postpartum fever. However, a recent study did not show any differences in postoperative morbidity.
- If IV ZDV is indicated, start the infusion 4 hours before beginning the CS and continue until the umbilical cord is clamped.
- Take a maternal sample for plasma viral load and CD4 lymphocyte count at delivery.

Vaginal delivery

- Offer vaginal delivery to women taking HAART with a viral load of <50 copies/ml.
- When a woman presents in labour with her recent viral load of <50 copies/ml, confirm the delivery plans.
- Advise women on HAART to continue their oral HAART regimen through labour.
- Do not perform invasive procedures such as FBS and fetal scalp electrodes.
- If labour progress is normal, avoid amniotomy unless delivery is imminent.
- Consider amniotomy and use of oxytocin for augmentation of labour.
- Although the limited data on rupture of membranes in women taking HAART is reassuring, leave the membranes intact for as long as possible.
- HIV infection alone is not an indication for continuous EFM.
- If instrumental delivery is indicated, low-cavity forceps are preferable to ventouse.
- Avoid mid-cavity and rotational instrumental deliveries.

Women diagnosed with HIV during labour

- If the woman's HIV status is unknown, request a rapid test for HIV.
- Seek urgent advice from the HIV physicians regarding optimum HAART; HAART regimen is likely to include IV ZDV and oral nevirapine (an antiretroviral with rapid placental transfer and of proven benefit in reducing transmission).
- Deliver by CS at least 2 hours after administration of nevirapine.
- Repeat a confirmatory test together with samples for CD4 count, viral load, and resistance testing.
- Inform the paediatricians.

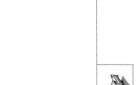

Postpartum management

Maternal

- In the absence of other interventions, breastfeeding doubles the risk of transmission.
- Risk of transmission through breastfeeding where the mother has a viral load of <50 copies/ml is uncertain.
- All women who are HIV positive in resource-rich settings should avoid breastfeeding.
- Pharmacological agents are better than no treatment at suppressing lactation in the first postpartum week. Give cabergoline 1 mg orally within 24 hours of birth.
- Advise women taking HAART to continue.
- Specialist advice about contraception – there are many interactions between hormonal contraception and HAART.
- MMR and varicella zoster immunization for susceptible individuals with CD4 counts above 200 and 400, respectively, for those found to be IgG-negative on antenatal testing.

What not to do

- HIV infection of itself is not an indication for continuous EFM.
- If instrumental delivery is indicated, avoid ventouse delivery.
- Avoid mid-cavity and rotational instrumental deliveries.
- Invasive procedures such as FBS and fetal scalp electrodes are contraindicated.
- If labour progress is normal, avoid amniotomy unless delivery is imminent.
- Avoid breastfeeding in all women who are HIV positive in resource-rich settings.

Neonatal

- Treat all neonates with antiretroviral therapy, ASAP after birth and certainly within 4 hours.
- Most neonates are treated with ZDV monotherapy (BD for 4 weeks).
- If a mother has resistance to ZDV, give an alternative monotherapy to the infant.
- Treat infants at high risk of HIV infection with HAART:
  - * Infants of untreated mothers.
  - * Mothers who have plasma viraemia > 50 copies/ml despite HAART.
- The only licensed antiretroviral drug available for IV use in sick or preterm infants is ZDV.
- Provide prophylaxis against PCP only for neonates at high risk of HIV infection.
- Test infants at 1 day, 6 weeks, and 12 weeks of age. If all these tests are negative and the baby is not being breastfed, the child is not HIV-infected.
- Repeat a confirmatory HIV antibody test at 18 months of age.

Management of HIV in Pregnancy. RCOG Green-top Guideline No. 39, June 2010.
British HIV Association and Children's HIV Association Guidelines for the Management of HIV Infection in Pregnant Women 2008.

CHAPTER 13 Hepatitis

Hepatitis A

- RNA virus.
- Infection does not have any teratogenic effects but there is an increased rate of miscarriage and premature labour, proportional to the severity of the illness.
- There have been case reports of possible vertical transmission.
- Breastfeeding can be continued and most children will have mild or asymptomatic infection.

- Consider hepatitis E if a pregnant woman develops acute hepatitis with a recent history of travel to an endemic area.

Hepatitis B

- DNA virus of Hepadna family.
- Vertical transmission occurs in 90% of pregnancies where the mother is hepatitis B e antigen positive and in about 10% of surface antigen positive, e antigen negative mothers.
- Mother – hepatitis B may exacerbate after the end of pregnancy. Most (>90%) of infected infants become chronic carriers. Refer to gastroenterologist and virologist for further management.
- Exposed contacts – offer an accelerated course of recombinant vaccine to all sexual and household contacts (0, 7, and 21 days or 0, 1, 2 months with a booster at 12 months). Vaccination provides some protection from disease when started up to 6 weeks after exposure. Advise to avoid unprotected penetrative sex, until vaccination has been successful (antiHBs titres >10 IU/l)
- Infant – vaccinate infants born to infectious mothers at birth and give hepatitis B specific immunoglobulin (HBIG) 200 IU IM. This reduces vertical transmission by 90%. Treating the mother in the last month of pregnancy with lamivudine may further reduce the transmission rate if she is highly infectious (HBVDNA $> 1.2 \times 10^9$ genomes/ml).
- Advise infected mothers to continue breastfeeding as there is no additional risk of transmission.
- Test infants for hepatitis B (HBsAg and anti-HBs) 4–6 weeks after the final dose of vaccine.

Hepatitis C

- RNA virus in the Flaviviridae family.
- Vertical spread occurs at a low rate of about 5% or less, but occurs at higher rates (up to 40%) if the woman is both HIV and HCV positive.
- Increased rate of transmission is seen in Japanese patients. Transmission risk correlates with the presence of detectable HCV RNA in the mother's blood.
- At present there is no known way of reducing the risk of vertical transmission. However, minimizing blood exposure from the mother to the child is expected to be beneficial, as in HIV infection.
- Breastfeeding – there is no evidence of additional risk of transmission except, perhaps, in women who are symptomatic with a high viral load.
- In women who are HIV negative but infected with HCV – most studies suggest that mode of delivery does not affect the transmission risk.

Care during pregnancy if hepatitis positive

- Confidentiality.
- Partner testing.
- Offer immunization of partner and other contacts if not immune.
- Refer to gastroenterologist and virologist.

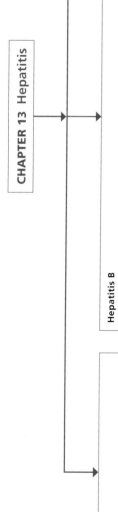

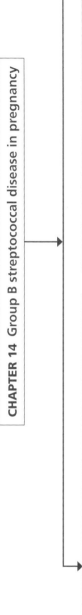

CHAPTER 14 Group B streptococcal disease in pregnancy

Background and prevalence

- Group B streptococcus (*Streptococcus agalactiae*) is the most common cause of severe early onset (< 7 days of age) infection in newborn infants.
- Incidence of early-onset GBS disease in the UK in the absence of screening or widespread intrapartum antibiotic prophylaxis (IAP) is 0.5/1000 births, which is similar to that seen in the USA after universal screening and IAP, despite comparable vaginal carriage rates.
- In 2001, 376 cases of early-onset GBS disease were identified in the UK, 39 of which were fatal. (There were 2519 neonatal deaths from all causes in the UK in 2000).

Screening for GBS in UK

- Screening and treatment with antibiotics are aimed to prevent early-onset GBS.
- Screening could be:
  * Universal bacteriological screening.
  * Risk factor based screening.
  * Universal screening with antibiotics to the at risk.
  * Antenatal screening and treatment have not demonstrated any effect on neonatal mortality and may carry disadvantages for the mother and baby.

Screening for GBS in UK

Universal – bacteriological screening

- Vaginal and rectal swabs from all women between 35 and 37 weeks of gestation.
- All women carrying GBS, and all women who labour before swabs are taken or for whom results are not available at the time of labour – IAP is given.
- Estimate – 27% of women receive IAP and this reduces the incidence of early-onset GBS disease by 86% (USA).

Risk factor-based screening

- IAP to all women with recognized risk factors:
  * Previous baby affected by GBS.
  * GBS bacteriuria detected during the current pregnancy.
  * Preterm labour.
  * Prolonged rupture of the membranes (PROM).
  * Fever in labour.
- Estimate – 25% of women receive IAP and this reduces the incidence of early-onset GBS disease by 50–69% (USA).

Universal screening with antibiotics to at risk

- Screen all women and offer IAP to the GBS carriers who also have a clinical risk factor (Canadian Task Force on Preventative Health Care).
- Estimate – 3.4% of women receive IAP and this reduces the incidence of early-onset GBS disease by 51%.

The US Centers for Disease Control and Prevention (CDC)

- The risk factor approach to screening is inferior to bacteriological screening. All pregnant women undergo bacteriological screening, with vaginal and rectal swabs taken for GBS culture at 35–37 weeks of gestation.
- All women colonized with GBS at 35–37 weeks (or labouring before this time) – offer IAP, usually in the form of high-dose intravenous penicillin or ampicillin. This has resulted in the fall of early-onset disease in the USA. It has significantly reduced the risk of early-onset but not late-onset disease (≥ 7 days after birth).

Potential risks of screening

- Anaphylaxis –
  * Severe anaphylaxis with penicillin – 1/10 000 women treated.
  * Fatal anaphylaxis with penicillin – 1/100 000 women treated.
  * If 30% of the UK pregnant population is treated with penicillin, this might result in 2 deaths/year as a result of penicillin anaphylaxis.
- Development of resistant organisms with the use of broad-spectrum antibiotics such as ampicillin.
- A possibility that exposure to antibiotics in the neonatal perinatal period may affect neonatal faecal flora, with a subsequent impact on immune development and later allergy.

CHAPTER 14 Group B streptococcal disease

55

Screening for GBS in UK – estimated effects

Universal – bacteriological screening

- Approximately 25% of mothers in the UK are likely to be GBS carriers. With the addition of women who present with other clinical risk factors for GBS disease, around 30% of all pregnant women would receive IAP with a bacteriological screening programme (approximately 204 000 women/year).
- The current incidence of early-onset GBS disease in the UK is 0.50/1000 births (approximately 340 babies/year).
- Estimate – IAP is 80% effective at preventing early-onset GBS disease, i.e., 272 babies developing early onset GBS disease are prevented.
- Therefore each year in the UK 204 000 women will be treated to prevent 272 babies developing early-onset GBS disease, i.e., 1.4 cases of disease may be prevented for every 1000 women treated.
- In practice, the numbers of women treated to prevent one case would be higher.
- To prevent one neonatal death from GBS would require at least 7000 colonized women to be given IAP, which would require at least 24 000 women to be screened.

Risk factor-based screening

- **Antenatal risk factors** – approximately 15% of all UK pregnancies have one or more of the following risk factors:
  * Intrapartum fever.
  * PROM > 18 hours.
  * Prematurity < 37 weeks.
  * Previous infant with GBS.
- Approximately 60% of UK early-onset GBS cases have such risk factors.
- 2 cases of disease and 0.21 deaths from GBS disease occur for every 1000 pregnancies with one or more of these factors.
- NNT – Approximately 625 women with one or more of these risk factors need to be treated to prevent one case of disease and 5882 women need to be treated to prevent one death.

GBS in pregnancy – recommendations in UK

Antenatal screening and prophylaxis

- Do not routinely screen (either bacteriological or risk based) for antenatal GBS carriage. (Until it is clear that antenatal screening for GBS carriage does more good than harm and that the benefits are cost effective.)
- Do not provide antenatal prophylaxis with oral penicillin, as it does not reduce the likelihood of GBS colonization at the time of delivery.

Intrapartum antibiotic prophylaxis (IAP)

- Consider IAP if:
  * GBS is detected incidentally.
  * GBS bacteriuria is found in the current pregnancy – it is associated with a higher risk of neonatal disease. Give antibiotics at the time of diagnosis as well as IAP.
  * Previous baby with neonatal GBS disease - subsequent infants born to these women are probably at increased risk of GBS disease.
  * Presence of known risk factors (stronger in the presence of ≥ 2 risk factors) – intrapartum fever (> 38°C); prematurity; PROM (>18 hours) at term.
- There is no good evidence to support IAP:
  * If GBS was detected in a previous pregnancy where the neonate was unaffected.
  * For women undergoing planned CS in the absence of labour and with intact membranes. The risk of neonatal GBS disease is extremely low.
  * For women with PPROM unless they are in established labour. Antibiotics specifically for GBS colonization are not necessary prior to labour. If these women are known to be colonized with GBS, consider IAP, especially if labour occurs prior to 37 weeks.

- Give penicillin ASAP after the onset of labour. Clindamycin if allergic to penicillin.
- Avoid broad-spectrum antibiotics such as ampicillin, due to the concerns regarding increased rates of neonatal gram-negative sepsis.
- If chorioamnionitis is suspected, give broad-spectrum antibiotics including an agent active against GBS.
- To optimize the efficacy of IAP, give the first dose at least 2 hours prior to delivery.

Management of the newborn infant

Sick infants

- Take blood cultures before antibiotics are commenced.
- Consider CSF cultures.
- Give broad-spectrum antibiotics, which provide cover against early-onset GBS disease and other common pathogens.

Well infant with risk factor, with or without IAP

- Some clinicians recommend treatment, while others will prefer to observe, because the balance of risks and benefits of treatment is uncertain.
- 90% of cases present clinically before 12 hours of age, the risk of disease in infants who remain well without treatment beyond this time may not be substantially elevated above that of the infant with no risk factors. Prolonged observation of well infants is therefore not indicated.
- The argument for using prophylactic treatment in well infants is stronger in the presence of multiple risk factors but is still unproven.

Low-risk term infants

- Do not give routine postnatal antibiotic prophylaxis to low-risk term infants.
- The incidence of early-onset GBS disease in term infants without antenatal risk factors in the UK is 0.2 cases/1000 births. If postnatal antibiotic treatment was completely effective and there were no adverse effects, 5000 infants would need to be treated to prevent a single case and at least 80000 infants would have to be treated to prevent a single death from early-onset GBS disease.

Previous infant with GBS disease

- The risk of GBS disease is unquantified but is probably significantly increased.
- Either clinically evaluate after birth and observe for at least 12 hours, or take blood cultures and commence penicillin until the culture results are available.
- There is insufficient evidence to suggest that neonatal treatment should be given if IAP has been given.

Routine neonatal surveillance cultures

- Most infants who develop early-onset GBS disease present with illness soon after birth, before culture results become available.
- Postnatal antibiotic treatment has not been shown to eradicate carriage of GBS or to influence the risk of late-onset GBS disease. It is therefore unnecessary to perform routine surface cultures or blood cultures on well infants, whether they received antibiotic prophylaxis or not.

What not to do

- Routine screening (either bacteriological or risk based) for antenatal GBS carriage.
- Antenatal prophylaxis with oral penicillin.
- There is no good evidence to support IAP:
  * When GBS was detected in a previous pregnancy and baby was well.
  * For women undergoing planned CS in the absence of labour and with intact membranes. The risk of neonatal GBS disease is extremely low in these circumstances.
  * For women with preterm rupture of membranes unless they are in established labour.
- It is unnecessary to perform routine surface cultures or blood cultures on well infants, whether they received antibiotic prophylaxis or not.
- Routine postnatal antibiotic prophylaxis in low-risk term infants.

- Breastfeeding does not increase the risk of neonatal GBS disease.

Guideline comparator

CDC – prevention of perinatal GBS disease: a public health perspective (MMWR 2002) Recommendations:

- Universal culture-based screening for vaginal and rectal GBS colonization of all pregnant women at 35–37 weeks' gestation. At the time of labour or rupture of membranes, give IAP to women identified as GBS carriers.
- Colonization during a previous pregnancy is not an indication for IAP in subsequent deliveries.
- No need for routine IAP for GBS in colonized women undergoing planned CS who have not begun labour or had rupture of membranes.
- Penicillin is the first-line agent for IAP with ampicillin an acceptable alternative.
- Women whose culture results are unknown at the time of delivery – manage on the risk-based approach (risk factors are delivery at < 37 weeks' gestation, duration of membrane rupture >18 hours, or temperature > 38.0°C).
- Women with negative vaginal and rectal GBS screening cultures within 5 weeks of delivery do not require IAP for GBS even if obstetric risk factors develop.
- Women with GBS bacteriuria during their current pregnancy or who previously gave birth to an infant with GBS disease – give IAP.
- In the absence of GBS UTI, do not use antibiotics before the intrapartum period to treat asymptomatic GBS colonization.
- Do not routinely use antibiotic prophylaxis for newborns whose mothers received IAP for GBS infection. However, therapeutic use of these agents is appropriate for infants with clinically suspected sepsis.

SOGC recommendations:

- Offer all women screening for GBS disease at 35–37 weeks' gestation with culture from swabs from vagina and the rectal area.
- Treat the following women intrapartum at time of labour or rupture of membranes with IV antibiotics:
  - * All women positive by GBS culture screening done at 35–37 weeks.
  - * Women with an infant previously infected with GBS.
  - * Women with GBS bacteriuria in this pregnancy.
- Treat women at < 37 weeks' gestation with IV antibiotics unless there has been a negative GBS vaginal/rectal swab culture within 5 weeks.
- Treat women with intrapartum fever with IV antibiotics.
- If a woman is GBS positive by culture screening or by history of bacteriuria, with prelabour rupture of membranes at term, treat with GBS antibiotic prophylaxis and initiate induction of labour with IV oxytocin.
- If GBS culture result is unknown and the woman has ruptured membranes at term for > 18 hours, treat with GBS antibiotic prophylaxis.

Extrapolation of practice from the USA to the UK may be inappropriate.

- There have been no RCTs comparing antenatal screening, whether bacteriological or risk factor-based, with no antenatal screening. No RCTs have compared the different screening strategies.
- A decreased incidence of neonatal sepsis due to GBS has not been accompanied by a decrease in neonatal sepsis as a whole nor in neonatal mortality.
- No study has yet been able to demonstrate that screening for GBS has any impact on neonatal sepsis as a whole.
- The incidence of early-onset GBS disease in the UK in the absence of systematic screening or widespread IAP is 0.5/1000 births, which is similar to that seen in the USA after screening and antibiotic prophylaxis, despite comparable vaginal carriage rates.

Prevention of Early Onset Neonatal Group B Streptococcal Disease. RCOG Guideline No. 36; November 2003.
Prevention of Perinatal Group B Streptococcal disease. CDC; http://www.cdc.gov/mmwr/preview/mmwrhtml/rr5111a1.htm
The Prevention of Early-Onset Neonatal Group B Streptococcal Disease. SOGC Clinical Practice Guidelines; No. 149, September 2004.

CHAPTER 15 Viral rash in pregnancy

A rash illness is defined as a rash compatible with a systemic viral illness

Advice and information on rash illness for pregnant women at booking

- Enquire if women have had a rash illness or had contact with a rash illness during current pregnancy. Advise women to inform an HCP urgently:
  * if they develop a rash at any time in pregnancy; or
  * if they have contact at any time in pregnancy with someone who has a rash.
- Advise to avoid any antenatal clinic or maternity setting until clinically assessed, to avoid exposing other pregnant women.
- If a woman gives a history of chickenpox or shingles and has had contact with either of these during pregnancy, reassure her that she is not at any risk. Refer all women with uncertain or no known history of chickenpox for investigations and further management.

Pregnant woman in significant contact with a rash illness

- Contact with a maculopapular or non-vesicular rash illness:
  * Assess for risk for measles, rubella, and parvovirus and arrange appropriate investigation and treatment. Investigate for parvovirus B19 and rubella infection, irrespective of whether they develop a rash or not, unless there is satisfactory evidence of past rubella infection (i.e., two documented vaccinations, or one documented vaccination and one prior positive rubella antibody test, or two positive antibody tests). See Chapter 17 Rubella infection in pregnancy and Chapter 20 Parvovirus infection in pregnancy.
  * Other viruses responsible for non-vesicular rash are cytomegalovirus, enterovirus, herpes virus 6 &7, and Epstein–Barr virus.
- Contact with a vesicular rash illness:
  * Chickenpox or shingles. See Chapter 21 Chickenpox in pregnancy.

Maculopapular rashes in pregnancy

- Take history and examine the woman.
- Check the appearance of the rash – vesicular or non-vesicular. If the nature of the rash is unclear – investigate for both vesicular and non-vesicular rash.
- Although parvovirus B19 and rubella infections predominantly have a specific impact on the fetus if infection occurs in the first 20 weeks of gestation, investigate even after 20 weeks since:
  * Specific diagnosis would help in managing potential risk to contacts.
  * It would confirm the date of infection related to gestational age.
  * Estimate of the gestation may be wrong.
  * Mother may be reassured that a specific diagnosis has been reached or excluded, and this may be helpful in the management of subsequent exposure.
  * Measles infection can affect the pregnancy at any stage.
- Assess for clinical features suggesting streptococcal and meningococcal infection, measles, enterovirus, syphilis, and infectious mononucleosis (EBV or CMV). Investigate for rubella and parvovirus B19 if any doubt or failure to confirm by laboratory investigations.

Pre-existing immunity

- Offer rubella antibody test at booking.
- Offer rubella-susceptible women of childbearing age MMR vaccine post delivery.
- Do not offer unselected screening of pregnant women for past infection with parvovirus B19 as neither vaccine nor prophylaxis are available.
- Do not offer unselected screening of pregnant women for adequate immunity to measles. Satisfactory evidence of protection includes documentation of having received two doses of measles-containing vaccine or a positive antibody test for measles. Offer all seronegative women of childbearing age MMR vaccine post delivery.
- Antenatal screening for VZV susceptibility – insufficient evidence to recommend the introduction of routine antenatal screening in the UK. At present it is good practice to establish and record whether there is a firm history of chickenpox or shingles at booking.

- Contact is defined as being in the same room for a significant period of time (≥ 15 minutes) or face-to-face contact. Use a less stringent definition of contact in other settings, where exposure is less well defined, especially for measles.
- For parvovirus B19 infections household exposure is the most important source of infections in pregnancy followed by occupational exposure.

- **Investigate for rubella and parvovirus B19 infection in all pregnant women presenting with a non-vesicular rash compatible with a systemic viral infection, irrespective of a prior history of rubella vaccination or previous positive rubella antibody tests because there is a remote possibility of past laboratory or documentation error, failed immunization, or symptomatic re-infection.**
- **Cases of measles and rubella are notifiable diseases; report them to the local Health Protection Unit.**
- Patients who have spent their childhood years in other countries may not have had the same exposure to natural infection or vaccination opportunities as those growing up in the UK; consequently, the risk estimates presented here may not apply to these groups as they may have a higher or lower level of susceptibility.

Inadvertent immunization during pregnancy

- MMR and chickenpox vaccines are live vaccines; therefore do not give them to women known to be pregnant. However, if women have been inadvertently immunized with these vaccines during pregnancy, do not recommend termination.

Occupational exposure

- Do not recommend exclusion of pregnant women susceptible to measles, chickenpox, or rubella from settings that may suggest a higher rate of exposure (e.g., nurseries and schools).
- Rubella is now rare in children.
- Exposure to measles and chickenpox is as likely to occur in the wider community. However, should there be a case or an outbreak of measles, undertake an individual risk assessment.
- Parvovirus B19 – see Chapter 20 Parvovirus infection in pregnancy.

Investigations

- Test to establish the initial diagnosis on blood samples.
- Further tests may be necessary to confirm the diagnosis. The need for more invasive tests such as amniocentesis is uncommon, and is only required in rare situations as advised by a specialist.
- If investigation is commenced some weeks after rash or contact, it may not be possible to confirm or refute a particular diagnosis.

- FMU referral – for counselling, serial USS, investigations, treatment, and follow-up where appropriate.

See Chapter 17 Rubella infection in pregnancy; Chapter 20 Parvovirus infection in pregnancy; Chapter 21 Chickenpox in pregnancy.

Guidance on Viral Rash in Pregnancy Investigation, Diagnosis and Management of Viral Rash Illness, or Exposure to Viral Rash Illness, in Pregnancy; HPA; Jan 2011.

	Rubella	Parvovirus B19	CMV	Chickenpox
Proportion seronegative in young adult females	3.6% of nulliparous women, rising to nearly 9%	40–50%	–	1.2–14%, varies with country of origin
Infectivity – risk transmission from close contact	High (90%)	Medium (50%)		High (70–90%)
Incubation period	14–21 days		28–60 days	10–21 days
Infectivity period (days pre and post rash onset)	7 days pre to 10 days post onset of rash	10 days pre to day of onset of rash		2 days pre onset of rash until all lesions crusted
Risk of intrauterine infection by (gestational age)	<11 weeks – 90% 11–16 weeks – 55% >16 weeks – 45%	<4 weeks – 0% 5–16 weeks – 15% >16 weeks – 25–70%	Primary infection – 30–40%; Secondary infection – 1%	<28 weeks – 5–10% 28–36 weeks – 2.5% >36 weeks – 50%
Risk of adverse outcome for the pregnant woman	Arthritis	Arthropathy	Pneumonia, hepatitis	Pneumonitis. Case fatality rate for pneumonitis in mother is 10%
Risk of adverse fetal outcome	<11 weeks – 90% 11–16 weeks – 20% 16–20 weeks – minimal risk of deafness >20 weeks – no increased risk	<20 weeks – 9% excess fetal loss; 3% hydrops fetalis, of which about 50% die	Congenital infection – 10–15% Infants (85–90%) with no signs or symptoms at birth – 5–15% develop sequelae such as sensorineural hearing loss	Congenital varicella syndrome risk: < 13 weeks 0.4% 13–20 weeks 2% Neonatal chickenpox risk: 4 days prior to 2 days post delivery is 20%
Risk to the neonate	None	None	Late sequelae	Risk of severe disseminated haemorrhagic chickenpox
Interventions and benefit	Termination of pregnancy	Fetal hydrops – intrauterine transfusion reduces odds of death to 0.14	TOP Hyperimmune globulin Ganciclovir	VZIG to exposed mother and neonate attenuates illness. IV aciclovir or valaciclovir within 24 hrs of rash onset for mother IV Aciclovir for infected neonates
Number of infections in pregnancy per year	2–3 in pregnancy	1 in 512 pregnancies or seroconversion of 1.5–13% among susceptibles	Congenital CMV infection in the UK is ≈ 3/1000	2–3/1000 pregnancies, 6/10000 deliveries or 2000 maternal infections/year
Number of babies born with congenital defects	Approx 1 per year	2–8 fetal hydrops/100000 pregnancies (14–56 cases/year) 12–48/100000 spontaneous abortion (84–336 cases/year)	2133 infections in pregnancy/year	Approx 10 babies born with congenital damage per year, England and Wales

CHAPTER 16 Genital herpes in pregnancy

Background and prevalence

- Incidence of genital herpes in pregnancy – around 2% (USA).
- Neonatal herpes – caused by HSV-1 or HSV-2.
- Carries high morbidity and mortality.
- Incidence in the UK – 1 in 60 000 live births annually.
- Most commonly acquired at or near the time of delivery due to a direct contact with infected maternal secretions. Some cases of postnatal transmission have been reported.
- Factors which influence transmission – type of maternal infection (primary or recurrent), presence of transplacental maternal neutralizing antibodies, duration of rupture of membranes before delivery, use of fetal scalp electrodes and mode of delivery.

Primary infection – risk is greatest with a newly acquired infection (primary genital herpes) in the third trimester, particularly within 6 weeks of delivery, as viral shedding may persist and the baby is likely to be born before the development of protective maternal antibodies.

Recurrent genital herpes – associated with a very low risk of neonatal herpes.

- Recurrent herpes at the time of delivery which is commonly asymptomatic or unrecognized may cause localized forms of neonatal herpes, affecting the CNS, skin, eye, and mouth.
- Transplacentally acquired HSV antibodies do not prevent neurogenic virus spread to the brain of the neonate.

Prevention during pregnancy

- Reassure women with a history of genital herpes – the risk of transmission to the neonate is very small in the event of HSV recurrence during pregnancy, even if genital lesions are present at delivery.
- Women with no history of genital herpes – may reduce their risk of acquiring herpes during pregnancy and transmission to the neonate by using condoms or abstaining from sexual intercourse during the third trimester.
- Women can acquire genital herpes through orogenital contact if their partners have orolabial herpes (cold sores).
- Due to the prevalence of asymptomatic or unrecognized HSV infection, asking pregnant woman at screening visit whether she or her partner has ever had genital herpes is not an accurate way of determining her risk of acquiring primary HSV infection in pregnancy.

Fetal infection

- Disease localized to skin, eye, and mouth – has the best prognosis; death is unusual. With antiviral treatment neurological and/or ocular morbidity is < 2%.
- Local CNS disease (encephalitis alone) – infants with local CNS disease often present late (between 10 days and 4 weeks postnatally); with treatment, mortality is around 6% and neurological morbidity is 70%.
- Disseminated infection with multiple organ involvement – has the worst prognosis; with antiviral treatment, mortality is around 30%; 17% have long-term neurological sequelae. More common in preterm infants and occurs almost exclusively as a result of primary infection in the mother.
- Congenital herpes – very rarely may occur as a result of transplacental intrauterine infection. The skin, eyes, and CNS may be affected and there may be IUGR/fetal death.

Herpes infection in pregnancy

- Refer to a GUM physician.
- Confirm the diagnosis by viral culture or PCR.
- Advise on management and screening for other STIs.
- Type-specific HSV antibody test – can help to differentiate between primary and recurrent infection. Offer it to women presenting with a first episode of genital herpes in the third trimester.
- The presence of antibodies of the same type as the HSV isolated from genital swabs will confirm this episode to be a recurrence rather than a primary infection.

Screening programme

- Universal serum screening, targeted screening, and no screening – Although screening strategies reduce cases of neonatal transmission, medical resource costs are very high.
- As there is a very low incidence of neonatal herpes in the UK, it seems unlikely that such a screening programme would be cost-effective at the present time.
- Do not offer type-specific screening for HSV antibodies in pregnancy to identify women susceptible to acquiring genital herpes in pregnancy.

Management – primary episode in pregnancy

Before 6 weeks of delivery

- Oral or IV aciclovir in standard doses is associated with a reduction in the duration and severity of symptoms and viral shedding.
- Safety data have not shown any evidence of teratogenicity. Although these data are reassuring, the number of pregnancies evaluated was insufficient to draw definite conclusions and aciclovir is not licensed for use in pregnancy. Use it with caution in pregnancies less than 20 weeks of gestation.
- Use IV aciclovir for disseminated HSV infection.
- Do not offer daily suppressive aciclovir from 36 weeks of gestation to reduce the likelihood of HSV lesions at term for women who experience a primary episode of genital herpes earlier in the current pregnancy since there is insufficient evidence to recommend its use in this respect.

At the time of delivery

- If the baby is delivered vaginally, the risk of neonatal herpes is 41%. **Advise CS to all women presenting with primary episode of genital herpes at the time of delivery, or within 6 weeks of the expected date of delivery as it may have some protective effect.**
- Women who opt for a vaginal birth – avoid rupture of membranes and invasive procedures. One study reported that CS was not protective when the membranes had been ruptured for > 4 hours. Invasive procedures, such as fetal scalp electrode and FBS, have been associated with neonatal transmission.
- Consider IV aciclovir intrapartum to the mother and subsequently to the neonate. Its use in labour for preventing neonatal herpes has not been assessed but consider it on the assumption that exposure of the fetus to HSV will be reduced.
- Neonate – inform neonatologist; evaluate clinically and consider treatment with IV aciclovir.

Management – recurrent episode in pregnancy

Pregnancy

- Majority of recurrent episodes are short lasting and resolve within 7–10 days.
- Supportive treatment – saline baths and analgesia. Antiviral treatment is rarely indicated.
- Antenatal swabbing does not predict the shedding of virus at the onset of labour. Cultures during late gestation to predict viral shedding at term are also not indicated.
- **Secondary infection is not an indication for delivery by CS.**
- For women who would opt for CS if HSV lesions were detected at the onset of labour, daily suppressive aciclovir from 36 weeks until delivery may reduce the risk of HSV lesions at term.
- A meta-analysis of the use of acyclovir suppression: reduced the risk of clinical HSV recurrence (OR 0.25), asymptomatic HSV shedding (OR 0.09), and delivery by CS (OR 0.3).

At the onset of labour

- Risk of neonatal herpes with vaginal delivery is 1–3%. This needs to be balanced against the risks to the mother of CS. A cost–benefit analysis – 1583 CS would need to be performed to prevent one case of herpes-related mortality or morbidity, at a cost of US$2.5 million/case averted.
- **Do not recommend CS routinely. Individualize the mode of delivery.**
- Expedite the delivery in women with confirmed rupture of membranes at term.
- Avoid invasive procedures in labour.
- PPROM – risk of neonatal transmission is very small and is likely to be outweighed by the morbidity and mortality associated with premature delivery.

HIV-positive women

- These women are at increased risk of more severe and frequent symptomatic recurrent episodes of genital herpes during pregnancy and of asymptomatic shedding of HSV at term.
- As co-infection with HSV and HIV results in an increased replication of both viruses, there are concerns that genital reactivation of HSV may increase the risk of perinatal transmission of both HIV and HSV.
- Consider use of daily suppressive aciclovir to prevent HSV lesions at term.

Management of Genital Herpes in Pregnancy. RCOG Green-top Guideline No. 30; September 2007.
Please refer to: Management of Genital Herpes in Pregnancy. RCOG. BASHH joint guidlines; October 2014.

CHAPTER 17 Rubella infection in pregnancy

Prevalence and background

- Mode of transmission – respiratory droplet.
- Incubation period – 12 to 23 days.
- Infectious period is from 7 days before to 5–7 days after rash.
- Incidence (2005–2009) – 13 cases of rubella infection in pregnancy (8 were born outside UK); and 6 cases of congenital rubella syndrome (CRS) (5 mothers born outside the UK).
- **Routine antenatal testing for rubella antibody – to determine susceptibility and to identify those who require vaccine post delivery.**
- Re-infection – rubella infection in someone who has previously had either documented natural rubella virus infection or successful rubella immunization. Maternal re-infection is usually subclinical and diagnosed by changes in antibody concentration (IgG and/or IgM). The risk of CRS with subclinical maternal re-infection in the first 16 weeks is < 10%, and probably <5% (8% SOGC). No case of CRS has been reported when maternal re-infection occurred >12 weeks of pregnancy.

Risk of vertical transmission

- Fetal infection rate is about 80% with maternal infection in the first trimester; drops to 25% in the late second trimester and increases again in third trimester being nearly 100% beyond 36 weeks.
- The risk of CRS – 90% at <11 weeks; 33% at 11–12 weeks; 11% at 13–14 weeks; 24% at 15–16 weeks; and 0% >16 weeks.
- Risk to the fetus of primary rubella in the first 16 weeks of gestation is substantial, with worst outcome in the first trimester.
- Infection between 16 and 20 weeks is associated with a minimal risk of deafness only and rubella prior to the conception or after 20 weeks carries no documented risk.
- Beyond 20 weeks, FGR seems to be the only sequelae of third trimester infection.
- Advise to avoid contact with rubella throughout the first two trimesters of pregnancy, even in IgG-positive pregnant women.

Maternal infection

- Asymptomatic in 25–50% of cases, some may experience mild prodromal symptoms such as low-grade fever, sore throat, coryza, headaches or malaise, and tender lymphadenopathy. These last 1–5 days before the onset of the scarletiniform rash, which may be mildly pruritic.
- Rash characteristically begins on the face and spreads to the trunk and extremities. It usually resolves within 3 days in the same order in which it appeared.
- Polyarthritis and polyarthralgia – last about 1–4 weeks.
- Treatment of acute infection is supportive; prognosis is generally excellent.

Neonatal manifestations

- Vertical transmission – spontaneous abortion, fetal infection, stillbirth, FGR, CRS.
- Audiological anomalies (60–75%) – sensorineural deafness.
- Cardiac defects (10–20%) – pulmonary stenosis, patent ductus arteriosus, VSD.
- Ophthalmic defects (10–25%) – retinopathy, cataracts, microphthalmia, pigmentary and congenital glaucoma.
- Central nervous system (10–25%) – mental retardation, microcephaly, meningoencephalitis.
- Others – thrombocytopenia, hepatosplenomegaly, radiolucent bone disease, characteristic purpura (blueberry muffin appearance).
- Late manifestations – DM, thyroiditis, growth hormone deficit, behavioural disorder.

Diagnosis of maternal infection

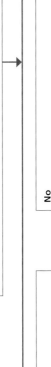

Contact with rubella or suspected rubella – Check whether the woman has a history of:
- rubella vaccine × 1 AND at least 1 rubella antibody positive test ≥10 IU/ml; OR
- rubella vaccine × 2; OR
- rubella antibody-positive tests × 2 (at least one ≥10 IU/ml).

Yes
- Reassure that rubella risk is remote and
- Advise to contact GP if rash develops.

No
- Test serum for rubella-specific IgG and IgM. Presence of a rubella infection is diagnosed by:
  * A 4-fold rise in rubella IgG antibody titre between acute and convalescent serum.
  * A positive serological test for rubella-specific IgM antibody.
- Serological tests are best performed within 7–10 days after the onset of the rash and repeated 2–3 weeks later.

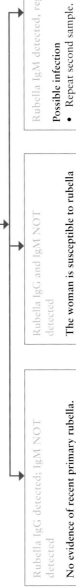

Rubella IgM detected, regardless of IgG

Possible infection
- Repeat second sample.
- Reference testing is recommended.
- Investigate both samples for rubella IgG and IgM plus avidity as appropriate.

→ **Possible infection**

Rubella IgG and IgM NOT detected

The woman is susceptible to rubella
- Repeat test 1 month after last contact or if illness develops.
- 2-dose course of MMR vaccine postpartum.

Rubella IgG detected; IgM NOT detected

No evidence of recent primary rubella.
- Reassure and advise to contact GP if rash develops (HPA).
- SOGC Guidelines differ.

- Booking sera or other earlier serum samples may be available and may aid in the diagnosis.
- Do not use methods on oral fluid alone for confirming or excluding rubella infection in pregnancy.
- A positive rubella culture – from nasal, blood, throat, urine, or cerebrospinal fluid may be positive from 1 week before to 2 weeks after the onset of the rash.

Diagnostic difficulty: late presentation with unknown immune status – Problems arise when investigation commences 4 weeks or more after the onset of rash.
- If rubella-specific IgG is detected and specific IgM is not detected – rubella cannot be excluded serologically unless past sera can be tested to determine whether seroconversion has occurred recently.
- Assess the probability of infection based on recent epidemiology of rubella in the community, past history of vaccine and testing, characteristics of illness.

- Do not diagnose rubella in pregnant woman on the basis of a single positive rubella-specific IgM. Interpret the results in relation to full clinical and epidemiological information.
- Unless seroconversion has been shown, test further by alternative rubella-specific IgM tests. Test an acute sample and a sample taken 10–14 days later for rubella IgG, and measure the strength of binding of specific IgG (avidity). IgG avidity is low soon after a primary infection, but matures over a few weeks to become more strongly binding.
- If rubella-specific IgM positivity reflects a recent rubella episode (whether primary or re-infection), the degree of reactivity will usually change over the period of a few weeks, rather than persisting at a similar level.

Diagnosis of fetal infection

- PCR on CVS or amniocentesis. Given the low but definite risk to the fetus of maternal rubella re-infection in the first 16 weeks of pregnancy, there may be occasions when consideration is given to further fetal investigation by PCR to ascertain if fetal infection has occurred.
- USS diagnosis of CRS is extremely difficult. Biometric data can aid in the diagnosis of FGR but are not a good tool for diagnosing CRS.

CHAPTER 17 Rubella infection in pregnancy

Management of primary or re-infection (SOGC)

- Depends on the gestation of pregnancy and state of immunity.
- Since the effects of CRS vary with the gestational age at the time of infection, establish accurate gestational dating, as it is critical to counselling.

Known immune

≥ 12 weeks of gestation

- No further testing as CRS has not been reported after maternal re-infection beyond 12 weeks' gestation.
- **Reassure.**

< 12 weeks of gestation

- If a significant rise in IgG titre without detection of IgM – re-infection is likely.
- Fetal risk for congenital infection after maternal re-infection during the first trimester is about 8%.
- **Offer counselling.**

Non-immune or immunity unknown

Gestation ≤ 16 weeks

- Acute and convalescent IgG and IgM – positive IgM or significant rise in IgG – recent acute infection.
- High risk of CRS.
- **TOP is advised.**

Gestation 16–20 weeks

- CRS is rare (< 1%) and may be manifested by sensorineural deafness (often severe).
- **Reassure.**

Gestation > 20 weeks

- No studies have documented CRS after 20 weeks.
- **Reassure.**

- Primary failure of the rubella vaccine occurs in < 5% of immunizations.
- Rubella vaccine virus has the potential to cross the placenta and infect the fetus. However, there has been no report of CRS in the offspring of women inadvertently vaccinated during early pregnancy. Therefore, do not advise pregnancy termination for these patients.
- Given the potential risks to the fetus, advise women not to become pregnant for a period of 28 days after immunization.
- Vaccine can be given safely to postpartum women who are breastfeeding and to the children of pregnant women, since infection is not transmitted from recently immunized individuals.
- Counsel and offer women wishing to conceive to have their antibody status determined and undergo rubella vaccination if needed.

- There are no data supporting the use of immunoglobulin in pregnant women with acute infection in order to diminish the fetal response to disease.
- The Centers for Disease Control recommend limiting its use to women with known rubella exposure who decline TOP.

Rubella in Pregnancy. SOGC Clinical Practice Guidelines; No. 203; February 2008.
Health Protection Agency. http://www.hpa.org.uk/Topics/InfectiousDiseases/InfectionsAZ/Rubella/
Clinical knowledge summaries: http://www.cks.nhs.uk/rubella

Background and prevalence

- The most common cause of intrauterine infection – 0.2% to 2.2% of all live births.
- A common cause of sensorineural hearing loss and mental retardation.
- Primary infection – mild or asymptomatic. Some – malaise, persistent fever, myalgia, cervical lymphadenopathy, and less commonly, pneumonia and hepatitis. Rarely, it may present with a generalized maculopapular rash.
- After the primary infection, the virus becomes dormant and exists in a latent state, from which it can be reactivated resulting in recurrent infection.
- Transmission – through droplet spread.

Recommendations for seronegative pregnant women

- Advise good personal hygiene, avoid intimate contact with salivary secretions and urine from young children, and hand washing after changing diapers and wiping secretions.
- No effective and safe immunization is available.
- **Do not routinely test (serological) pregnant women for CMV to identify those who have acquired primary infection during pregnancy.**
- Test (serological antibodies) for CMV only in women who develop influenza-like symptoms during pregnancy or following detection of sonographic findings that are suggestive of CMV infection which cannot be explained by other causes.

Investigations – diagnosis of maternal infection

- Clinical diagnosis of primary CMV infection is unreliable because it is asymptomatic in 90% of cases and clinical signs, when present, are often non-specific.
- Seroconversion – the de novo appearance of virus-specific IgG in the serum of a pregnant woman who was previously seronegative (saved maternal serum) is diagnostic.
- When the immune status before pregnancy is unknown, determination of primary CMV infection is based on detection of specific IgM antibody. However, IgM can also be detected in 10% of recurrent infections and can be detected for months after primary infection. Therefore, the group of women designated CMV-IgM positive could include women with primary infection acquired before pregnancy and a few women with recurrent infections.
- The IgG avidity assay can help distinguish primary infection from past or recurrent infection. IgG of low avidity is produced during the first months after onset of infection, whereas subsequently a maturation process occurs by which IgG antibody of increasingly higher avidity is generated. An avidity index > 60% is highly suggestive of past or secondary infection, while an avidity index < 30% is highly suggestive of a recent primary infection (duration < 3 months).

Risk of transmission

- Congenital infection is due to transplacental transmission of CMV.
- Transmission to the fetus may occur due to primary or secondary infection.
- The probability of intrauterine transmission following **primary infection during pregnancy is 30% to 40%, compared with only 1% following secondary infection.**
- The risk of serious fetal injury is greatest after primary maternal infection in the first trimester or early in the second trimester.
- Prevalence of congenital CMV infection in the UK is ≈ 3/1000.
- Seroconversion occurs in 1% to 4% of all pregnancies and is higher in women who are of low socioeconomic status or who have poor personal hygiene.
- Modes of transmission – transplacental, perinatal ingestion or aspiration of cervicovaginal secretions at the time of delivery, and ingestion of breast milk.

Risks – newborn/congenital infection

- Asymptomatic at birth: most of the congenitally infected infants (85–90%) have no signs or symptoms at birth, but 5% to 15% of them will develop sequelae such as sensorineural hearing loss, delay of psychomotor development, and visual impairment.
- Symptomatic at birth:
  * 10–15% of congenitally infected infants will have symptoms at birth – FGR, microcephaly, hepatosplenomegaly, petechiae, jaundice, chorioretinitis, thrombocytopenia, and anaemia.
  * The risk of any sequelae in infants with symptomatic congenital CMV at birth is 90%.
  * 20% to 30% of them will die, mostly of disseminated intravascular coagulation, hepatic dysfunction, or bacterial superinfection.

Fetus – prenatal diagnosis of fetal infection

USS

- It is helpful but not diagnostic because CMV has features in common with other intrauterine infections and these abnormalities are observed in < 25% of infected fetuses. Fetal USS is neither sensitive nor specific to congenital CMV infection.
- Congenital CMV infection findings – IUGR, cerebral ventriculomegaly, microcephaly, intracranial calcifications, ascites/pleural effusion, hydrops fetalis, hyperechogenic bowel, liver calcifications, oligohydramnios/polyhydramnios.

Amniocentesis

- CMV isolation from amniotic fluid by culture and PCR testing – high sensitivity and specificity – the gold standard.
- Quantitative PCR to detect high CMV viral load in the amniotic fluid is also used to determine fetuses at risk of clinical sequelae.
- Perform amniocentesis at least 7 weeks after the onset of maternal infection and after 21 weeks of gestation because a detectable quantity of the virus is not secreted to the amniotic fluid until 5 to 7 weeks after fetal infection and replication of the virus in the kidney.

Cordocentesis

- Do not test for IgM from cord blood. This is due to the risk associated with cordocentesis and because many fetuses infected by CMV do not develop specific IgM until late in pregnancy, resulting in poor sensitivity.

Diagnosed as fetal infection – prognostic markers

- Positive results of amniotic fluid tests do not discriminate between infants who will have symptoms at birth and those who will not.
- There is no method of antenatal diagnosis that will reliably identify infected fetuses at risk of adverse outcome.

- Serial USS every 2 to 4 weeks to look for signs of CMV infection. USS detected abnormalities may aid in determining the prognosis of the fetus, but the absence of sonographic findings does not guarantee a normal outcome.
- Fetal MRI may improve the prognostic evaluation, especially when brain abnormalities are detected by USS. But there is no evidence to support its routine use or benefit over ultrasound.

- Viral load in amniotic fluid – the CMV DNA load in amniotic fluid samples is significantly higher in symptomatic fetuses than asymptomatic fetuses. However, a great deal of overlap exists between the two groups; thus the role of quantitative determination of CMV DNA in the amniotic fluid as a prognostic factor still awaits confirmation.

Management options

- There is no effective therapy; can consider TOP once fetal infection is detected by USS or amniocentesis or once a fetus is suspected to be affected.

- Postnatal therapy – there is some evidence suggesting a beneficial role for ganciclovir in neonates with symptomatic congenital CMV infection with some hearing improvement.
- Ganciclovir is associated with significant haematological toxicity and requires 6 weeks of intravenous therapy; so its routine use remains controversial.
- Treat the infants with CNS signs at birth with ganciclovir according to the protocol from the Collaborative Antiviral Study Group (RCOG).

- A recent study of women with confirmed primary CMV infection evaluated the use of CMV-specific hyperimmune globulin for the treatment and prevention of fetal CMV infection. In the prevention group, 16% had infants with congenital CMV infection, compared with 40% who did not receive hyperimmune globulin. No adverse effects of hyperimmune globulin were observed. Further studies are necessary.
- A study investigated whether oral maternal valaciclovir in the treatment of symptomatic intrauterine CMV infection could achieve therapeutic fetal concentrations; there was no statistically significant difference in poor outcome between the treatment and non-treatment arms. Valaciclovir therapy remains confined to clinical trials until further evidence is available.

Summary – maternal diagnosis

↓

Serological tests – IgG, IgM

- Seroconversion (the appearance of CMV-specific IgG antibody in a previously seronegative woman).

- Detection of specific IgM antibody associated with low IgG avidity.

- Detectable IgG antibodies without IgM before pregnancy and a significant rise of IgG titre with or without the presence of IgM and with high IgG avidity – **recurrent infection.**

  - Although it is accepted that amniocentesis in primary infection is warranted because of the high risk of fetal infection, there is no consensus on whether to perform amniotic fluid viral studies in cases of secondary infection, when the risk of fetal infection is low. However, there are several cases of secondary infection with severe sequelae described in the literature; therefore, it may be considered even in cases of secondary infection.

FMU – prenatal fetal diagnosis

Amniocentesis
5–7 weeks after infection/after 21 weeks of gestation
+
USS signs

→ **Negative**: Fetal infection unlikely. Repeat USS in 4–6 weeks.

→ **Positive**:
- TOP if USS suggestive of fetus being affected.
- Serial USS every 2 weeks for signs of fetal infection. Consider quantitative viral DNA in amniotic fluid.

Cytomegalovirus Infection in Pregnancy. SOGC Clinical Practice Guidelines; No. 240, April 2010.
https://www.gov.uk/government/publications/viral-rash-in-pregnancy
McCarthy FP, Jones C, Rowlands S, Giles M. Primary and secondary cytomegalovirus in pregnancy. The Obstetrician & Gynaecologist 2009;11:96–100.

CHAPTER 18 CMV infection in pregnancy

69

CHAPTER 19 Toxoplasmosis in pregnancy

Background and prevalence

- Zoonotic infection caused by the parasite *Toxoplasma gondii*. Pregnant women and individuals with a depressed immune system are at higher risk.
- Primary host – cat; secondary host – human, cattle.
- Following the acute active phase of infection the parasite persists for years (probably lifelong) in the form of latent cysts located throughout the body, especially in cardiac and skeletal muscle and CNS.
- Incidence – about 2/1000 pregnancies in UK.
- Incidence of congenital toxoplasmosis for England and Wales – 3.4/100 000 live births.
- Toxoplasma screening is not part of routine screening for women in the UK.

Source of infection

- Ingestion of cysts in undercooked meat or raw meat; raw cured meat, such as salami or Parma ham; unpasteurized goats' milk.
- Hand-to-mouth contact with faeces of infected cats, contaminated soil, poorly washed garden produce; direct contamination of cuts and grazes; contact with infected sheep.
- Prevention – take general hygiene precautions to avoid ingesting the parasite.
- Provide appropriate health information about toxoplasmosis to all pregnant women.

Risk of vertical transmission

- Less than half of the cases are transmitted to the fetus. Even when transmission occurs, the majority of babies (90–95%) have no symptoms.
- Lower risk of transmission if maternal infection is acquired in the early stages of pregnancy but the outcome can be severe such as miscarriage, stillbirth or birth defects.
- Higher risk of transmission if acquired later in pregnancy but the clinical outcome is less severe (subtle neurological, ocular or systemic signs) or the child may be asymptomatic.
- Infection acquired 2–3 months prior to conception can very rarely (a few case reports) present a risk of damage to the fetus.
- Risk of transmission in the first trimester is 10–15%, rising to 70–80% in the third trimester.

Maternal infection

- Majority are asymptomatic.
- If symptomatic – usually mild to moderate and non-specific flu-like symptoms: fatigue, malaise, myalgia, sore throat, low-grade fever, and lymphadenopathy (often involving the posterior cervical region). Symptoms can last from a few weeks to several months.
- Incubation period is 5–23 days. It can take 4–8 weeks for the infection to pass to the baby.

- There is no vaccine available.
- If a non-pregnant woman of childbearing age is diagnosed with a recently acquired *T. gondii* infection, advise the woman to wait 6 months (from the date that the acute infection was diagnosed or documented) before attempting to become pregnant. Reassure that subsequent pregnancies are not at risk.

Neonatal infection

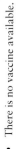

- The classical triad – hydrocephalus, cerebral calcification, and chorioretinitis strongly indicates congenital toxoplasmosis.
- Many children are born either with more subtle signs or are born apparently normal. In the latter, clinical features can present in the first weeks or months of life but may not be apparent for several years or even decades.
- The range of presentations that may occur months or years after birth include:
  * Chorioretinitis, hydrocephalus, cerebral calcification, seizures.
  * Hepatosplenomegaly, jaundice, rash, mental retardation, deafness, spasticity.
  * Cataracts, strabismus, blindness.
- Babies who are badly affected are at risk of blindness, deafness, seizures or brain damage. Some babies may be stillborn or die a few days after birth.

Investigations for suspected maternal infection

- To find whether or not a pregnancy is at risk from toxoplasma infection:
  - ☆ Is there evidence of past infection of toxoplasma – IgG assays.
  - ☆ Is the infection recent – IgM, IgA assays.
  - ☆ When did infection occur in relation to conception – IgG avidity assays.

Negative for IgG and IgM:

- Reassure and advise on precautions aimed to reduce the risk of infection for the remainder of the pregnancy.

IgG is positive and IgM is negative:

- Reassure that the pregnancy is not at risk.
- Pre-conceptional blood (if available) can be tested to assess if infection occurred prior to pregnancy.
- The incidence of congenital toxoplasmosis in women infected before pregnancy has been shown to be extremely low (approaching zero); treatment and prenatal diagnosis of fetal infection are not indicated unless the mother is immunocompromised.

IgG and IgM positive – infection occurred during pregnancy and fetus is at risk.

- Further laboratory tests to provide a more precise estimate of the duration of infection (IgG avidity test); comparison of IgG and IgM levels in sequential samples to confirm the original result and to allow comparison for possible changes in titre.
- IgG avidity – can discriminate between infections acquired recently and those acquired several months earlier or more.
- A detailed history of the women can be helpful in revealing clinical features which may help in timing the onset of infection.

Referral to FMU – results diagnostic or highly suggestive of an infection acquired during gestation or shortly before conception.

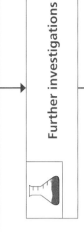

Further investigations

1. Detection of the parasite and/or specific antibody

Cordocentesis:

- Detection of the parasite and specific anti-toxoplasma IgM/IgA.
- However, negative serological findings are not reliable in excluding congenital infection.

Amniocentesis:

- The level of detection in amniotic fluid is good and has fewer risks to the fetus compared to cordocentesis. Perform amniocentesis at 18 weeks of gestation (the optimal time) or later. Sensitivity and specificity for amniotic fluid obtained before 18 weeks of gestation have not been studied, and it may be associated with a higher risk to the fetus. At 18 weeks – it has sensitivity of 64% for the diagnosis of congenital infection in the fetus, an NPV of 88%, and a specificity and PPV of 100%.
- Also indicated in women who have evidence of fetal damage by USS examination, or are significantly immunosuppressed and thus at risk of reactivation of their latent infection (with the exception of women with AIDS).
- Amniocentesis does not show how badly the baby is affected.

2. Ultrasound scan

- Ultrasound may reveal the presence of fetal abnormalities (e.g., ventriculomegaly or hepatic or brain calcifications, hydrocephalus, splenomegaly, and ascites).
- Recent studies – In women who were infected in the first trimester, received spiramycin treatment, had normal ultrasounds but congenitally infected fetuses – 2-year follow-up revealed that their outcomes were similar to those of infected children born to mothers who had acquired the infection during the second and third trimesters. In such circumstances, TOP was not indicated. CT for brain calcifications, and MRI for other abnormalities in the fetus.

Rx

3. Treatment – to prevent vertical transmission of the parasite

< 18 weeks

- **Spiramycin** – the protection is more distinct in women infected during their first trimester. The incidence of congenital infection is reduced by 60%. Spiramycin does not readily cross the placenta and thus is not reliable for treatment of infection in the fetus.
- There is no evidence that spiramycin is teratogenic.

≥ 18 weeks

- Because of the high transmission rates observed after 18 weeks of gestation, treat with **pyrimethamine, sulfadiazine, and folinic acid** to prevent fetal infection and treat the infected fetus if transmission has occurred.
- Pyrimethamine is not used earlier because it is potentially teratogenic.

Fetal USS and amniocentesis ≥ 18 weeks

Fetal USS and amniocentesis ≥ 18 weeks

PCR negative and USS negative

- **Continue spiramycin** – administer until delivery even in those patients with negative results of amniotic fluid PCR, because of the theoretical possibility that fetal infection can occur later in pregnancy from a placenta that was infected earlier in gestation.

PCR positive +/- USS positive

- **Pyrimethamine, sulfadiazine, and folinic acid** – for pregnant women in whom the possibility of fetal infection is high or fetal infection has been established.
- Pyrimethamine – produces reversible, usually gradual, dose-related depression of the bone marrow. Monitor patients who receive pyrimethamine with full blood cell counts frequently. Folinic acid is used for reduction and prevention of the haematological toxicities of the drug.

PCR negative and USS negative

- Consider switching to spiramycin. Or continue with pyrimethamine, sulfadiazine, and folinic acid.

Neonatal infection

- Clinical and ophthalmological examination.
- USS of the brain.
- Frequently it is not possible to detect these changes and diagnosis has to be based solely on laboratory findings.

Cord blood and matched maternal sample for serological tests:

- Since maternal IgG is transferred passively to the fetus in utero, detection of IgG in the neonate is of limited value unless levels are significantly elevated compared to maternal titres.
- Comparison of maternal and neonatal IgG by immunoblot may be helpful since detection of a neonatal immune response to any antigens not recognized by the maternal immune response would imply this IgG is unique to the neonate.
- Detection of neonatal IgM and IgA is diagnostic for neonatal infection. However, IgM and IgA may only be present in 50–60% of congenitally infected children in the first month of life but may appear subsequently. Therefore monitor the child serologically throughout the first year of life by which time any passively acquired maternal IgG antibodies will decline. The disappearance of IgG within the first year of life excludes congenital infection. Persistence of positive IgG after 12 months confirms infection.

- Up to 9 in 10 infected babies seem normal at birth. But about 8 in 10 of these babies will have health problems months or even years later. These include eye infections, hearing problems, and learning difficulties.
- About 1 in 10 babies with toxoplasmosis have severe infection that is obvious at the time of birth.
- Retinochoroiditis is the most common long-term health problem. It can permanently damage a baby's eyesight.
- Treat babies with toxoplasmosis with antibiotics for a year after birth.
- Early treatment of congenital toxoplasmosis appears to decrease the frequency of chorioretinitis and be associated with the disappearance of cerebral opacities.

Montoya JG & Remington JS. Management of *Toxoplasma gondii* infection during pregnancy. Clinical Infectious Diseases 2008;47:554–566.

Investigation of Toxoplasma Infection in Pregnancy. HPA QSOP 59 Health Protection Agency.

CHAPTER 20 Parvovirus infection in pregnancy

Background and prevalence

- Parvoviridae family of single-stranded DNA viruses (genus Erythrovirus).
- Spreads through respiratory secretions, close contact, and (rarely) by blood transfusion.
- Outbreaks usually occur every 4–5 years and may last up to 6 months.
- The virus targets rapidly growing erythroid progenitor cells in bone marrow, fetal liver, umbilical cord, and peripheral blood.
- Infection – common with 50–60% of adults having been infected.
- Incubation period – 4 to 14 days after exposure.
- Incidence in the UK is not precisely known.
- Risk of acquiring parvovirus infection in pregnancy is 1:400; during an endemic year there would be 2 cases of fetal hydrops and 12 miscarriages/IUD per 100000 pregnancies.
- Women at increased risk – mothers of preschool and school-age children, workers at day care centres, and school teachers. Nursery school teachers have a 3-fold increased risk of acute infection and other school teachers have a 1.6-fold increased risk.

- Transplacental transmission occurs in 17–33% of women. Fetus is most vulnerable when infected in the second trimester, with the peak risk at 17–24 weeks' gestation, although it may also occur in late gestation.
- First trimester loss is rare (3%).
- Most fetuses infected have spontaneous resolution with no adverse outcomes.
- The estimated fetal loss rate during pregnancy is about 5–10%. The loss rate of fetuses < 20 weeks' gestation is 15% and > 20 weeks' gestation is 2.3%.
- The consequences usually develop 3–5 weeks after the onset of maternal infection.
- Permanent congenital abnormality and/or congenital anaemia have rarely been identified as a consequence of intrauterine infection.
- Currently no licensed vaccine and preventive measures are available.
- There is no evidence to suggest that re-infection is a risk to the fetus.

Maternal infection

- Asymptomatic – 20–25% of adults.
- Erythema infectiosum (fifth disease) – children initially present with flu-like symptoms, fever, and headache, followed 1 to 4 days later by a 'slapped cheek' rash that becomes lacy in appearance and after about 1 week may spread to the trunk and limbs.
- Adults with parvovirus B19 (B19V) infection usually do not have an extensive rash. Minor febrile illness, a rash, and arthralgia may begin around day 15, by which time the person is usually no longer infectious. The rash is clinically indistinguishable from rubella.
- Arthropathy – symmetrical polyarthralgia affects hands, wrists, ankles, and knees. Most common symptom in adults; affects up to 80% and may last several weeks to months.
- Although the illness is usually self-limiting, the person may become severely ill with aplastic crisis, which may be fatal if left untreated.
- Myocarditis: case reports of acute myocarditis leading to heart failure.

Fetal infection

- Fetal loss – spontaneously or as a consequence of non-immune fetal hydrops (NIFH).
- NIFH – parvovirus B19 infection accounts for 8–10% of NIFH.
- NIFH – risk is 3% if infection occurs between 9 and 20 weeks, of which about half die.
- Fetal anaemia, combined with the shorter half life of fetal red blood cells, leads to severe anaemia, hypoxia, and high output cardiac failure.
- Other possible causes of death include fetal viral myocarditis leading to cardiac failure, and impaired hepatic function caused by direct damage of hepatocytes and indirect damage due to hemosiderin deposits.
- Fetal loss is most likely when infection occurs at 9–16 weeks.
- There is no evidence that it is teratogenic in human pregnancy; therefore maternal infection with parvovirus B19 is not an indication for TOP.

Suspected parvovirus B19 infection

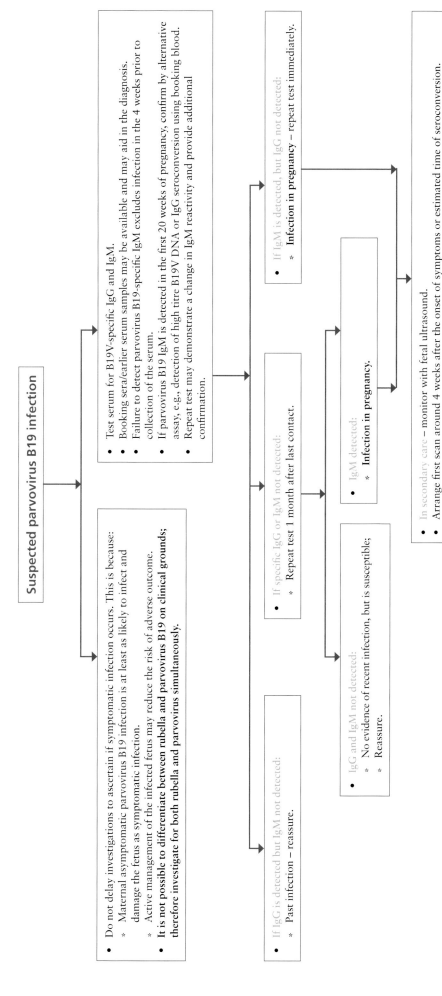

- Do not delay investigations to ascertain if symptomatic infection occurs. This is because:
  * Maternal asymptomatic parvovirus B19 infection is at least as likely to infect and damage the fetus as symptomatic infection.
  * Active management of the infected fetus may reduce the risk of adverse outcome.
- **It is not possible to differentiate between rubella and parvovirus B19 on clinical grounds; therefore investigate for both rubella and parvovirus simultaneously.**

- Test serum for B19V-specific IgG and IgM.
- Booking sera/earlier serum samples may be available and may aid in the diagnosis.
- Failure to detect parvovirus B19-specific IgM excludes infection in the 4 weeks prior to collection of the serum.
- If parvovirus B19 IgM is detected in the first 20 weeks of pregnancy, confirm by alternative assay, e.g., detection of high titre B19V DNA or IgG seroconversion using booking blood.
- Repeat test may demonstrate a change in IgM reactivity and provide additional confirmation.

- If IgG is detected but IgM not detected:
  * Past infection – reassure.

- If IgM is detected, but IgG not detected – repeat test immediately.
  * **Infection in pregnancy.**

- If specific IgG or IgM not detected:
  * Repeat test 1 month after last contact.

- IgG and IgM not detected:
  * No evidence of recent infection, but is susceptible;
  * Reassure.

- IgM detected:
  * **Infection in pregnancy.**

- In secondary care – monitor with fetal ultrasound.
- Arrange first scan around 4 weeks after the onset of symptoms or estimated time of seroconversion.
- Following this, scan every 1–2 weeks until 30 weeks of gestation or up to 8–12 weeks after.
- Fetal hydrops initially presents on USS with ascites and thickening and enlargement of the fetal heart. Refer to FMU.

FMU – further assessment
- Doppler assessment of the middle cerebral artery; parvovirus B19V DNA detection in amniotic fluid or fetal blood by PCR.
- Presence of IgM in fetal blood is not reliable for the diagnosis of fetal infection, as the fetus does not begin to make its own IgM until 22 weeks' gestation.
- Fetal blood sampling and intrauterine transfusion (IUT) of erythrocytes – the fetal mortality rate with IUT is 18%, compared with 50% in fetuses who do not receive IUT. More than 7-fold reduction in fetal death with IUT has been reported.
- Early delivery of the baby if it is near full term.
- Use of corticosteroids to accelerate lung maturity is not contraindicated and should be considered.

Parvovirus B19 Infection in Pregnancy. SOGC Clinical Practice Guidelines; No. 119, September 2002.
Health Protection Agency: http://www.hpa.org.uk/Topics/InfectiousDiseases/InfectionsAZ/ParvovirusB19/
Clinical knowledge summaries: http://www.cks.nhs.uk/parvovirus_b19_infection

CHAPTER 21 Chickenpox in pregnancy

Background and prevalence

- Herpes varicella-zoster virus (VZV) – primary infection.
- DNA virus. Highly infectious.
- Transmission – respiratory droplets; direct contact with vesicle fluid; indirect via fomites.
- Primary infection – fever, malaise, and a pruritic rash. Rash – crops of maculopapules which become vesicular and crust over before healing. The incubation period is 1–3 weeks and the disease is infectious 48 hours before the rash appears and continues to be infectious until the vesicles crust over. The vesicles usually crust within 5 days.
- Following the primary infection, the virus remains dormant in sensory nerve root ganglia and can be reactivated to cause shingles – a vesicular erythematous skin rash in a dermatomal distribution.
- Primary VZV infection in pregnancy is uncommon, as > 90% of the antenatal population are seropositive for VZV IgG antibody. Women from tropical and subtropical areas are more likely to be seronegative for VZV IgG and are more susceptible to the development of chickenpox.
- Incidence 3/1000 pregnancies.
- Risk of acquiring infection from an immunocompetent individual with herpes zoster in non-exposed sites (for example, thoracolumbar) is remote. However, disseminated zoster or exposed zoster (such as ophthalmic) in any individual or localized zoster in an immunosuppressed patient can be infectious when the lesions are active until they have crusted over.

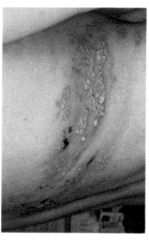

Shingles.

Risks or complications

Maternal

- Pneumonia, hepatitis, encephalitis, and rarely death.
- Pneumonia – up to 10%; severity increases in later gestation.
- Mortality rates of 20–45% were reported in the pre-antiviral era but have fallen to 3–14% with antiviral therapy and improved intensive care.
- Case fatality rate of < 1% but five times higher in pregnancy than in the non-pregnant adult.

First 28 weeks of pregnancy

- Risk of spontaneous miscarriage is not increased
- Fetal varicella syndrome – infection between 3 weeks to 28 weeks:
  * < 20 weeks – incidence of 0.9%; risk is in the first trimester (0.55%).
  * 20–28 weeks – extremely rare (1 case reported).
  * > 28 weeks – no cases reported.
- Characterized by – skin scarring in a dermatomal distribution; eye defects (microphthalmia, chorioretinitis, cataracts); hypoplasia of the limbs; and neurological abnormalities (microcephaly, cortical atrophy, mental restriction, and dysfunction of bowel and bladder sphincters). It does not occur at the time of initial fetal infection but results from a subsequent herpes zoster reactivation in utero.

Fetal/neonatal

Rest of pregnancy

- May have no fetal or neonatal effect other then the development of shingles in the first few years.
- This is due to reactivation of the virus after a primary infection in utero.

At term – varicella of the newborn

- If infection occurs 1–4 weeks before delivery, up to 50% of babies are infected and approximately 23% develop clinical varicella despite high titres of passively acquired maternal antibody.
- Severe chickenpox can occur if the infant is born within 7 days of onset of the mother's rash or if the mother develops the rash up to 7 days after delivery when cord blood VZV IgG is low.
- It can also occur from contact with a person with chickenpox or shingles.
- The route of infection – transplacental, ascending vaginal or from direct contact with lesions during or after delivery.

A. Woman seen preconceptually

- Determine the varicella immune status of women by:
  * Past history of chickenpox.
  * If no history or uncertain history of previous infection – check serum for varicella antibodies.
- There is no national screening recommendation in the UK.

In the non-immune

- Varicella vaccination (live attenuated virus) pre-pregnancy or postpartum. If vaccinated, advise to avoid pregnancy for 3 months and to avoid contact with other susceptible pregnant women and neonates if a post-vaccination rash occurs.
- Varicella vaccine – since its introduction, the incidence of primary infection (chickenpox) has fallen by 90% and the mortality has decreased by two-thirds.
- Immunity from the vaccine may persist for up to 20 years.

B. Pregnant women at booking visit

- Ask about previous chickenpox/shingles – a previous history of chickenpox is 97–99% predictive of the presence of serum varicella antibodies.
- A history of chickenpox can be a less reliable predictor of immunity in individuals born and raised overseas and it may be appropriate to undertake serum testing routinely in this group of women.

- Women who
  * Have no history or an uncertain history of previous infection.
  * Are seronegative for VZV IgG.
  Advise to avoid contact with chickenpox and shingles during pregnancy and to inform HCPs of a potential exposure.

Although it is shown that antenatal varicella screening by history and serological testing for VZIG antibody in those with a negative history followed by postpartum vaccination is cost effective, this is not currently part of a UK screening programme.

C. Pregnant woman with history of contact with chickenpox or shingles

- Elicit history to confirm the significance of the contact and the susceptibility of the patient.
- History regarding the type of VZV infection; the timing of the exposure; the closeness and duration of contact. **Significant contact** – contact in the same room for 15 minutes or more, face-to-face contact, and contact in the setting of a large open ward. Any close contact during the period of infectiousness is significant.
- Check the susceptibility of the woman – by eliciting a past history of chickenpox or shingles.

- If there is a definite past history of chickenpox, it is reasonable to assume that the woman is immune to varicella infection.

- At least 80–90% of women will have VZ IgG – reassure.

- Test serum VZV IgG:
  * if the woman's immunity to chickenpox is unknown,
  * if there is any doubt about previous infection, or
  * if there is no previous history of chickenpox or shingles.

- **If the pregnant woman is not immune and she has had a significant exposure – give VZIG ASAP.**
- VZIG prevents or attenuates the disease if given within 10 days of significant exposure by 50%. It has no therapeutic benefit once chickenpox has developed. It is not known whether it reduces the risk of FVS.
- If VZIG is given, manage the pregnant woman as potentially infectious from 8 to 28 days after VZIG (8–21 days if no VZIG given).
- Advise women to inform their HCP early if a rash develops. Maternal death has been reported following the development of varicella pneumonia despite the administration of VZIG.
- A second dose of VZIG may be required if a further exposure is reported and 3 weeks have elapsed since the last dose.
- VZIG – manufactured from the plasma of human blood donors, therefore limited and expensive. Rare anaphylactoid reactions have occurred in individuals with hypogammaglobulinaemia who have IgA antibodies or in those that have atypical reactions to blood transfusion. No case of blood-borne infection has been reported.

D. The pregnant woman who develops chickenpox

- Advise women to:
  - * Immediately contact their GP.
  - * Avoid contact with susceptible individuals until the lesions have crusted over, usually about 5 days after the onset of the rash.
- Symptomatic treatment and hygiene to prevent secondary bacterial infection of the lesions.

Oral aciclovir (800 mg five times a day for 7 days):

- If women present within 24 hours of the onset of the rash and if > 20 weeks of gestation.
- It reduces the duration of fever and symptomatology in immunocompetent adults if commenced within 24 hours of the rash.
- Be cautious at < 20 weeks of gestation. There is no increase in the risk of fetal malformation with aciclovir in pregnancy, although there is a theoretical risk of teratogenesis in the first trimester.

Refer/admission to hospital (but NOT to a maternity ward)

- Women who develop: chest symptoms, neurological symptoms, haemorrhagic rash or bleeding, a dense rash with or without mucosal lesions.
- Women with significant immunosuppression.
- Women at greater risk of pneumonitis are – smokers, women with chronic lung disease, those on corticosteroids, those in latter half of pregnancy. These women have a more extensive or haemorrhagic rash.

- MDT: obstetrician or fetal medicine specialist, virologist and neonatologist, respiratory physician and intensive care specialist.
- Women should be nursed in isolation from babies or susceptible pregnant women or non-immune staff.

Investigations – prenatal diagnosis of fetal risks

- Refer to an FMU at 16–20 weeks or 5 weeks after infection, for discussion and detailed USS.
- Prenatal diagnosis is possible with detailed USS if it shows any limb deformity, microcephaly, hydrocephalus, soft-tissue calcification, and IUGR.
- A time lag of at least 5 weeks after the primary infection is needed.
- Fetal MRI can be useful to look for morphological abnormalities.

- Do not advise routine amniocentesis because the risk of FVS is very low, even when amniotic fluid is positive for VZV DNA.
- VZV DNA can be detected by PCR in amniotic fluid. It has a high sensitivity but a low specificity for FVS.

- If amniotic fluid is PCR positive and USS is normal at 17–21 weeks, the risk of FVS is low.
- If repeat USS is normal at 23–24 weeks – risk of FVS is remote.

- A negative result in amniotic fluid and a normal USS from 23 weeks onwards suggest a low risk of FVS.

- If USS shows features compatible with FVS and the amniotic fluid is positive – the risk of FVS is very high.

Timing and mode of delivery

- Delivery during the viraemic period may be extremely hazardous.
- Maternal risks – bleeding, thrombocytopenia, DIC, and hepatitis.
- Neonatal – high risk of varicella infection with significant morbidity and mortality.
- Supportive treatment and IV aciclovir – resolution of the rash, immune recovery, and transfer of protective antibodies from the mother to the fetus.
- Consider delivery in women to facilitate assisted ventilation in cases where varicella pneumonia is complicated by respiratory failure.
- General anaesthesia may exacerbate varicella pneumonia. There is theoretical risk of transmitting the varicella virus from skin lesions to the CNS via spinal anaesthesia. Epidural anaesthesia may be safer than spinal anaesthesia, because the dura is not penetrated.

Neonatal varicella

- Maternal rash – the risk of varicella of the newborn is highest if maternal disease occurs up to 7 days before or after delivery. The risk is greatest when the onset of the rash is 5 days before and up to 2 days after delivery.
- Avoid elective delivery until 5–7 days after the onset of maternal rash to allow for the passive transfer of antibodies from mother to child.

- Neonatal contact with chickenpox in the first 7 days of life.
- If the mother is immune – no intervention is required; the risk to the neonate is minimal because it is protected by passively acquired maternal antibodies. This may not apply to the baby who delivers before 28 weeks or weighs < 1 kg who may lack maternal antibodies.
- If mother is not immune or if the neonate is premature – give VZIG.
- If mother is not immune – consider aciclovir prophylaxis as it may provide some protection from infection with an associated reduction in the chance of transmission to the newborn.

- Maternal shingles around the time of delivery is not a risk to the neonate because it is protected by transplacentally acquired maternal antibodies.
- This may not apply to the baby who delivers before 28 weeks or weighs < 1 kg who may lack maternal antibodies.

- VZIG is indicated:
  - ★ If birth occurs within the 7 days following the onset of the maternal rash, or if the mother develops the chickenpox rash within the 7 days after birth.
  - ★ For non-immune neonates that are exposed to chickenpox or shingles (other than maternal) in the first 7 days of life.
- Neonatal ophthalmic examination.
- Test neonatal blood for VZV IgM antibody and for VZV IgG antibody after 7 months.
- Approximately 50% of the neonates exposed to maternal varicella will develop chickenpox despite the VZIG but mortality rates are lower than previously reported.
- VZIG may prolong the incubation period of the virus for up to 28 days and therefore monitor the exposed neonates that are given VZIG for signs of infection for this time period.
- Neonatal infection – Aciclovir can be given following discussion with a neonatologist and virologist. VZIG is of no benefit once neonatal chickenpox has developed.

Chickenpox in Pregnancy. RCOG Green-top Guideline No. 13; September 2007.
http://www.patient.co.uk/health/chickenpox-in-children-under-12
Shingles at a glance: http://www.healingrosacea.com
Please refer to: Chickenpox in Pregnancy. RCOG. Green-top Guideline No. 13; January 2015 for updated version.

CHAPTER 22 Measles in pregnancy

Background

- Measles in pregnancy is relatively uncommon but can be associated with severe maternal morbidity as well as fetal loss and PTD.
- No evidence of any association with congenital infection and damage to fetus.
- Clinical features and complications of measles include disseminated rash, coryza, conjunctivitis, pneumonia, otitis media and encephalitis.

Risks or complications

- Although rare, neonatal measles can be associated with subacute sclerosing panencephalitis (SSPE) with a short onset latency and fulminant course.
- Human normal immunoglobulin (HNIG) may not prevent measles, but may attenuate the illness. There is no evidence that it prevents IUD or PTD.

Investigations of suspected measles

- Test for serum measles-specific IgM and IgG – recent measles infection can be confirmed or excluded by testing for measles-specific IgM on a serum sample taken more than 4 days, but within 1 month, after the onset of rash.
- Oral fluid confirms the diagnosis by detection of viral RNA.

Management of confirmed measles

- Continue management of the pregnancy as normal.
- Although no congenital infection or damage is anticipated, consider follow-up of the infant.

Neonates born to measles-infected mothers

Offer human normal immunoglobulin (HNIG) immediately after birth or postnatal exposure to neonates born to mothers in whom the rash appears 6 days before to 6 days after birth.

CHAPTER 23 Malaria in pregnancy

Background and prevalence

- Malaria is caused by a bite from a parasite-infected (species of *Plasmodium*) mosquito. There are five species of *Plasmodium* – *P. falciparum*, *P. vivax*, *P. malariae*, *P. ovale*, or *P. knowlesi*.
- After a period of pre-erythrocytic stage in the liver, the blood stage begins, which causes the disease. Parasitic invasion of the erythrocyte consumes haemoglobin and alters the red cell membrane resulting in *Plasmodium falciparum* infected erythrocytes that cytoadhere inside the small blood vessels of brain, kidneys, and other organs. Cytoadherence and rosetting interfere with microcirculatory flow and metabolism of vital organs.
- Hallmark of falciparum malaria in pregnancy is parasite sequestration in the placenta. Sequestered parasites evade host defence mechanisms, e.g., splenic processing and filtration. It is not known to occur in the benign malarias due to *P. vivax*, *P. ovale*, and *P. malariae*.
- *P. falciparum* causes greater morbidity and mortality than non-falciparum infections.
- Most commonly imported into the UK with approximately 1500 cases/year. The highest risk groups are immigrants and relatives who assume they are immune.
- Average 5–15 deaths/year (mortality rate approximately 0.5–1.0%) – 79% due to *P. falciparum*.
- USA: pregnant women comprised 1.6% of malaria cases during 2008. In the UK, the prevalence of imported malaria in pregnancy is unknown.
- Estimated mortality is 2–10 times higher in pregnant women than in non-pregnant women in endemic areas.

Complications in pregnancy

Obstetric

- Risks of systemic infection (like any severe febrile illness):
  * maternal and fetal mortality   * miscarriage
  * stillbirth   * premature birth
- The parasitization itself:
  * FGR and low birth weight   * fetal anaemia
  * interaction with HIV   * susceptibility of the infant to malaria

Medical – more common and severe in pregnant women:
  * hypoglycaemia   * pulmonary oedema
  * severe anaemia   * secondary bacterial infection
  * thrombocytopenia   * disseminated intravascular coagulation

- The clinical manifestations in pregnancy depend on premunition; that is, the degree of naturally acquired host immunity to malaria.
- Maternal mortality or complications are more common in women with low premunition and complications are likely to be equivalent or worse in women who are not immune.

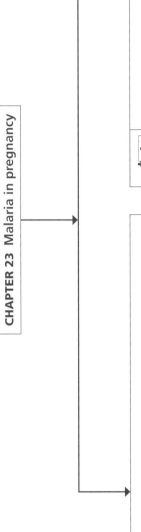

Prevention of malaria infection in pregnancy

The 'ABCD' of malaria prevention

- Awareness of risk
- Chemoprophylaxis
- Bite prevention
- Diagnosis and treatment which must be prompt

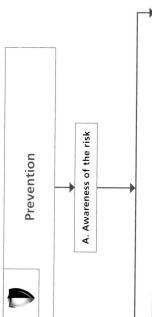

Prevention

A. Awareness of the risk

- Inform women about bite prevention measures. The risk period is from dawn to dusk. Other mosquito-borne diseases, such as dengue, are caused by a daytime-biting mosquito, so advise applying mosquito bite prevention measures 24 hours a day.
- Educate about the symptoms of malaria (such as a fever or flu-like illness) to enable women to realize that they need to seek medical attention without delay and to state that they have travelled to a malaria endemic area.
- A fever or flu-like illness while travelling or upon returning home, up to 1 year or more, may indicate malaria and requires medical attention.
- Despite applying effective anti-mosquito measures and good compliance to chemoprophylaxis, women can still contract malaria.

- Educate women about possible preventive measures – 'think malaria leaflets'.
- Advise pregnant women about the risks of travel to malaria endemic countries and to consider postponing their trip, unless travel is unavoidable.
- If travel is unavoidable, advise woman to seek guidance from a centre with expertise on malaria risks and avoidance strategies.
- The risk of malaria is dependent on a variety of factors, including the level of transmission in the area of travel and the time of year (rainy or dry season), the presence of drug-resistant strains, whether rural or urban stays are planned, length of travel, and the availability and likelihood of uptake of malaria prevention interventions.

B. Bite prevention

Mosquito sprays

- Insect sprays active against mosquitoes are useful.
- Pyrethroids kill mosquitoes and are the preferred ingredient in sprays, while permethrin both repels and kills mosquitoes.

Bed nets

- Long pyrethroid insecticide-treated bed nets offer a protective efficacy of up to 50%.
- The net needs reimpregnating every 6 months.
- Nets are recommended by WHO for all pregnant women in malaria-endemic areas.

Herb-based remedies

- There is no evidence that any of the following offers sufficient protection from malaria – herbal remedies, homeopathy, buzzers, wrist and ankle bands, vitamin B1, garlic, yeast extracts, tea tree oil, and bath oils.
- While citronella has repellent properties, the effects are too short-lasting to recommend its use.

Repellents

- A solution of 20% DEET applied to the exposed areas twice daily (second and third trimesters) – no adverse effects noted in the woman or fetus.
- No specific data on the safety of DEET in the first trimester of pregnancy but it has been used by millions with no apparent adverse effects.
- As the consequences of malaria in pregnancy can be devastating and higher concentrations give longer protection, 50% DEET is recommended.
- Alternatives when 50% DEET is not tolerated – PMD, IR3535, picaridin 20%; all less effective than DEET and require more frequent applications.

Clothing and room protection

- Clothing that covers the body and forms a barrier from biting mosquitoes will reduce the risk of malaria. Clothes can be impregnated with permethrin. Alternatively, permethrin or DEET can be spayed on to the clothes.
- Room protection: electrically heated device that vaporizes synthetic pyrethroids from a mat tablet can kill mosquitoes.
- While mosquito coils could be used as an alternative, they are not as effective and are not recommended indoors.

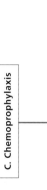

C. Chemoprophylaxis

Provide information on:

- Risks and benefits of chemoprophylaxis vs the risks of malaria.
- There is no malaria prophylaxis regimen that is 100% protective.
- Background medical problems may affect the choice of chemoprophylactic agent.
- Causal prophylaxis is directed against liver schizont stage, which takes approximately 7 days to develop so the drugs (atovaquone–proguanil (Malarone)) need to be continued for 7 days after leaving a malarious area.
- Suppressive prophylaxis (mefloquine) is directed against the red blood cell stages of the parasite and is continued for 4 weeks after leaving a malarious area.
- www.hpa.org.uk/HPA/Topics/InfectiousDiseases/InfectionsAZ

Suspected malaria – emergency standby treatment

- Provide written instructions to pregnant travellers in the event of suspected malaria without access to medical care.
- Advise women to seek diagnosis and treatment at a health facility at the earliest opportunity for a full medical evaluation.
- Advise to start standby treatment if malaria is suspected (flu-like illness) and temperature 38°C or above.
- Drugs that are highly efficacious and well tolerated are likely to be the best candidate drugs for stand-by emergency treatment. Quinine may be efficacious in most parts of the world but it is not well tolerated. The only recommended treatment in the UK for pregnant women is quinine and clindamycin.
- Advise to repeat the full dose if a dose is vomited within 30 minutes, and half the dose if the dose is vomited after 30–60 minutes.
- Advise to complete the treatment and to commence mefloquine 1 week after the last treatment dose.
- Coartem (Riamet) or atovaquone–proguanil (Malarone) (if not used as prophylaxis) could be used as standby emergency treatment.

Chemoprophylaxis – pre-conception

- Prophylaxis is not 100% effective and malaria is associated with increased risk of miscarriage.
- Chloroquine and proguanil are not effective in chloroquine-resistant areas.
- To avoid any potential adverse drug effects from preconceptual and first-trimester exposure, advise women to wait for complete excretion of the drug, before becoming pregnant.
- Unplanned conception while taking malaria prophylaxis is not a reason to recommend TOP, owing to the low risk of teratogenicity.

Chemoprophylaxis – pregnant or breastfeeding women

- Mefloquine is the drug of choice in the second and third trimesters for chloroquine-resistant areas. It is the only drug considered safe for prophylaxis in pregnant travellers.
- Mefloquine does not increase the risk of stillbirth or congenital malformation at prophylactic doses.
- Use of mefloquine in the first trimester may be justified in areas of high risk of acquiring falciparum.
- If travel to a chloroquine-resistant area is essential and mefloquine cannot be tolerated or is contraindicated, consider atovaquone and proguanil.
- Contraindications to mefloquine – current or previous history of depression, neuropsychiatric disorders, epilepsy, or hypersensitivity to quinine or mefloquine.

- Atovaquone and proguanil (Malarone) are not recommended, due to insufficient data on their safety in pregnancy.
- Doxycycline and primaquine are contraindicated.
- Doxycycline – disturbs bone growth of the fetus and causes irreversible teeth coloration when given in the third trimester, and congenital cataract has been reported.
- Primaquine can cause haemolysis, particularly in G6PD deficiency. Fetal red blood cells are more sensitive to haemolysis and the G6PD status of the fetus cannot be determined.

CHAPTER 23 Malaria in pregnancy

83

Diagnosis of malaria in pregnancy

History

- If pyrexia of unknown origin, enquire about history of travel to any malaria endemic areas.
- For the non-falciparum malarias, the history of travel may be > 1 year before the onset of symptoms and, for any woman who has taken prophylaxis, compliance does not rule out the diagnosis of malaria.
- No specific symptoms or signs.
- May present with a flu-like illness.
- Symptoms – fever/chills/sweats, headache, muscle pain, nausea, vomiting, cough, general malaise.
- When the leading symptoms are jaundice, respiratory and gastrointestinal, it can lead to misdiagnosis. Misdiagnosis and delay of treatment are the most common reasons for death from malaria.

Examination

- Signs – jaundice, elevated temperature, perspiration, pallor, splenomegaly, respiratory distress

Investigations

- Malaria blood film – microscopic examination (gold standard) of thick and thin blood films for parasites. It allows species identification and estimation of parasitaemia.
- Rapid detection tests detect specific parasite antigen or enzyme – may miss low parasitaemia, which is more likely in pregnant women; relatively insensitive in *P. vivax* malaria; less sensitive than malaria blood film.
- If a positive rapid diagnostic test – arrange further microscopy to confirm the species, stage of parasites, and to quantify parasitaemia.

Assess severity of malaria

- Clinical condition is the most important indicator of severity.
- Severity of malaria determines the treatment and predicts the case fatality rate.

Uncomplicated malaria

- Uncomplicated malaria – < 2% parasitized red blood cells in a woman with no signs of severity and no complicating features.
- Fatality rates are approximately 0.1% for *P. falciparum*.
- Drug treatment:
  * *P. falciparum* – oral quinine and oral clindamycin or Riamet or atovaquone–proguanil.
  * Vomiting but no signs of severe or complicated malaria – IV quinine plus IV clindamycin. When the patient is well enough to take oral medication, switch to oral quinine and clindamycin.

Severe and complicated malaria

- Pregnant women with ≥ 2% parasitized red blood cells are at higher risk of developing severe malaria. However, the parasitaemia of severe malaria can be < 2%.
- Clinical manifestations – prostration, impaired consciousness, respiratory distress (acute respiratory distress syndrome), pulmonary oedema, convulsions, circulatory collapse/shock, abnormal bleeding, DIC, jaundice, haemoglobinuria.
- Laboratory tests – severe anaemia (haemoglobin < 8.0 g/dl), thrombocytopenia, hypoglycaemia (< 2.2 mmol/l), acidosis (pH < 7.3), renal impairment (creatinine > 265 μmol/l), hyperlactataemia (correlates with mortality), 'Algid malaria' – gram-negative septicaemia (lumbar puncture to exclude meningitis).
- In pregnancy, fatality rates are high (15–20% in non-pregnant women compared with 50% in pregnancy).
- Treatment – artesunate IV, switch to oral artesunate plus clindamycin once able to tolerate oral. If oral artesunate is not available – 3-day course of Riamet or atovaquone–proguanil or 7-day course of quinine and clindamycin.
  * Alternatively – IV quinine in 5% dextrose plus IV clindamycin. When the patient is well enough to take oral medication switch to oral quinine and oral clindamycin. Quinine can result in severe and recurrent hypoglycaemia in late pregnancy.

DDx

Differential diagnosis

In a patient with a history of travel to the tropics and non-specific symptoms and signs – consider investigating other travel-related infections, according to the region visited. These include influenza-like illnesses including H1N1, severe acute respiratory syndrome, avian influenza, HIV, meningitis/encephalitis, viral haemorrhagic fevers, hepatitis, dengue fever, scrub and murine typhus, and leptospirosis.

- In a febrile patient, 3 negative smears 12–24 hours apart rules out the diagnosis of malaria.
- Women who have taken prophylaxis may have their parasitaemia suppressed below the level of microscopic detection.
- Pregnant women with a high background immune level may have negative peripheral blood thick films but parasites may remain sequestered in the placenta (for example, a recently arrived woman from a high malaria-endemic country with an unexplained anaemia).

Treatment of malaria in pregnancy

Hospitalize

- Treat malaria in pregnancy as an emergency. Hospitalize women with *P. falciparum*, as the clinical condition can deteriorate rapidly. While non-falciparum malaria can be managed on an outpatient basis, admission ensures compliance. The risk of vomiting or rapid deterioration is an indication for parenteral therapy.
- Quinine has significant adverse effects – cinchonism with tinnitus, headache, nausea, diarrhoea, altered auditory acuity, and blurred vision. This can lead to non-compliance. Hospitalization is useful, as compliance with quinine and clindamycin can be observed and this may lead to improved cure rates.
- Admit women with uncomplicated malaria to hospital and women with severe and complicated malaria to an intensive care unit (ICU).
- Seek advice from infectious disease specialists for severe and recurrent cases.

Treatment

- Vomiting is associated with treatment failure – use an antiemetic. After the antiemetic has had time to take effect, repeat the dose. Repeat vomiting after an antiemetic is an indication for parenteral therapy.
- Fever – treat with antipyretics.
- Monitor blood films every 24 hours but clinical deterioration is an indication for a repeat blood film.
- IV artesunate is the treatment of choice for severe falciparum malaria. Use IV quinine if artesunate is not available.
- Quinine and clindamycin for uncomplicated *P. falciparum* (or mixed, e.g., *P. falciparum* and *vivax*).
- Chloroquine for *P. vivax, P. ovale* or *P. malariae*.
- Do not use primaquine in pregnancy.
- Anaemia – in *P. falciparum* malaria, 90% of women with low premunition develop anaemia. Treat mild and moderate anaemia with ferrous sulphate and folic acid.

Management of pregnancy-related complications of severe malaria

Hypoglycaemia – commonly asymptomatic, may be associated with fetal bradycardia and other signs of fetal distress.

- In the most severely ill women, it is associated with lactic acidosis and high mortality.
- In patients on quinine, abnormal behaviour, sweating, and sudden loss of consciousness are the usual manifestations.
- Hypoglycaemia may be profound, recurrent, and intractable in pregnancy. Monitor glucose levels regularly while taking quinine treatment.

Pulmonary oedema – high mortality of > 50%.

- May develop suddenly and unexpectedly. It can develop immediately after childbirth.
- The first indication of impending pulmonary oedema is an increase in the respiratory rate.
- Ensure that the pulmonary oedema has not resulted from iatrogenic fluid overload and monitor UOP and CVP to keep right arterial pressure < 10 cm H$_2$O.
- In some women, ARDS can develop in addition to the pulmonary oedema.

Severe anaemia – associated with maternal morbidity, an increased risk of PPH, and perinatal mortality. Women who go into labour when severely anaemic or fluid-overloaded may develop acute pulmonary oedema after separation of the placenta.

- Monitor haemoglobin and transfuse as necessary. Transfuse slowly, preferably with packed cells and IV frusemide. Alternatively, consider exchange transfusion.

Secondary bacterial infection – principally Gram-negative septicaemia.

- Suspect if the patient becomes hypotensive.
- Blood cultures if the patient shows signs of shock or fever returns after apparent fever clearance.
- Start broad-spectrum antibiotics (such as ceftriaxone) immediately. Once the results of blood culture and sensitivity testing are available, give the appropriate antibiotic.

Management of obstetric problems and management with acute malaria

- Fetal compromise – MDT care (intensive care specialist, infectious disease specialist, obstetrician, neonatologist) to plan optimal management.
- IUGR and FHR abnormalities – effective and prompt treatment of malaria reduces the systemic effects of parasitaemia and reduces the adverse effects on the fetus, such as fetal distress, PTD, and stillbirth. In severe malaria, monitor with CTG, particularly in the presence of fever.
- PTL – the risk of PTD in women with histological evidence of past placental malaria infection compared with women without infection is more than doubled (RR 2.33). Tocolysis and prophylactic steroids are indicated.
- Acute malaria can cause thrombocytopenia in pregnancy, an increased mean blood loss but no confirmed increased risk of PPH.
- Uncomplicated malaria in pregnancy is not a reason for IOL. In severe malaria, the role of early CS for the viable fetus is unproven.
- There is usually no need for thromboprophylaxis. It should be weighed up against the risk of haemorrhage and withheld if the platelet count is falling or < 100 × 10⁹/l.

Treatment for recurrence

- Treatments in pregnancy may have lower efficacy than in non-pregnant patients; this could result from lowered concentrations of antimalarials in pregnancy.
- Malaria in pregnancy is unique due to the ability of *P. falciparum* to sequester in the placenta. PCR confirmed prolonged submicroscopic carriage with subsequent recurrence has been reported for months following drug treatment for uncomplicated *P. falciparum*.
- Most recurrence is around days 28–42 but can be later.
- Repeat blood film if symptoms or fever return.
- Alternatively, weekly screening by blood film can provide early detection and treatment of malaria. This can reduce maternal deaths from malaria.

- Infections that recur following treatment are likely to be less sensitive to drugs.
- A highly effective 7-day treatment has more chance of cure.
- Options for treatment of recurrent infection in pregnancy are limited but if quinine and clindamycin have failed as first-line treatment, consider an alternative.
- Atovaquone–proguanil–artesunate and dihydroartemisinin–piperaquine have been used in pregnant women with multiple recurrent infections with good effect.
- Atovaquone–proguanil (Malarone) is highly effective against uncomplicated *P. falciparum* malaria even when it is not combined with artesunate.
- WHO recommends regimen of 7 days of artesunate and clindamycin.

Antenatal care after recovery from an episode of malaria

Maternal

- Regular antenatal care, monitor haemoglobin, platelets, and glucose.
- Pre-eclampsia – in malaria-endemic countries there is an increased risk of PET when the infection affects the placenta. The risk of PET in UK pregnant women treated for malaria is not known but may be lower than in malaria endemic countries.

Fetus

- IUGR – monitor fetal growth. If IUGR is identified – appropriate obstetric management. In endemic settings, malaria in pregnancy is responsible for > 50% of FGR but most babies born to women with infection during pregnancy will be of normal birth weight. No additional fetal surveillance will prevent the FGR.
- Effective antimalarial treatment to clear the placenta of parasites is the most important step in preventing this complication followed by prophylaxis to prevent recurrence.

Newborn – risk of vertical transmission

- Prevalence of congenital malaria is 8–33%.
- Vertical transmission of malaria occurs either during pregnancy or at the time of birth. Higher risk if there is infection at the time of birth and the placenta and cord are blood film-positive for malaria.
- Peripartum malaria – placental histology and placenta, cord and baby blood films to detect congenital malaria.
  * A negative placental blood film reduces the risk of congenital malaria significantly.
  * Placenta and cord-positive blood films have higher chance of congenital malaria than placenta-positive, cord-negative blood films.
- In the presence of positive placental blood films, fever in the infant could indicate malaria; a blood film from the baby is required for confirmation.
- Infection of the newborn can occur despite appropriate treatment in the mother during pregnancy. Antimalarial drugs can clear peripheral parasitaemia more quickly than from the placenta. Screen all neonates whose mothers developed malaria in pregnancy with microscopy of thick and thin blood films at birth and weekly blood films for 28 days.

The Prevention of Malaria in Pregnancy. RCOG Green-top Guideline No. 54A; April 2010.
The Diagnosis and Treatment of Malaria in Pregnancy. RCOG Green-top Guideline No. 54B; April 2010.

Background and prevalence

- Important cause of maternal death in the UK.
- 2006–2008 – sepsis was the leading cause of direct maternal deaths in the UK, with 13 deaths due to group A streptococcal infection (GAS).
- Severe sepsis with acute organ dysfunction has a mortality rate of 20 to 40%, which increases to 60% if septic shock develops.
- Sepsis – infection plus systemic manifestations of infection.
- Severe sepsis – sepsis plus sepsis-induced organ dysfunction or tissue hypoperfusion.
- Septic shock – persistence of hypoperfusion despite adequate fluid replacement.
- **Common organisms**
  * Most common – Group A beta-haemolytic *Streptococcus* and *E. coli.*
  * Mixed infections with gram-positive and gram-negative organisms, especially in chorioamnionitis.
  * Coliform infection in urinary sepsis, preterm PROM, and cervical cerclage.
  * Anaerobes such as *Clostridium perfringens* are less common with *Peptostreptococcus* and *Bacteroides* spp. predominating.
- UTI and chorioamnionitis are common infections associated with septic shock.

Risk factors for severe sepsis

- Risk factors – obesity; impaired glucose tolerance/diabetes; immunosuppression (HIV or immunosuppressive drugs); anaemia; vaginal discharge; history of pelvic infection; history of GBS; amniocentesis and other invasive procedures; cervical cerclage; prolonged SROM; GAS infection in close contacts; Black or other minority ethnic groups.

Risks or complications

Fetus:

- The direct effect of infection in the fetus.
- The effect of maternal illness/shock.
- The effect of maternal treatment.
- Risk of neonatal encephalopathy and cerebral palsy is increased in the presence of intrauterine infection

History and examination

- Signs and symptoms of sepsis in pregnant women may be less distinctive than in the non-pregnant population and are not necessarily present in all cases.

Symptoms:

- * Fever or rigors.
- * Constant severe abdominal pain and tenderness unrelieved by analgesia – genital tract sepsis.
- * Offensive vaginal discharge (offensive smell suggests anaerobes; serosanguineous suggests streptococcal infection).
- * Productive cough.
- * Urinary symptoms.
- * Diarrhoea or vomiting – may indicate exotoxin production (early toxic shock).
- * Rash (generalized streptococcal maculopapular rash or purpura fulminans).
- * PTL – severe infection.
- * Toxic shock syndrome caused by staphylococcal or streptococcal exotoxins – nausea, vomiting, and diarrhoea; exquisite severe pain out of proportion to clinical signs due to necrotizing fasciitis; a watery vaginal discharge; generalized rash; and conjunctival suffusion.

Clinical signs: pyrexia, hypothermia, tachycardia, tachypnoea, hypoxia, hypotension, oliguria, impaired consciousness, and failure to respond to treatment.

Diagnostic criteria for sepsis

Infection, documented or suspected, and the following:

- **General variables:**
  * Fever (> 38°C); hypothermia (core temperature < 36°C).
  * Tachycardia (> 100 beats per minute); tachypnoea (> 20 breaths per minute).
  * Impaired mental state.
  * Significant oedema or positive fluid balance (> 20 ml/kg over 24 hours).
  * Hyperglycaemia in the absence of diabetes (plasma glucose > 7.7 mmol/l).
- **Inflammatory variables:**
  * WBC count > 12×10^9/l; WBC count < 4×10^9/l; CRP > 7 mg/l.
  * Normal WBC count with > 10% immature forms.
- **Haemodynamic variables:**
  * Arterial hypotension (SBP < 90 mmHg; MAP < 70 mmHg or SBP decrease > 40 mmHg.
- **Tissue perfusion variables:**
  * Raised serum lactate ≥ 4 mmol/l; increased capillary refill time or mottling.
- **Organ dysfunction variables:**
  * Arterial hypoxaemia (PaO_2/FIO_2 < 40 kPa). Severe sepsis if < 33.3 kPa in the absence of pneumonia or < 26.7 kPa in the presence of pneumonia.
  * Oliguria (UOP < 0.5 ml/kg/hr for at least 2 hours, despite adequate fluid resuscitation).
  * Creatinine rise of > 44.2 mmol/l. Sepsis is severe if creatinine level > 176 mmol/l.
  * Coagulation abnormalities (INR > 1.5 or APTT > 60 s).
  * Thrombocytopenia (platelet count < 100×10^9/l).
  * Hyperbilirubinaemia (plasma total bilirubin > 70 mmol/l).
  * Ileus (absent bowel sounds).

MDT – consultant microbiologist or infectious disease physician; critical care and obstetric anaesthetists.

Investigations

- Blood cultures, throat swabs, mid-stream urine, high vaginal swab, consider cerebrospinal fluid.
- Nose swab for MRSA screening.
- Serum lactate within 6 hours of the suspicion of severe sepsis. Serum lactate ≥ 4 mmol/l is indicative of tissue hypoperfusion.
- Relevant imaging.
- Arterial blood gas to assess for hypoxia.

Management – maternal

- Regular observations using MEOWS chart.
- Broad-spectrum antibiotics within 1 hour of recognition of severe sepsis. Empirically, give broad-spectrum antimicrobials active against gram-negative bacteria, and capable of preventing exotoxin production from gram-positive bacteria.
- Find and treat the source of sepsis.
- Hypotension and/or a serum lactate > 4 mmol/l – give an initial minimum 20 ml/kg of crystalloid or an equivalent. If hypotension is not responding, give vasopressors to maintain mean arterial pressure (MAP) > 65 mmHg.
- Persistent hypotension despite fluid resuscitation (septic shock) and/or lactate > 4mmol/l:
  a. achieve a CVP of ≥ 8 mmHg.
  b. achieve a central venous oxygen saturation (ScvO₂) ≥ 70% or mixed venous oxygen saturation (ScvO₂) ≥ 65%.
- In critically ill woman, consider delivery if beneficial to the mother or the baby or to both.

Transfer to ICU

- Liaise with critical care team, obstetric consultant, and the consultant obstetric anaesthetist.
- **Indications for transfer to ICU:**
  * Cardiovascular hypotension or raised serum lactate persisting despite fluid resuscitation, suggesting the need for inotropic support.
  * Respiratory – pulmonary oedema; mechanical ventilation; airway protection.
  * Renal dialysis.
  * Significantly decreased conscious level.
  * Multi-organ failure; uncorrected acidosis; hypothermia.
- Give IVIG for severe invasive streptococcal or staphylococcal infection if other therapies have failed. IVIG has an immunomodulatory effect, neutralizes the superantigen effect of exotoxins, and inhibits production of tumour necrosis factor (TNF) and interleukins. It is effective in exotoxic shock (i.e., toxic shock due to streptococci and staphylococci) but with little evidence of benefit in gram-negative (endotoxin related) sepsis. Congenital deficiency of immunoglobulin A is the main contraindication.

Antenatal and intrapartum care

- Consider antenatal corticosteroids for fetal lung maturity if preterm delivery is anticipated.
- EFM:
  * In labour – continuous EFM if maternal pyrexia (temperature > 38.0°C once, or 37.5°C on two occasions 2 hours apart) and sepsis without pyrexia.
  * Intrauterine infection is associated with abnormal fetal heart monitoring; however, EFM is not a sensitive predictor of early onset neonatal sepsis.
  * Changes in CTG, such as changes in baseline rate and variability or new onset decelerations – reassess maternal MAP, hypoxia, and acidaemia. These changes may be early signs for derangements in maternal end-organ systems.
- Insufficient evidence regarding FBS in the presence of maternal sepsis to guide practice.
- Avoid epidural/spinal anaesthesia; general anaesthetic is usually required for CS.
- Deliver – if chorioamnionitis.
- Delivery in the setting of maternal instability increases the maternal and fetal mortality rates if infection is not intrauterine. Individualize based on severity of maternal illness, duration of labour, gestational age, and viability.

- Group A β-haemolytic *Streptococcus* and MRSA are easily transmitted via the hands of HCP and via close contact in households.
- Invasive group A streptococcal infections are notifiable.

Newborn

- Inform neonatologist.
- Give prophylactic antibiotics to the baby.
- **If mother has GAS infection in the peripartum period:**
  * Isolate in a single room with en suite facilities to minimize the risk of spread to other women.
  * Warn close household contacts to seek medical attention if any symptoms develop; provide antibiotic prophylaxis if needed.
  * Consider antibiotic prophylaxis for HCPs who have been exposed to respiratory secretions from infected mother.

Bacterial Sepsis in Pregnancy. RCOG Green-top Guideline No. 64a; 1st edition; April 2012.

CHAPTER 25 Antenatal care

1. Antenatal information

2. Provision and organization of care

3. Lifestyle considerations

4. Management of common symptoms of pregnancy

5. Clinical examination of pregnant women

6. Screening for infections

7. Screening for haematological conditions

8. Screening for fetal anomalies

9. Screening for clinical conditions

10. Fetal growth and wellbeing

11. Management of specific clinical conditions

1. Antenatal information

First contact

- Folic acid supplementation.
- Food hygiene, including how to reduce the risk of food-acquired infection.
- Lifestyle advice, including smoking cessation, and the implications of recreational drug use and alcohol consumption in pregnancy.
- Discuss risks and benefits of antenatal screening tests.

At booking (ideally by 10 weeks)

- Nutrition and diet, including vitamin D supplementation for women at risk of vitamin D deficiency.
- Exercise including pelvic floor exercises.
- Place of birth; pregnancy care pathway.
- Breastfeeding, including workshops; participant-led antenatal classes.
- Further discussion of all antenatal screening; discussion of mental health issues.

≤ 36 weeks

- Preparation for labour and birth, coping with pain in labour and the birth plan; recognition of active labour.
- Care of the new baby; breastfeeding information.
- Vitamin K prophylaxis; newborn screening tests.
- Postnatal self-care; awareness of 'baby blues' and postnatal depression.

At 38 weeks

- Options for management of prolonged pregnancy.

- Provide information in a form that is easy to understand and accessible to pregnant women with additional needs, such as physical, sensory or learning disabilities, and to pregnant women who do not speak or read English.
- At each antenatal appointment, offer consistent information and clear explanations, and provide women with an opportunity to discuss issues and ask questions.
- Offer women participant-led antenatal classes, including breastfeeding workshops.
- Respect women's decisions even when this is contrary to the views of the HCP.
- Inform women about the purpose of any test before it is performed. Make sure that the woman has understood this information and has sufficient time to make an informed decision. Make clear the right of a woman to accept or decline a test.
- Provide all women with written information about the likely number, timing, and content of antenatal appointments associated with different options of care and give an opportunity to discuss this schedule.

2. Provision and organization of care

Who provides care – midwife and GP-led models of care to women with an uncomplicated pregnancy.
Continuity of care – there should be continuity of care throughout the antenatal period.

- A system of clear referral paths – so that pregnant women who require additional care are managed and treated by the appropriate specialist teams when problems are identified. Place of antenatal appointments – ANC should be readily and easily accessible to all pregnant women and should be sensitive to the needs of individual women and the local community.
- The environment in which antenatal appointments take place should enable women to discuss sensitive issues such as domestic violence, sexual abuse, psychiatric illness, and recreational drug use.

Gestational age assessment

- Offer an early USS between 10 and 13 weeks 6 days to determine gestational age and to detect multiple pregnancies. This will ensure consistency of gestational age assessment and reduce the incidence of IOL for prolonged pregnancy.
- Use CRL measurement to determine gestational age. If the CRL is above 84 mm, use head circumference to estimate the gestational age.

Frequency of antenatal appointments

- For a woman who is nulliparous with an uncomplicated pregnancy, a schedule of 10 appointments is adequate.
- For a woman who is parous with an uncomplicated pregnancy, a schedule of 7 appointments is adequate.
- Longer appointments are needed early in pregnancy to allow comprehensive assessment and discussion.
- Wherever possible, appointments should incorporate routine tests and investigations to minimize inconvenience to women.

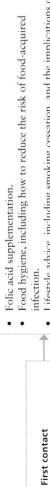

3. Lifestyle considerations

Working during pregnancy

- Inform maternity rights and benefits.
- Reassure that it is safe to continue working during pregnancy.
- Ascertain woman's occupation during pregnancy to identify those who are at increased risk through occupational exposure.

Exercise – beginning or continuing a moderate course of exercise during pregnancy is not associated with adverse outcomes.

Sexual intercourse – is not known to be associated with any adverse outcomes.

Nutritional supplements

- Dietary supplementation with folic acid, before conception and throughout the first 12 weeks, reduces the risk of having a baby with a neural tube defect. The recommended dose is 400 µg per day.
- Do not offer iron supplementation routinely. It does not benefit the mother's or the baby's health and may have unpleasant maternal side effects.
- Avoid vitamin A supplementation (> 700 µg) as it might be teratogenic. Liver and liver products may contain high levels of vitamin A, therefore avoid.
- Maintain adequate vitamin D stores during pregnancy and breastfeeding. Offer 10 µg of vitamin D per day. Women at greatest risk of vitamin D deficiency are:
  * Women of South Asian, African, Caribbean or Middle Eastern origin.
  * Women who have limited exposure to sunlight, such as women who are predominantly housebound, or usually remain covered when outdoors.
  * Women who eat a diet particularly low in vitamin D, such as women who consume no oily fish, eggs, meat, vitamin D-fortified margarine.
  * Women with a pre-pregnancy BMI > 30 kg/m².

Prescribed medicines – use as little as possible during pregnancy and limit to circumstances in which the benefit outweighs the risk.

Over-the-counter medicines – use as little as possible during pregnancy, since only a few over-the-counter medicines have been established as being safe to be taken in pregnancy.

Complementary therapies – only a few complementary therapies have been established as being safe and effective during pregnancy; do not assume that such therapies are safe and use as little as possible during pregnancy.

Air travel – see Chapter 66 Air travel in pregnancy

Car travel – the correct use of seatbelts (that is, three-point seatbelts 'above and below the bump, not over it').

Travelling abroad – if planning to travel abroad, discuss considerations such as flying, vaccinations, and travel insurance with their midwife or doctor.

Smoking – See Chapter 63: Smoking in pregnancy

Alcohol consumption – see Chapter 62: Alcohol consumption in pregnancy

Cannabis – the direct effects of cannabis on the fetus are uncertain but may be harmful. Cannabis use is associated with smoking, which is known to be harmful; therefore discourage women from using cannabis during pregnancy.

Food-acquired infections

- To reduce the risk of listeriosis: advise to drink only pasteurized or UHT milk; not to eat ripened soft cheese such as Camembert, Brie, and blue-veined cheese (there is no risk with hard cheeses, such as Cheddar, or cottage cheese and processed cheese); not to eat paté (of any sort, including vegetable); not to eat uncooked or undercooked ready-prepared meals.
- To reduce the risk of salmonella infection: advise to avoid raw or partially cooked eggs or food that may contain them (such as mayonnaise); avoid raw or partially cooked meat, especially poultry.

4. Management of common symptoms of pregnancy

Nausea and vomiting and heartburn

- Most cases of nausea and vomiting in pregnancy resolve spontaneously within 16–20 weeks and are not usually associated with a poor pregnancy outcome.
- **Heartburn** – offer information regarding lifestyle and diet modification or antacids to women whose heartburn remains troublesome.

Backache – exercising in water, massage therapy, and group or individual back care classes might help to ease backache during pregnancy.

Constipation – offer information regarding diet modification, such as bran or wheat fibre supplementation.
Haemorrhoids – in the absence of evidence of the effectiveness of treatments for haemorrhoids in pregnancy, offer information concerning diet modification. If clinical symptoms remain troublesome, consider standard haemorrhoid creams.
Varicose veins – these are a common symptom of pregnancy that does not cause harm and compression stockings can improve the symptoms but will not prevent varicose veins from emerging.

Vaginal discharge

- An increase in vaginal discharge is a common physiological change that occurs during pregnancy. If it is associated with itching, soreness, offensive smell or pain on passing urine there may be an infective cause so consider investigations.
- A 1-week course of a topical imidazole is an effective treatment for vaginal candidiasis.
- The effectiveness and safety of oral treatments for vaginal candidiasis in pregnancy are uncertain, therefore do not offer.

5. Clinical examination of pregnant women

Measurement of weight, height, and BMI at the booking appointment. Repeated weighing during pregnancy should be confined to circumstances in which clinical management is likely to be influenced.

Breast and pelvic examination

- Do not perform routine breast examination for the promotion of postnatal breastfeeding.
- Do not perform routine antenatal pelvic examination, as it does not accurately assess gestational age, nor does it accurately predict preterm birth or cephalopelvic disproportion.

Female genital mutilation – identify pregnant women who have had female genital mutilation early in ANC through sensitive enquiry. Antenatal examination will then allow planning of intrapartum care.
Domestic violence – be aware of the symptoms or signs of domestic violence and give women the opportunity to disclose domestic violence in an environment in which they feel secure.

Prediction, detection, and initial management of mental disorders

- At a woman's first contact with services, ask about:
  - Past or present severe mental illness including schizophrenia, bipolar disorder, psychosis in the postnatal period, and severe depression.
  - Previous treatment by a psychiatrist/specialist mental health team, including inpatient care.
  - A family history of perinatal mental illness.
- Do not use other specific predictors, such as poor relationship with her partner, for the routine prediction of the development of a mental disorder.
- Ask two questions to identify possible depression – During the past month, have you often been bothered by feeling down, depressed or hopeless?; bothered by having little interest or pleasure in doing things? Consider a third question if the woman answers 'yes' to either of the initial questions – Is this something you feel you need or want help with?
- After identifying a possible mental disorder in a woman, consider further assessment. If any significant concerns, refer to her GP for further assessment. If the woman has, or is suspected to have, a severe mental illness, refer to a specialist mental health service, including, a specialist perinatal mental health service.
- Inform the woman's GP if a current mental disorder or a history of significant mental disorder is detected.

6. Screening for fetal anomalies

Structural anomalies

- Offer USS screening for fetal anomalies between 18 weeks and 20 weeks 6 days.
- Provide information about the purpose and implications of the anomaly scan. The purpose of the scan is to identify fetal anomalies and allow: parents to prepare for any treatment/disability/palliative care/TOP; manage birth in a specialist centre.
- Inform on the limitations of routine USS screening and that detection rates vary by the type of fetal anomaly, the woman's BMI, and the position of the unborn baby at the time of the scan.
- If an anomaly is detected during the anomaly scan – inform women of the findings to enable them to make an informed choice as to whether they wish to continue with the pregnancy or have a TOP.
- Fetal echocardiography involving the four-chamber view of the fetal heart and outflow tracts is recommended as part of the routine anomaly scan.
- Do not offer routine screening for cardiac anomalies using NT.
- When routine USS screening is performed to detect NTDs, alpha-fetoprotein testing is not required.

Screening for Down syndrome

- Offer screening for Down syndrome by the end of the first trimester (13 weeks 6 days), but provision should be made to allow later screening for women booking later in pregnancy.
- Offer the 'combined test' (NT, beta-hCG, PAPP-A) between 11 weeks 0 days and 13 weeks 6 days. For women who book later in pregnancy offer the most clinically and cost-effective serum screening test (triple or quadruple test) between 15 weeks 0 days and 20 weeks 0 days.
- When it is not possible to measure NT, owing to fetal position or raised BMI, offer serum screening (triple or quadruple test) between 15 weeks 0 days and 20 weeks 0 days.
- Screen-positive result for Down syndrome – provide rapid access to appropriate counselling.
- The routine anomaly scan (at 18 weeks 0 days to 20 weeks 6 days) should not be routinely used for Down syndrome screening using soft markers.
- The presence of an isolated soft marker, with the exception of increased nuchal fold, on the routine anomaly scan, should not be used to adjust the a prior risk for Down syndrome.
- The presence of an increased nuchal fold (6 mm or above) or two or more soft markers on the routine anomaly scan – refer to a fetal medicine specialist.

7. Screening for haematological conditions

Anaemia – screen at booking and at 28 weeks. This allows enough time for treatment if anaemia is detected.

- Investigate haemoglobin levels outside the normal UK range for pregnancy (11 g/100 ml at first contact and 10.5 g/100 ml at 28 weeks) and consider iron supplementation.

Blood grouping and red-cell alloantibodies

- Test for blood group and rhesus D status at booking.
- Offer routine antenatal anti-D prophylaxis to all non-sensitized pregnant women who are rhesus D-negative.
- Screen for atypical red-cell alloantibodies at booking and again at 28 weeks, regardless of their rhesus D status.
- Women with clinically significant atypical red-cell alloantibodies – refer to a specialist centre for further investigation and subsequent antenatal management.
- If a pregnant woman is rhesus D-negative, consider partner testing to determine whether the administration of anti-D prophylaxis is necessary. See Chapter 6: Fetal haemolytic disease.

Haemoglobinopathies

- Provide pre-conception counselling and carrier testing to women who are identified as being at higher risk of haemoglobinopathies using the Family Origin Questionnaire.
- Inform about screening for sickle cell diseases and thalassaemias, including carrier status and its implications.
- Offer screening for sickle cell diseases and thalassaemias to all women at booking. The type of screening depends upon the prevalence and can be carried out in either primary or secondary care.
- Where prevalence of sickle cell disease is high (fetal prevalence > 1.5 cases per 10000 pregnancies), offer laboratory screening to identify carriers of sickle cell disease and/or thalassaemia.
- Where prevalence of sickle cell disease is low (fetal prevalence ≤ 1.5 cases per 10000 pregnancies), offer screening for haemoglobinopathies using the Family Origin Questionnaire.
- If the Family Origin Questionnaire indicates a high risk of sickle cell disorders, offer laboratory screening (preferably high-performance liquid chromatography).
- If the mean corpuscular haemoglobin is < 27 picograms, offer laboratory screening.
- If the woman is identified as a carrier of a clinically significant haemoglobinopathy then screen the father of the baby after counselling without delay.

8. Screening for clinical conditions

Others

Preterm birth – do not offer routine screening for preterm labour.

Placenta praevia – because most low-lying placentas detected at the routine anomaly scan will have resolved by the time the baby is born, offer repeat scan only to woman whose placenta extends over the internal cervical os at 32 weeks. If the transabdominal scan is unclear, offer a transvaginal scan.

Pre-eclampsia

- BP measurement and urinalysis for protein at each antenatal visit to screen for PET.
- At booking appointment, determine the following risk factors for PET:
  * Age ≥ 40 years, nulliparity, BMI ≥ 30 kg/m².
  * Pregnancy interval of > 10 years.
  * Family history or previous history of PET.
  * Pre-existing vascular disease such as HT or renal disease.
  * Multiple pregnancy.
- Consider more frequent BP measurements if any of the above risk factors are present.
- The presence of significant HT and/or proteinuria – need for increased surveillance.
- HT in which there is a single DBP of 110 mmHg or two consecutive readings of 90 mmHg at least 4 hours apart and/or significant proteinuria (1+) – increase surveillance.
- If the SBP is > 160 mmHg on two consecutive readings at least 4 hours apart, consider treatment.
- Warn all pregnant women to seek immediate advice if they experience symptoms of PET: severe headache; problems with vision, such as blurring or flashing before the eyes; severe pain just below the ribs; vomiting; sudden swelling of the face, hands and feet.

Gestational diabetes mellitus (GDM)

- Screen for GDM using risk factors in a healthy population. At booking appointment, determine the risk factors for GDM:
  * BMI > 30 kg/m².
  * Previous macrosomic baby weighing ≥ 4.5 kg.
  * Previous GDM.
  * Family history of diabetes (first-degree relative with DM).
  * Family origin with a high prevalence of diabetes: South Asian (specifically women whose country of family origin is India, Pakistan or Bangladesh); black Caribbean; Middle Eastern.
- Offer women with any one of these risk factors testing for GDM.
- Inform that:
  * In most women, GDM responds to changes in diet and exercise.
  * 10–20% of women will need oral hypoglycaemic agents or insulin therapy if diet and exercise are not effective.
  * A diagnosis of GDM may lead to increased monitoring and interventions during both pregnancy and labour.
- Do not offer screening for GDM using fasting plasma glucose, random blood glucose, glucose challenge test, and urinalysis for glucose.

9. Screening for infections

Hepatitis B – offer serological screening for hepatitis B so that effective postnatal interventions can be provided to infected women to decrease the risk of mother-to-child transmission.

Hepatitis C – do not offer routine screening for hepatitis C virus because there is insufficient evidence to support its clinical and cost effectiveness.

HIV – offer screening for HIV infection early in ANC because appropriate antenatal interventions can reduce mother-to-child transmission of HIV infection.

Rubella – offer rubella susceptibility screening to identify women at risk of contracting rubella infection and to enable vaccination in the postnatal period for the protection of future pregnancies.

Cytomegalovirus – the available evidence does not support routine CMV screening in pregnant women.

Group B streptococcus – do not offer routine antenatal screening for GBS because evidence of its clinical and cost effectiveness remains uncertain.

Syphilis – offer screening for syphilis because treatment of syphilis is beneficial to the mother and baby.

Toxoplasmosis – do not offer routine screening because the risks of screening may outweigh the potential benefits. Inform women of primary prevention measures to avoid toxoplasmosis infection, such as: washing hands before handling food; thoroughly washing all fruit and vegetables, including ready-prepared salads, before eating; thoroughly cooking raw meats and ready-prepared chilled meals; wearing gloves and thoroughly washing hands after handling soil and gardening; avoiding cat faeces in cat litter or in soil.

Asymptomatic bacteriuria – offer routine screening for asymptomatic bacteriuria by MSU culture early in pregnancy. Identification and treatment of asymptomatic bacteriuria reduces the risk of pyelonephritis.

Asymptomatic bacterial vaginosis – do not offer routine screening for bacterial vaginosis because the evidence suggests that the identification and treatment of asymptomatic bacterial vaginosis does not lower the risk of preterm birth and other adverse reproductive outcomes.

Chlamydia trachomatis – do not offer *Chlamydia* screening as part of routine ANC.

10. Fetal growth and wellbeing

Examination

- Measure SFH at each antenatal appointment from 24 weeks.
- Assess fetal presentation by abdominal palpation at 36 weeks or later, when presentation is likely to influence the plans for the birth. Do not routinely assess presentation by abdominal palpation before 36 weeks because it is not always accurate and may be uncomfortable.

Fetal heart

- Do not offer routine formal fetal-movement counting.
- Auscultation of the fetal heart may confirm that the fetus is alive but is unlikely to have any predictive value and routine listening is therefore not necessary. However, when requested by the mother, auscultation of the fetal heart may provide reassurance.
- The evidence does not support the routine use of antenatal EFM (CTG) for fetal assessment in women with an uncomplicated pregnancy.

USS

- Confirm suspected fetal malpresentation by an USS.
- Do not offer USS estimation of fetal size for suspected large-for-gestational-age babies in a low-risk population.
- Do not offer routine Doppler USS in low-risk pregnancies.
- The evidence does not support the routine use of USS scanning after 24 weeks of gestation.

11. Management of specific clinical conditions

Pregnancy after 41 weeks

- Prior to formal IOL, offer a vaginal examination for membrane sweeping.
- Women with uncomplicated pregnancies, offer IOL beyond 41 weeks.
- From 42 weeks, women who decline IOL, offer increased antenatal monitoring consisting of at least twice-weekly CTG and USS estimation of maximum amniotic pool depth.

Breech presentation at term

- Offer external cephalic version to women who have an uncomplicated singleton breech pregnancy at 36 weeks. Exceptions include women in labour and women with a uterine scar or abnormality, fetal compromise, ruptured membranes, vaginal bleeding, and medical conditions.
- Where it is not possible to schedule an appointment for external cephalic version at 37 weeks, schedule it at 36 weeks.

Antenatal Care: Routine Care for the Healthy Pregnant Woman. NICE Clinical Guideline 62; March 2008.

Prevalence and background

- New hypertension presenting after 20 weeks without significant proteinuria.
- Incidence of PIH – 4.2–7.9%.
- Up to 10% of pregnancies are complicated by hypertensive disorders and there is evidence that the rate may be increasing.

History

- Any severe headache, severe pain just below ribs, problems with vision such as blurring or flashing before eyes, vomiting, sudden swelling of face, hands or feet.

Full assessment in a secondary care facility

Investigations

- BP and proteinuria
- Proteinuria – an automated reagent-strip reading device or urinary protein:creatinine ratio (uPCR).

Risks or complications

- **Fetal** – higher rate of perinatal mortality, preterm birth, and LBW.
- **Maternal** – See Chapter 27 Pre-eclampsia (PET) and eclampsia

Risk factors

- PET or gestational HT disease during a previous pregnancy, chronic HT, chronic kidney disease, type 1 or type 2 diabetes, autoimmune disease such as SLE or APA syndrome.
- Give 75 mg of aspirin daily from 12 weeks until delivery.
- Do not use the following to prevent hypertension in pregnancy: * Nitric oxide donors. * Diuretics. * Progesterone. * Supplements of magnesium. * Restricting salt intake. * Antioxidants (vitamins C and E). * Fish or algal oils. * Garlic.
- The following risk factors require additional assessment and follow-up: nulliparity, age ≥40 years, pregnancy interval of > 10 years, family history of PET, multiple pregnancy, BMI ≥35, pre-existing vascular disease.

- **Any proteinuria** – See Chapter 27 Pre-eclampsia (PET) and eclampsia.

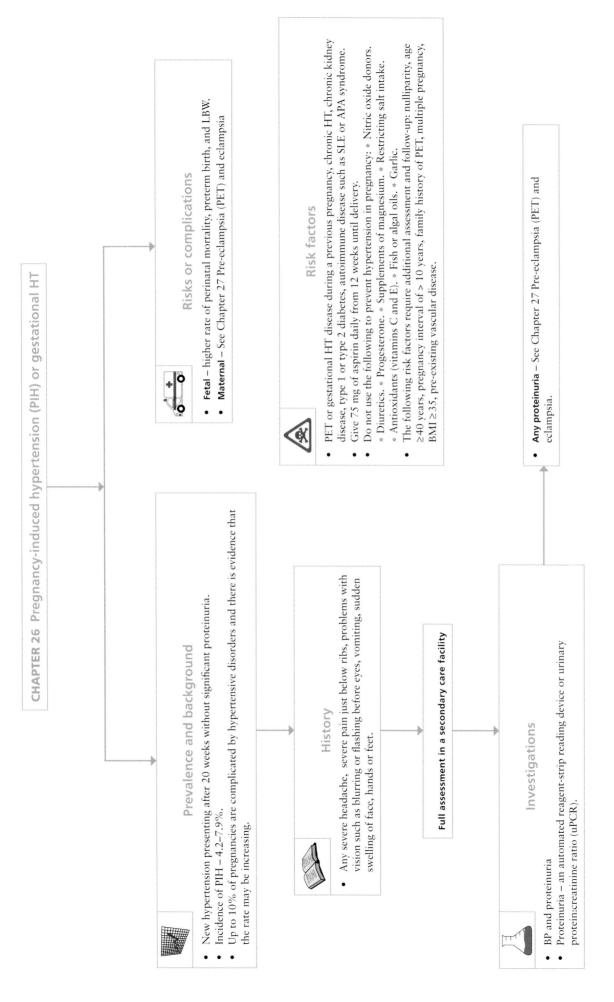

BP

Mild hypertension
(BP 140/90–149/99 mmHg)

- Outpatient monitoring.
- BP weekly.
- Test for proteinuria at each visit.
- Routine antenatal blood tests.
- If < 32 weeks or at high risk of PET – test for proteinuria and measure BP 2 times/week.

Moderate hypertension
(BP 150/100–159/109 mmHg)

- Outpatient monitoring,
- Oral labetalol to keep BP < 150/100 mmHg.
- BP, proteinuria at least 2 times a week.
- Test RFT, FBC, LFTs.
- No further blood tests if no subsequent proteinuria.

Severe hypertension
(BP ≥ 160/110 mmHg)

- **Inpatient care** until BP ≤ 159/109.
- Oral labetalol to keep BP < 150/100.
- BP at least 4 times a day.
- Proteinuria daily.
- Test RFT, FBC, LFTs at presentation and then weekly.

Mild or moderate hypertension

- If < 34 weeks – USS for fetal growth and AFV, UtAD.
- If USS normal – do not repeat after 34 weeks unless clinically indicated.
- Do not carry out USS for fetal growth and AFV, UtAD if diagnosis is confirmed after 34 weeks, unless otherwise clinically indicated.
- CTG only if fetal activity abnormal.

- USS for fetal growth and AFV + UtAD at diagnosis – If conservative management is planned: repeat every 2 weeks.
- CTG – carry out at diagnosis. If the results of all fetal monitoring are normal, do not routinely repeat CTG more than weekly.
- Repeat CTG if – change in fetal movement, vaginal bleeding, abdominal pain, deterioration in maternal condition.

- Alternative antihypertensives – nifedipine or methyldopa. Only offer after considering side-effect profiles for the woman, fetus, and newborn baby.
- Care plan – the timing and nature of fetal monitoring; fetal indications for birth and if and when corticosteroids should be given; when discussion with neonatal paediatricians and obstetric anaesthetists should take place.

Timing of birth

- Women whose BP is < 160/110 mmHg, with or without antihypertensive treatment:
  * Do not offer birth before 37 weeks.
  * After 37 weeks – timing of birth, and maternal and fetal indications for birth should be agreed between the woman and the senior obstetrician.
- Offer birth to women with refractory severe PIH after a course of corticosteroids (if required) has been completed.

Intrapartum care

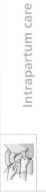

Mild and moderate hypertension

- Measure BP hourly.
- Continue antenatal hypertensive treatment.
- Carry out haematological and biochemical monitoring according to criteria from antenatal period.
- Do not routinely limit duration of second stage of labour if BP is stable.

Severe hypertension

- Measure BP continually.
- Continue antenatal hypertensive treatment.
- If BP controlled within target ranges, do not routinely limit duration of second stage of labour.
- If BP does not respond to initial treatment, advise operative vaginal delivery in second stage.

Postnatal care

- Measure BP :
  * Daily for first 2 days after birth.
  * At least once 3–5 days after birth.
  * As clinically indicated if anti-HT treatment changed.
- If methyldopa was used during pregnancy, stop within 2 days of birth.
- Continue antenatal antihypertensive treatment:
  * Start antihypertensive treatment if BP ≥ 150/100.
  * If BP falls to < 130/80, reduce anti-HT treatment.
  * If BP falls to < 140/90, consider reducing anti-HT treatment.
- If breastfeeding – avoid diuretic treatment for hypertension.
- Assess wellbeing of baby, especially adequacy of feeding, at least daily for first 2 days after birth.

Follow-up care

- At transfer to community care, write a care plan that includes who will provide follow-up care, frequency of BP monitoring, thresholds for reducing or stopping treatment, indications for referral to primary care for BP review.
- If antihypertensive treatment is to be continued – review 2 weeks after transfer to community care.
- Postnatal review at 6–8 weeks.
- If antihypertensive treatment is to be continued after 6–8 weeks postnatal review – specialist assessment.

What not to do

- Use of the following to prevent hypertension in pregnancy: * Nitric oxide donors. * Diuretics. * Progesterone. * Supplements of magnesium. * Restricting salt intake. * Antioxidants (vitamins C and E). * Fish or algal oils. * Garlic.
- Bed rest in hospital as a treatment.

Mild or moderate hypertension -
- USS for fetal growth and AFV, UmAD if diagnosis is confirmed after 34 weeks.
- Repeat USS after 34 weeks unless clinically indicated.

Severe hypertension
- Routine repeat USS more than every 2 weeks.
- Routine repeat CTG more than weekly.

Hypertension in Pregnancy: The management of hypertensive disorders during pregnancy; NICE CGN 107, August 2010.

CHAPTER 27 Pre-eclampsia (PET) and eclampsia

Prevalence and background

- PET – HT presenting after 20 weeks with significant proteinuria (> 0.3 g in 24 hours).
- Severe PET – PET with severe HT and/or with symptoms, and/or biochemical and/or haematological impairment.
  1. There is consensus on severe HT – severe HT (DBP ≥ 110 mmHg or SBP ≥ 170 mmHg on 2 occasions), together with significant proteinuria (at least 1 g/litre).
  2. There is less agreement on degree of moderate HT, which together with other symptoms or signs constitute severe PET. A DBP ≥ 100 mmHg on 2 occasions and significant proteinuria with at least two signs or symptoms of imminent eclampsia. (Although some women who present with eclampsia have no prodromal signs.)
- Eclampsia – the occurrence of one or more convulsions superimposed on PET.
- HELLP syndrome – haemolysis, elevated liver enzymes, and low platelet count.
- Rates for PET – 1.5% to 7.7%.
- The rate depends on parity: the rate for primigravid women is 4.1% and in women in their second pregnancy 1.7%.
- In the UK – severe PET – 5/1000 maternities; eclampsia – 5/10000 maternities.

Risks or complications

Maternal:

- HT in pregnancy is one of the leading causes of maternal death in the UK.
- One-third of severe maternal morbidity is as a consequence of hypertensive conditions.
- 5% of women with severe PET or eclampsia are admitted to intensive care (UK).
- Case fatality rate – 1.8% and a further 35% of women experience a major complication.
- Long-term consequences for women with a diagnosis of HT during pregnancy – chronic HT and an increase in lifetime cardiovascular risk.

Fetal:

- 5% of stillbirths in infants without congenital abnormality occur in women with PET.
- PTB rate – 1 in 250 (0.4%) women in their first pregnancy give birth before 34 weeks due to PET and 8–10% of all PTBs result from hypertensive disorders.
- Half of women with severe PET deliver preterm.
- SGA (FGR arising from placental disease) – 20–25% of PTBs and 14–19% of term births in women with PET.

Risk factors for pre-eclampsia

Very high

History of:
- Severe eclampsia.
- Pre-eclampsia needing birth before 34 weeks.
- PET with baby's birth weight < 10th centile.
- Intrauterine death.
- Placental abruption.

- Aspirin 75 mg/day from 12 weeks until birth.
- USS – fetal growth and AFV + UmAD:
  * Start at 28–30 weeks, or at least 2 weeks before previous gestational age of onset of hypertensive disorder if earlier than 28 weeks.
  * Repeat at least 4 weeks later.

High

- Hypertensive disease during previous pregnancy.
- Chronic kidney disease.
- Autoimmune disease such as systemic lupus erythematosus or antiphospholipid syndrome.
- Type 1 or type 2 diabetes.
- Chronic hypertension.

Moderate

- First pregnancy.
- Age ≥ 40 years.
- Pregnancy interval > 10 years.
- BMI ≥ 35 kg/m² at first visit.
- Family history of pre-eclampsia.
- Multiple pregnancy.

- If at least two moderate risk factors, or
- At least one high risk factor for pre-eclampsia.

- Aspirin 75 mg/day from 12 weeks until birth.
- If fetal activity abnormal carry out CTG.

Prevention

- **Women at high risk and with more than one moderate risk factor for PET – 75 mg of aspirin daily from 12 weeks until the birth of the baby.**
- Do not use the following solely with the aim of preventing hypertensive disorders during pregnancy: * Nitric oxide donors. * Progesterone. * Diuretics. * LMWH. * Magnesium. * Folic acid antioxidants (vitamins C and E). * Fish oils or algal oils. * Garlic. * Salt restriction during pregnancy.
- Advice on rest, exercise, and work for women at risk of hypertensive disorders during pregnancy is the same as for healthy pregnant women.

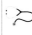

Symptoms and assessment of proteinuria

Clinical features of severe PET (in addition to HT and proteinuria) are:

- **Symptoms** – severe headache, problems with vision, such as blurring or flashing before the eyes, severe pain just below the ribs (epigastric pain), vomiting, sudden swelling of the face, hands or feet, convulsions, abdominal pain or general malaise.
- Increasing oedema is not in itself a sign to determine management.
- **Signs** – liver tenderness, clonus, papilloedema.
- Maternal tendon reflexes, although useful to assess magnesium toxicity, are not of value in assessing the risk of convulsion although the presence of clonus may be.
- **Investigations** – platelet count falling to < 100 x 10⁹/l; abnormal liver enzymes (ALT or AST > 70 IU/l); HELLP syndrome.

Investigations

Maternal

- **FBC, LFT, and RFTs.**
- Uric acid – rise confirms the diagnosis of PET and confers an increased risk to the mother and baby but do not use the levels in themselves for clinical decision making.
- Renal function is generally maintained in PET until the late stage unless HELLP syndrome develops. If creatinine is elevated early in the disease process, suspect underlying renal disease. In severe disease, serum creatinine can be seen to rise and is associated with a worsening outcome but renal failure is uncommon in the developed world and when it does occur it is usually associated with haemorrhage, HELLP syndrome or sepsis.
- A falling platelet count is associated with worsening disease and is itself a risk to the mother. However, it is not until the count is < 100 × 10⁹/l that there may be an associated coagulation abnormality. Consider delivery if platelet count is < 100. Clotting studies are not required if the platelet count is > 100 × 10⁹/l.
- An AST or ALT level of > 75 IU/l is seen as significant and a level > 150 IU/l is associated with increased morbidity to the mother.
- A diagnosis of HELLP syndrome needs confirmation of haemolysis, either by LDH levels, or by blood film to look for fragmented red cells.

Blood pressure (BP)

- When taking BP, the woman should be rested and sitting at a 45° angle. The BP cuff should be of the appropriate size and placed at the level of the heart. Use multiple readings to confirm the diagnosis. Korotkoff phase 5 is the appropriate measurement of DBP.
- Automated methods need to be used with caution, as they may give inaccurate BP readings in PET.

Proteinuria

- Use an automated reagent-strip reading device or a spot urinary protein:creatinine ratio (uPCR) for estimating proteinuria.
- Automated reagent-strip reading device – if result of 1+ or more, use a spot uPCR or 24-hour urine collection to quantify proteinuria.
- Diagnose significant proteinuria if the uPCR is > 30 mg/mmol or a validated 24-hour urine collection result shows > 300 mg protein.

Fetal

- The main pathology affecting the fetus, apart from prematurity, is placental insufficiency leading to IUGR.
- IUGR occurs in around 30% of PET pregnancies.
- Ultrasound assessment of fetal size, at the time of the initial presentation to assess fetal growth. Growth restriction is usually asymmetrical so measurement of the abdominal circumference (AC) is the best method of assessment.
- Reduced liquor volume is also associated with placental insufficiency and FGR. Serial estimations of liquor volume can detect fetal compromise.
- Umbilical artery Doppler assessment (UmAD), using absent or reversed-end diastolic flow, improves neonatal outcome. Serial investigations of this and other fetal vessels can be used to follow pregnancies and optimize delivery.

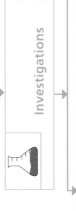

Management of PET pregnancy

Mild hypertension (140/90 to 149/99 mmHg)

- Admit to hospital.
- No antihypertensive treatment.
- Measure BP – at least four times a day.
- Do not repeat quantification of proteinuria.
- Blood tests monitor – twice a week: kidney function, electrolytes, FBC, transaminases, bilirubin.

Moderate hypertension (150/100 to 159/109 mmHg)

- Admit to hospital.
- Antihypertensive treatment – with oral labetalol as first-line treatment to keep: DBP between 80 and 100 mmHg and SBP < 150 mmHg.
- Measure BP – at least four times a day.
- Do not repeat quantification of proteinuria.
- Blood tests monitor – three times a week: kidney function, electrolytes, FBC, transaminases, bilirubin.

Severe hypertension (160/110 mmHg or higher)

- Admit to hospital.
- Antihypertensive treatment – with oral labetalol as first-line treatment to keep: DBP between 80–100 mmHg and SBP < 150 mmHg.
- Measure BP > four times a day.
- Do not repeat quantification of proteinuria.
- Blood tests monitor – three times a week: kidney function, electrolytes, FBC, transaminases, bilirubin.

Consider referral to level 2 critical care.

- Only offer antihypertensive treatment other than labetalol after considering side-effect profiles for the woman, fetus, and newborn baby.
- Alternatives include methyldopa and nifedipine.
- Atenolol is associated with an increase in FGR.
- ACE inhibitors and ARBs are contraindicated because of unacceptable fetal adverse effects.
- Diuretics are relatively contraindicated and reserve it for pulmonary oedema.

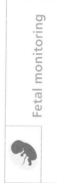

Fetal monitoring

Pre-eclampsia

- USS for fetal growth and AFV + UmAD at diagnosis – if conservative management is planned, repeat every 2 weeks.
- Do not routinely repeat USS more than every 2 weeks.
- CTG – carry out at diagnosis. If the results of all fetal monitoring are normal, do not routinely repeat CTG more than weekly.
- Repeat CTG if – change in fetal movement, vaginal bleeding, abdominal pain, deterioration in maternal condition.

Women at high risk of pre-eclampsia

- USS for fetal growth and AFV + UtAD starting at between 28 and 30 weeks (or at least 2 weeks before previous gestational age of onset if earlier than 28 weeks) and
- Repeat 4 weeks later.
- Only carry out CTG if fetal activity is abnormal, in women with previous:
  * Severe PET.
  * PET that needed birth before 34 weeks.
  * PET with a baby whose birth weight was < 10th centile.
  * Intrauterine death.
  * Placental abruption.

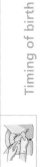

Timing of birth

Before 34 weeks

- Manage conservatively as it may improve the perinatal outcome at very early gestations but carefully balance with maternal wellbeing.
- Plan and document the maternal (biochemical, haematological, and clinical) and fetal thresholds for elective delivery before 34 weeks.
- Offer delivery after discussion with neonatal team and a course of corticosteroids has been given if:
  * Severe HT develops refractory to treatment.
  * Maternal or fetal indications develop.

34–36 weeks

- Deliver if PET with severe HT once BP has been controlled and a course of corticosteroids has been completed.
- Offer delivery if mild or moderate HT depending on maternal and fetal condition, risk factors, and availability of NICU.

After 37 weeks

- Deliver within 24–48 hours if PET is mild or moderate.

Mode of delivery

- **CS versus IOL** – choose mode of birth for women with severe HT, severe PET or eclampsia according to the clinical circumstances and the woman's preference.
- Decide the mode of delivery after considering the presentation of the fetus and the fetal condition, together with the likelihood of success of IOL after assessment of the cervix. Vaginal delivery is generally preferable but, if gestation is < 32 weeks, CS is more likely as the success of induction is reduced.
- After 34 weeks with a cephalic presentation, consider vaginal delivery.
- Manage third stage with 5 units IM Syntocinon or 5 units IV Syntocinon given slowly.
- Do not use Ergometrine or Syntometrine for prevention of PPH as this can further increase the BP.

Intrapartum care

See Chapter 26 Pregnancy-induced hypertension (PIH) or gestational HT

Postnatal investigation, monitoring, and treatment

Up to 44% of eclampsia occurs postpartum, especially at term, so assess women with signs or symptoms compatible with PET carefully.

Blood pressure

Women who did not take anti-HT treatment

- Measure BP:
  * At least 4 times a day while the woman is an inpatient.
  * At least once between D 3 and D 5 after birth.
  * On alternate days until normal if it was abnormal on D 3–5.
- Start anti-HT treatment if BP is ≥ 150/100 mmHg.
- Ask women about severe headache and epigastric pain each time BP is measured.

Women who took anti-HT treatment

- Measure BP:
  * At least 4 times a day while the woman is an inpatient.
  * Every 1–2 days for up to 2 weeks until the woman is off treatment and has no HT.
- Continue antenatal anti-HT treatment:
  * Consider reducing anti-HT treatment if BP < 140/90 mmHg.
  * Reduce anti-HT treatment if BPs < 130/80 mmHg.
- If a woman has taken methyldopa, stop within 2 days of birth.

Haematological and biochemical monitoring

Women with mild or moderate HT who have given birth, or after step-down from critical care:

- Measure platelet count, transaminases, and serum creatinine 48–72 hours after.
- Do not repeat if results are normal at 48–72 hours after.
- If indices are improving but stay within the abnormal range, repeat them as clinically indicated and at the postnatal review.
- If indices are not improving relative to pregnancy ranges, repeat them as clinically indicated.
- In women who have stepped down from critical care level, do not measure fluid balance if creatinine is within the normal range.

Postnatal care

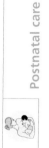

Community care

- **Transfer to community care if all of the following criteria are met:**
  - No symptoms of PET.
  - BP with or without treatment is ≤ 149/99 mmHg.
  - Blood test results are stable or improving.
- Write a care plan for women who are being transferred to community care: who will provide follow-up care, including medical review if needed, frequency of BP monitoring, thresholds for reducing or stopping treatment, indications for referral to primary care for BP review, self-monitoring for symptoms.
- **Women who are still on anti-HT treatment 2 weeks after transfer to community care – offer a medical review.**

Breastfeeding

- In women who still need anti-HT treatment in the postnatal period, avoid diuretics if the woman is breastfeeding or expressing milk.
- These anti-HT drugs have no known adverse effects on babies receiving breast milk: labetalol, nifedipine, enalapril, captopril, atenolol, metoprolol.
- There is insufficient evidence on the safety of breastfeeding with ARBs, amlodipine, ACE inhibitors other than enalapril and captopril.
- Assess the clinical wellbeing of the baby, especially adequacy of feeding, at least daily for the first 2 days after the birth.

Postnatal review (6–8 weeks after the birth)

- Offer all women a medical review.
- Offer women who still need anti-HT treatment a specialist assessment of their HT.
- Urinary reagent-strip test. Offer women who still have proteinuria (≥ 1+) a further review at 3 months to assess kidney function and consider referral for specialist kidney assessment.
- Up to 13% of women with PET will have underlying chronic or essential HT that was not suspected antenatally.

Follow-up care

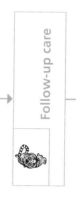

Long-term risk

- Long-term risk of cardiovascular disease – an increased risk of developing high BP and its complications in later life.
- Long-term risk of end-stage kidney disease – women who have no proteinuria and no HT at the postnatal review have a low absolute risk and no further follow-up is necessary.
- Thrombophilia and the risk of PET – do not routinely perform screening for thrombophilia in women who have had PET.

Risk of recurrence

- Women with PIH – risk in future pregnancy:
  - PIH – 1 in 6 (16%) to 1 in 2 (47%) pregnancies.
  - PET – 1 in 50 (2%) to 1 in 14 (7%) pregnancies.
- Women with PET – risk of developing in future pregnancy:
  - PIH – 1 in 8 (13%) to 1 in 2 (53%) pregnancies.
  - PET – up to 1 in 6 (16%) pregnancies.
  - No additional risk if interval before next pregnancy < 10 years.
- Women with severe PET, HELLP syndrome or eclampsia:
  - And if led to birth < 34 weeks – PET in a future pregnancy is about 1 in 4 (25%) pregnancies.
  - And if led to birth < 28 weeks – 1 in 2 (55%) pregnancies.

Medical management of severe HT, severe PET or eclampsia in a critical care setting

Anticonvulsants

- Give **IV magnesium sulphate** – if a woman has severe HT or severe PET, has or previously had an eclamptic fit.
- **Consider IV magnesium sulphate** to women with severe PET who are in a critical care setting if birth is planned within 24 hours.
- **Features of severe PET:**
  1. Severe HT and proteinuria or
  2. Mild or moderate HT and proteinuria with one or more of:
     * Severe headache.
     * Problems with vision – blurring or flashing before the eyes.
     * Severe pain just below the ribs or vomiting.
     * Papilloedema.
     * Liver tenderness.
     * Clonus (3 beats).
     * HELLP syndrome.
     * Platelet count < 100 × 10⁹/l.
     * Abnormal liver enzymes (ALT or AST > 70 IU/l).
- Regimen for administration of magnesium sulphate – loading dose of 4 g IV over 5 minutes, followed by an infusion of 1 g/hour maintained for 24 hours. Treat recurrent seizures with a further dose of 2–4 g given over 5 minutes.
- Do not use diazepam, phenytoin or lytic cocktail as an alternative to magnesium sulphate in women with eclampsia.
- Administration of magnesium sulphate reduces the risk of an eclamptic seizure with a 58% lower risk of an eclamptic seizure.
- More women need to be treated when PET is not severe (109) to prevent one seizure when compared with severe PET (60).
- If magnesium sulphate is given, continue for 24 hours following delivery or 24 hours after the last seizure, whichever is the later.
- Monitor urine output, maternal reflexes, respiratory rate, and oxygen saturation.

Antihypertensives

- Treat with – labetalol (oral or IV); hydralazine (IV); nifedipine (oral).
- Aim to keep SBP < 150 mmHg and DBP between 80 and 100 mmHg.
- Measure BP continually.
- Monitor response: to ensure that BP falls, to identify adverse effects for both the woman and the fetus, to modify treatment according to response.
- Consider using up to 500 ml crystalloid fluid before or at the same time as the first dose of IV hydralazine in the antenatal period.

Corticosteroids

- **For fetal lung maturation** –if delivery is likely within 7 days:
  * Give 2 doses of betamethasone 12 mg IM, 24 hours apart in women between 24 and 34 weeks.
  * Consider giving 2 doses of betamethasone 12 mg IM, 24 hours apart in women between 35 and 36 weeks.
- Do not use dexamethasone or betamethasone for the treatment of HELLP syndrome.

Fluid balance and volume expansion

- Pulmonary oedema has been a significant cause of maternal death.
- This is associated with inappropriate fluid management. Limit maintenance fluids to 80 ml/hour unless there are other ongoing fluid losses (for example, haemorrhage).
- Maintain the regime of fluid restriction until there is a postpartum diuresis, as oliguria is common with severe PET.
- Do not use volume expansion unless hydralazine is the antenatal antihypertensive.

Indications for referral to critical care levels women with severe HT or severe PET

Level 3

- Severe PET needing ventilation.

Level 2

Step-down from level 3 or severe PET with:
- Eclampsia.
- HELLP syndrome.
- Haemorrhage.
- Hyperkalaemia.
- Severe oliguria.
- Coagulation support.
- IV antihypertensive treatment.
- Initial stabilization of severe HT.
- Evidence of cardiac failure.
- Abnormal neurology.

Level 1

- PET with mild or moderate HT.
- Ongoing conservative antenatal management of severe preterm HT.
- Step-down treatment after the birth.

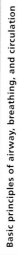
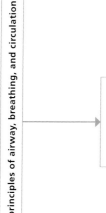

Management of eclampsia

Basic principles of airway, breathing, and circulation

- Call for help (anaesthetist and senior obstetrician).
- Aim to prevent maternal injury during the convulsion.
- Place the woman in the left lateral position and administer oxygen.
- Assess the airway and breathing and check pulse and BP.
- Pulse oximetry is helpful.

Anticonvulsants

- Magnesium sulphate is the therapy of choice
- Do not use diazepam and phenytoin as first-line drugs.
- Magnesium toxicity is unlikely with standard regimens so do not measure levels routinely. Magnesium sulphate is mostly excreted in the urine. Monitor urine output closely observed and if it becomes reduced < 20 ml/hour, stop magnesium infusion.
- Magnesium toxicity can be assessed by clinical assessment as it causes a loss of deep tendon reflexes and respiratory depression. If there is loss of deep tendon reflexes, stop magnesium sulphate infusion.
- Calcium gluconate 1 g (10 ml) over 10 minutes can be given if there is concern over respiratory depression.

Antihypertensives

- Treat with – labetalol (oral or IV); hydralazine (IV); nifedipine (oral).
- Aim to keep SBP < 150 mmHg and DBP between 80 and 100 mmHg.
- Up to 500 ml crystalloid fluid before or at the same time as the first dose of IV hydralazine.
- Measure BP continually. Monitor response: to ensure that BP falls; to identify adverse effects for both the woman and the fetus; to modify treatment according to response.

Repeated seizures

- Repeat magnesium sulphate.
- Alternative agents such as diazepam or thiopentone may be used, but only as single doses, since prolonged use of diazepam is associated with an increase in maternal death.
- If convulsions persist, intubation is necessary to protect the airway and maintain oxygenation.
- Transfer to intensive care facilities with intermittent positive pressure ventilation is appropriate in these circumstances.

Delivery

- Once stabilized, plan to deliver; however there is no particular hurry and a delay of several hours to make sure the correct care is in hand is acceptable, assuming that there is no acute fetal concern such as a fetal bradycardia.

The Management of Severe Pre-Eclampsia/Eclampsia. RCOG Guideline No. 10(A); March 2006.
Hypertension in Pregnancy: The Management of Hypertensive Disorders during Pregnancy; NICE CGN 107, August 2010.

Risks

Maternal

- Meconium-stained liquor (MSL), CS or PPH:
  * MSL is more common in preterm than term OC pregnancy (25% vs 12%) and preterm controls (18% vs 3%).
  * MSL may be more common in those with severe cholestasis (defined as bile acids > 40 μmol/l) compared with mild cholestasis.
  * CS rates are high, ranging from 10% to 36%.
  * PPH is reported to range from 2% to 22%.

Fetus

- Prematurity – increased, mainly iatrogenic (range 7–25%), risk of spontaneous premature delivery is only slightly increased compared with general population (range 4–12%).
- Stillbirth – risk in 'untreated' OC is unclear. Studies between 2001 and 2011 reported the PNM rate 5.7/1000. These are comparable to that of general population – PNM is reported as 8.3 in 2002 and 5.4 in 2008.

Differential diagnosis

DDx

- Other causes of pruritus (see Chapter 44 Pruritus in pregnancy).
- Other causes of abnormal LFTs:
  * Viral infections – hepatitis A, B, C, EBV, and CMV.
  * Liver autoimmune conditions – chronic active hepatitis and primary biliary cirrhosis.
  * PET and acute fatty liver of pregnancy in atypical cases.

Prevalence and background

- Prevalence – 0.7% of pregnancies. More common (1.2–1.5%) in women of Indian or Pakistani origin.
- It is a multifactorial condition, influenced by genetic and environmental aspects and varies among populations.
- OC is characterized by intense pruritus in the absence of a skin rash, with abnormal liver function tests (LFTs), neither of which have an alternative cause and both of which remit following delivery.
- It is a diagnosis of exclusion.

History and examination

- Pruritus – typically worse at night, often widespread and may involve the palms of the hands or the soles of the feet.
- Consequent sleep deprivation
- Evidence of cholestasis – pale stool, dark urine.
- Family history of OC.
- Skin inspection – no rash.
- Skin trauma from intense scratching may be seen (excoriations).

Investigations

- LFTs – abnormal transaminases, GGT, bilirubin, and/or bile salts.
  * Use pregnancy-specific reference ranges.
  * Isolated elevation of bile salts may occur.
  * Normal levels of bile salts do not exclude the diagnosis. Substantial number of women will have pruritus for days or weeks before the development of abnormal LFTs. If pruritus persists, LFTs should be measured every 1–2 weeks.
- Viral screen.
- Liver USS.
- Liver autoimmune screen (anti-smooth muscle, antimitochondrial antibodies) may be indicated.

Monitoring

Maternal

- LFTs weekly.
- Do not decide delivery based on the degree of abnormality of biochemical tests, as current data are not robust enough to demonstrate or exclude a correlation between levels of liver enzymes or bile salts and IUD.
- Bile salts may play a role in fetal demise. However, it is unclear whether bile acid concentrations are related to fetal outcome.

Fetus

- **No specific fetal monitoring for the prediction of fetal death can be recommended.**
- IUD is usually sudden and seems to be due to acute anoxia. There is no evidence of placental insufficiency. USS including UtAD assessment is not a reliable method for preventing fetal death.
- CTG – lack of predictability of future fetal wellbeing of a normal CTG is a major limitation of the use of this test.
- Amniocentesis – too invasive.
- Maternal detection of movements is simple, inexpensive, and not time-consuming but its role in monitoring pregnancy complicated by OC has not been evaluated.

Management

There is no evidence that any specific treatment improves maternal symptoms or neonatal outcomes.

Topical emollients and antihistamines

- Topical emollients are safe but their efficacy is unknown. Clinical experience suggests that for some women they may provide slight temporary relief of pruritus.
- Antihistamines such as chlorpheniramine may provide some welcome sedation at night but do not make a significant impact on pruritus.

Ursodeoxycholic acid

- There is lack of data concerning improvement in pruritus, protection against SB, and safety to the fetus.
- UDCA can displace more hydrophobic endogenous bile salts from the bile acid pool and thereby protect the hepatocyte membrane from their damaging toxicity and enhance bile acid clearance across the placenta from the fetus.
- As the pathophysiology of OC and the mechanism of fetal demise are uncertain, the possible role of UDCA is unclear.

S adenosyl methionine

- There is insufficient evidence to show whether it is effective for either control of maternal symptoms or improving fetal outcome.

Vitamin K

- OC can result in reduced absorption of dietary fats, due to failure of excretion of bile salts into the GIT and reduced micelle formation, leading to reduced absorption of fat-soluble vitamins including vitamin K, which is required for the manufacture of coagulation factors 2, 7, 9, 10.
- Daily supplementation of vitamin K aims to improve both maternal and neonatal levels and therefore reduce PPH and fetal or neonatal bleeding.

Dexamethasone

- Do not offer as first-line therapy for OC outside of RCT.
- Observational reports – results are conflicting.
- The general concern about adverse fetal and neonatal neurological effects of repeated courses of maternally administered dexamethasone limits the potential use of it.

Time and mode of delivery

- Stillbirths in OC have been reported across all gestations. As gestation advances, the risk of delivery (prematurity, respiratory distress, failed induction) versus the uncertain fetal risk of continuing the pregnancy (stillbirth) may justify IOL after 37 weeks.
- IOL at 37 weeks – while it is certain that delivery at 37 weeks will prevent a SB beyond that gestation, it is not known how high the risk of such an SB might be. Risks of perinatal (respiratory morbidity and admission to SCBU) and maternal morbidity are increased.
- Offer continuous fetal monitoring in labour.

Postnatal care

- Repeat LFTs – postnatal resolution of symptoms and of biochemical abnormalities is required to secure the diagnosis. In normal pregnancy, LFTs may increase in the first 10 days of the puerperium; in a pregnancy complicated by OC, defer routine measurement of LFTs beyond this time.
- Offer postnatal vitamin K for the babies.

Follow-up

- To ensure that LFTs have returned to normal, pruritus resolves, and to provide appropriate counselling.
- Reassure about the lack of long-term sequelae for mother and baby.
- Discuss contraceptive choices (avoid oestrogen-containing methods).
- Risk of recurrence is high.
- Increased incidence of OC in family members.

What not to do

- Any specific fetal monitoring modality for the prediction of fetal death.
- Dexamethasone or S adenosyl methionine for management.
- Decide delivery based on the degree of abnormality of biochemical tests.

Obstetric Cholestasis. RCOG Green-top Guideline No. 43; April 2011.

CHAPTER 29 Gestational diabetes mellitus (GDM)

Any degree of glucose intolerance with onset or first recognition during pregnancy

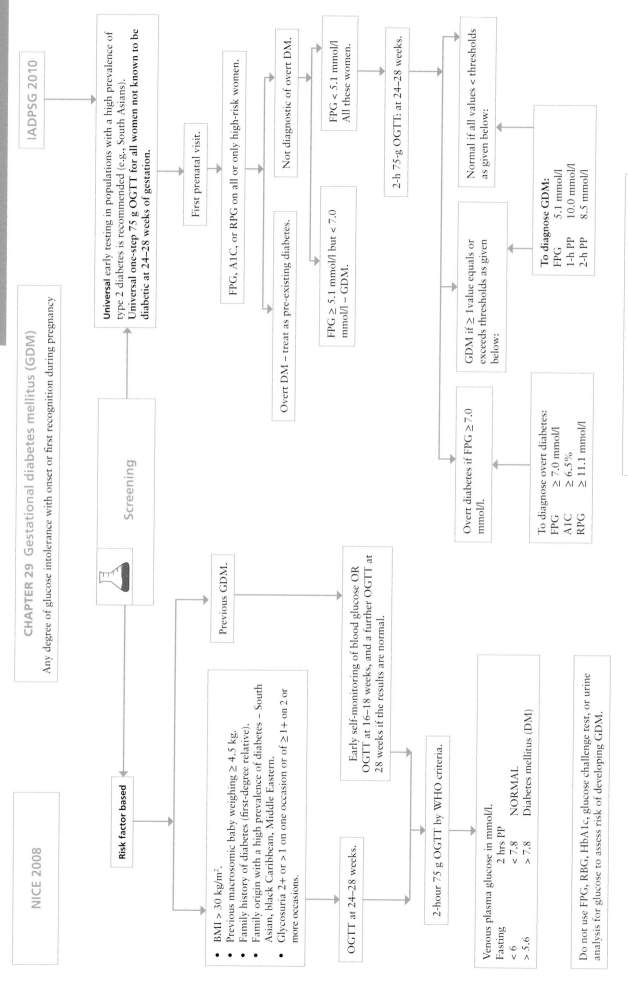

Prevalence and incidence

- Diabetes is a disorder of carbohydrate metabolism.
- GDM – defined as carbohydrate intolerance that develops first time in the pregnancy.
- Approximately 650 000 women give birth in England and Wales each year, and 2–5% of pregnancies involve women with diabetes.
- Diabetes in pregnancy is seen in 2–5% of pregnancies – 87.5% are GDM, 7.5% due to type 1 DM, and remaining 5% due to type 2 DM.
- The prevalence of type 1 and type 2 diabetes is increasing. Type 2 diabetes is increasing in minority ethnic groups (African, black Caribbean, South Asian, Middle Eastern, and Chinese family origin).
- The incidence of GDM is also increasing probably due to increasing rates of obesity.
- Risk factors – age, ethnicity, obesity, family history of DM, and past history of GDM.

Risks

Maternal

- Pre-eclampsia and preterm labour:
- Increased monitoring and interventions during pregnancy and labour.
- Likelihood of birth trauma, IOL, and CS.

Fetal

- Stillbirth, macrosomia, birth injury (shoulder dystocia), perinatal mortality, and postnatal adaptation problems such as neonatal hypoglycaemia and admission to the neonatal unit.
- Obesity and/or diabetes in later life.

Antenatal care

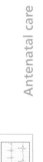

Joint diabetes and antenatal clinic – within 1 week

There is a continuous linear relationship between maternal BG and fetal growth. Good glycaemic control throughout pregnancy will reduce the risk of fetal macrosomia, trauma during birth, IOL or CS, neonatal hypoglycaemia, and perinatal death.

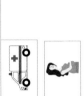

- **Lifestyle advice** – weight control, diet and exercise – most women respond to it.
  - Diet – carbohydrates from low glycaemic index sources, lean proteins including oily fish, and a balance of polyunsaturated fats and monounsaturated fats.
  - If pre-pregnancy BMI is > 27 kg/m² – advise to restrict calorie intake (to 25 kcal/kg/day or less) and to take moderate exercise (of at least 30 minutes daily).
  - Folic acid 5 mg/day.
- **Oral hypoglycaemic agents** – 10–20% will need oral hypoglycaemic agents if:
  * Diet and exercise fail to maintain BG targets during a period of 1–2 weeks.
  * USS suggests incipient fetal macrosomia (AC > 70th percentile) at diagnosis.
- Start treatment with oral hypoglycaemic agents but often insulin is needed to ensure adequate glycaemic control.
  - Both glibenclamide and metformin are effective treatments for GDM.
  - Offer metformin if blood sugar not controlled with changes in diet and exercise within 1–2 weeks.
  - Need for insulin is in about 20–30% of patients who were initially started on glibenclamide and metformin. Agents – regular insulin, rapid-acting insulin analogues.

Monitoring

Maternal

- Diabetes care team for assessment of glycaemic control every 1–2 weeks throughout pregnancy.
- Self-monitoring of blood glucose (BG) levels.
- FBG and BG levels 1 hour after every meal.
- Aim to keep FBG 3.5–5.9 mmol/l and 1-hour PP BG < 7.8 mmol/l; 2-hour PP 6.4 mmol/l.
- Women with insulin-treated diabetes – to test BG levels before going to bed at night.
- Do not use HbA1c routinely for assessing glycaemic control in the 2nd and 3rd trimesters of pregnancy.

Fetus

- USS monitoring of fetal growth and amniotic fluid volume every 4 weeks from 28 weeks.
- 38 weeks – start regular tests of fetal wellbeing in women who are awaiting spontaneous labour weekly.
- Risk of IUGR (macrovascular disease and/or nephropathy) – use an individualized approach to monitor fetal growth and wellbeing.

CHAPTER 29 Gestational diabetes mellitus (GDM)

Time and mode of delivery

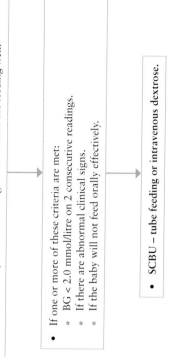

- Normally grown fetus – IOL or ELCS if indicated, after 38 completed weeks.
- USS diagnosed macrosomic fetus – discuss the risks and benefits of vaginal birth, IOL, and CS.
- During labour and birth, monitor capillary BG hourly and maintain it between 4 and 7 mmol/l.
- Commence IV dextrose & insulin infusion if BG is not maintained at 4–7 mmol/l.
- Diabetes is not a contraindication for VBAC.

Preterm labour

- Women with insulin-treated diabetes who are receiving steroids for fetal lung maturation – give additional insulin and closely monitor.
- Do not use betamimetic drugs for tocolysis.

Postnatal care

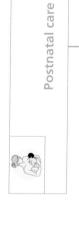

Neonatal

- Feed ASAP after birth (within 30 minutes) and then at frequent intervals (every 2–3 hours) until feeding maintains pre-feed blood glucose levels at a minimum of 2.0 mmol/litre. Test BG routinely at 2–4 hours after birth.
- Do not transfer babies to community care until they are at least 24 hours old, and not before they are maintaining BG levels and are feeding well.

- If one or more of these criteria are met:
  * BG < 2.0 mmol/litre on 2 consecutive readings.
  * If there are abnormal clinical signs.
  * If the baby will not feed orally effectively.

- **SCBU – tube feeding or intravenous dextrose.**

Maternal

- Discontinue hypoglycaemic treatment immediately after birth.
- BG to exclude persisting hyperglycaemia before women are transferred to community care.
- Warn women of the symptoms of hyperglycaemia.
- Lifestyle advice (including weight control, diet, and exercise).
- Discuss contraception.

Follow-up

- FPG (but not an OGTT) at the 6-week postnatal check and annually thereafter.
- Inform of risks of GDM in future pregnancy (including those with ongoing impaired glucose regulation) and offer women screening (OGTT or FPG) for diabetes when planning future pregnancy.
- Offer early self-monitoring of BG or an OGTT in future pregnancies (including those with ongoing impaired glucose regulation). Offer a subsequent OGTT if the test results in early pregnancy are normal.
- Remind of the importance of contraception and the need for pre-conception care when planning future pregnancies.

What not to do

- Betamimetic drugs for tocolysis.

Guideline comparator

ACOG

- Screen all pregnant women for GDM, whether by patient history, clinical risk factors, or a 50 g 1 hour GTT.
- The diagnosis of GDM can be made by 100 g 3 hour OGTT, for which there is evidence that treatment improves outcome.
- Diagnosis of GDM based on 'one-step screening and diagnosis test' as outlined by IADPSG (2010) is not recommended at this time because there is no evidence that diagnosis using these criteria leads to clinically significant improvements in the maternal or neonatal outcomes and it would lead to a significant increase in health care costs.
- Insulin therapy for women receiving medical/nutritional therapy whose FBG > 5.35; 1-h PP BG level > 7.75; or 2-h PP BG level > 6.65 mmol/l.
- Insulin is the first-line therapy. Most insulin regimens include intermediate-acting insulins, such as isophane (NPH), and short-acting insulins, such as regular recombinant (Humulin R), and the insulin analogues aspart (Novolog) and lispro (Humalog).
- American Family Physician guidelines – metformin (Glucophage) may be another option.
- The ADA – screen for congenital anomalies in women with GDM who present with evidence of pre-existing hyperglycaemia, such as an A1C level > 7%, a FBG > 6.65 mmol/l or a diagnosed GDM in the first trimester. Women with these findings are more likely to have unrecognized pre-gestational diabetes and are therefore at higher risk of fetal malformation from exposure to hyperglycaemia during organogenesis.
- ACOG – women with GDM who are on insulin or who have poor glucose control have the same antenatal monitoring as women with pre-gestational DM.
- If the estimated fetal weight exceeds 4500 g, CS may reduce the likelihood of brachial plexus injury in the infant.
- Postpartum – an OGTT at 3-year intervals has been shown to be a cost-effective strategy for screening.

SOGC

- A single approach of testing for GDM cannot be recommended at present as there is not enough evidence proving the beneficial effect of a large screening programme.
- Each of the following approaches is acceptable.
  * Routine screening of women at 24–28 weeks with the 50 g glucose challenge test (GCT), using a threshold of 7.8 mmol/l except in the women who are low risk.
  * Maternal age < 25.
  * Caucasian or other ethnic group with low prevalence of diabetes.
  * Pregnant BMI ≤ 27.
  * No previous history of GDM or glucose intolerance.
  * No family history of diabetes in first-degree relative.
  * No history of GDM-associated adverse pregnancy outcomes.
- The diagnostic test can be the 100 g OGTT or the 75 g OGTT, according to the American Diabetes Association (ADA) criteria. Use of the WHO criteria will approximately double the number of women diagnosed with GDM without an apparent clinical benefit.
  * Women at high risk for GDM – diagnostic test as early in pregnancy as possible and repeat it at 24–28 weeks if initial results are negative.
- Until evidence is available from large RCTs that show a clear benefit from screening for glucose intolerance in pregnancy, the option of not screening for GDM is considered acceptable. Conversely, there are no compelling data to stop screening when it is practised.
- Reassess glucose tolerance with a 75 g OGTT 6–12 weeks postpartum in order to identify women with persistent glucose intolerance.

Diabetes in Pregnancy: Management of Diabetes and its Complications from Pre-conception to the Postnatal Period; NICE CGN 63, March 2008. Please refer to updated guideline from February 2015.

International Association of Diabetes and Pregnancy Study Groups Recommendations 2010.

SOGC. Clinical Practice Guidelines: Screening for Gestational Diabetes Mellitus. J Obstet Gynaecol Can 2002;24(11):894–903.

ACOG Committee opinion. Screening and Diagnosis of GDM; No. 504, 2011.

ACOG Practice Bulletin. Clinical management guidelines for obstetrician-gynecologists. Number 30, September 2001; Gestational diabetes. Obstet Gynecol. 2001 Sep;98(3):525–538.

David C. Serlin and Robert W. Lash. Diagnosis and management of gestational diabetes mellitus. Am Fam Physician. 2009 Jul 1;80(1):57–62.

RCOG. Diagnosis and Treatment of Gestational Diabetes Scientific Advisory Committee Opinion Paper 23; January 2011.

CHAPTER 30 Antepartum haemorrhage (APH)

Definition and incidence

- Bleeding from or into the genital tract, after 24+0 weeks of pregnancy, before onset of labour.
- APH complicates 3–5% of pregnancies.
- Severity of APH – no consistent definitions. Presence of maternal shock and fetal compromise or demise are important indicators of volume depletion.

  Severity:
  * Spotting – staining, streaking or blood spotting noted.
  * Minor haemorrhage – blood loss < 50 ml that has settled.
  * Major haemorrhage – blood loss of 50–1000 ml, with no signs of clinical shock.
  * Massive haemorrhage – blood loss > 1000 ml and/or signs of clinical shock.
  * Recurrent APH – episodes of APH on more than one occasion.

- Advise women to report all vaginal bleeding.
- Women with APH presenting to a midwifery-led maternity unit, a GP or to an A&E should be assessed, stabilized if necessary, and transferred to a hospital maternity unit with facilities for resuscitation and performing emergency operative delivery.
- MDT – midwifery and obstetric staff, with immediate access to laboratory, theatre, neonatal and anaesthetic services should be available at these centres.

Clinical assessment

- To establish whether urgent intervention is required to manage maternal or fetal compromise.
- History to assess coexisting symptoms.
- The cardiovascular condition of the mother.
- Assess extent of vaginal bleeding.
- Assess fetal wellbeing.

No maternal compromise

History

- Enquire about pain associated with the haemorrhage. Consider placental abruption if the pain is continuous. Consider labour if the pain is intermittent.
- Assess risk factors for abruption and placenta praevia.
- Check fetal movements and auscultate the fetal heart.
- If the APH is associated with spontaneous or iatrogenic rupture of the fetal membranes, consider bleeding from a ruptured vasa praevia.
- Previous cervical smear history – most women with FIGO stage I cancer are asymptomatic; symptomatic pregnant women usually present with APH (mostly postcoital) or vaginal

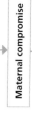

Risks or complications

- Obstetric haemorrhage remains one of the major causes of maternal death in developing countries. Cause of up to 50% of estimated 500 000 maternal deaths globally each year.
- In the UK, deaths from obstetric haemorrhage are uncommon. In the 2006–08 CEMACE report, haemorrhage was the sixth highest direct cause of maternal death (9 direct deaths; 3.9 deaths/million maternities). There were 4 deaths from APH in the more recent report.
- Maternal – anaemia, infection, maternal shock, renal tubular necrosis, consumptive coagulopathy, PPH, prolonged hospital stay, psychological sequelae, complications of blood transfusion.
- Fetal – fetal hypoxia, SGA and FGR, prematurity (iatrogenic and spontaneous), death.
- APH is a leading cause of perinatal mortality worldwide. Up to one-fifth of very preterm babies are born in association with APH, and the known association of APH with cerebral palsy can be explained by preterm delivery.

Causes of APH

- Placenta praevia – placenta that lies wholly or partly within the lower uterine segment – leading to haemorrhage as the lower segment forms or the cervix dilates. Incidence – 1:200.
- Placental abruption:
  * Premature separation of a normally implanted placenta from the uterine wall.
  * Incidence – 1:80. * PNM – 300/1000. * Risk of recurrence – 7–9%.
- Uncertain origin causes:
  * Cervical lesions – polyp, ectropion. * Vaginal lesions.
  * Localized placental abruption. * Marginal haemorrhage. * Excessive show.
- Unexplained:
  * Pregnancies complicated by unexplained APH are also at increased risk of adverse maternal and perinatal outcomes.
  * Meta-analysis – higher risk of PTD (OR 3.17), SB (OR 2.09), and fetal anomalies (OR 1.42).
  * An observational study – higher risk of smaller babies, PTD, IOL at term, admission to NICU, and development of hyperbilirubinaemia in babies.

Maternal compromise

- Undertake acute appraisal of maternal wellbeing and resuscitation if there is major or massive haemorrhage that is persisting or if the woman is unable to provide a history due to a compromised clinical state.
- Mother is the priority; stabilize her prior to establishing the fetal condition.
- Follow basic principles of resuscitation in all women presenting with collapse or major haemorrhage.
- Deliver.

Examination – to assess the amount and cause of APH.

- General examination – pulse and BP.
- Abdominal palpation – for tenderness or signs of an acute abdomen – tense or 'woody' feel to the uterus indicates a significant abruption; uterine contractions; soft, non-tender uterus may suggest a lower genital tract cause or bleeding from placenta or vasa praevia.
- Speculum examination – to identify cervical dilatation or lower genital tract cause of APH.
- Clinically suspicious cervix – refer for colposcopic evaluation.
- Vaginal examination – if placenta praevia is a possible diagnosis (previous scan shows a low placenta, there is a high presenting part on abdominal examination or the bleed has been painless), do not perform a digital vaginal examination until an USS has excluded placenta praevia.
- It can provide information on cervical dilatation if APH is associated with pain or uterine activity.

Investigations

Maternal – to assess the extent and physiological consequences of the APH

- Major haemorrhage – FBC, U&Es, LFTs, coagulation screen, and 4 units of blood cross-matched. The initial haemoglobin may not reflect the amount of blood lost. The platelet count, if low, may indicate a consumptive process seen in relation to significant abruption; this may be associated with a coagulopathy.
- Minor haemorrhage – FBC and 'Group & Save (G&S)'.
- The Kleihauer test in rhesus D (RhD)-negative women to quantify FMH. It is not a sensitive test for diagnosing abruption.
- USS – to confirm or exclude placenta praevia if the placental site is not already known.
- Placental abruption is a clinical diagnosis and there are no sensitive or reliable diagnostic tests available. USS for the detection of retroplacental clot (abruption) has poor sensitivity, specificity, and positive and negative predictive values – 24%, 96%, 88%, and 53% respectively. USS fails to detect three-quarters of cases of abruption. However, when the USS suggests an abruption, the likelihood that there is an abruption is high.

Fetal

- CTG for FHR. Use USS to establish fetal heart if fetal viability cannot be detected using auscultation.
- MOH can result in fetal hypoxia and abnormalities of the FHR pattern.
- If active obstetric intervention in the interests of the fetus is not planned, for example at gestations < 26+0 weeks, do not offer continuous monitoring of the FHR.
- Preterm pregnancies with placental abruption and a normal CTG consider expectant management. Deliver if abnormal CTG.
- **Suspected vasa praevia** – various tests exist that can differentiate between fetal and maternal blood, but are often not applicable. In the event of a significant bleed related to vasa praevia, signs of fetal compromise would be identifiable on FHR monitoring, deliver irrespective of the results of such a test.

Antenatal management

Should women be hospitalized?

- Women presenting with spotting who are no longer bleeding and where placenta praevia has been excluded can go home after a reassuring initial clinical assessment.
- Admit all women with APH heavier than spotting and ongoing bleeding in hospital at least until the bleeding has stopped.
- Advise woman to contact the maternity unit if she has any further bleeding, pain or a reduction in FMs.
- Individualize care – for example, if a woman presents with spotting and has a past history of IUFD resulting from placental abruption, then hospitalization would be appropriate.

Corticosteroids

- Offer a single course of corticosteroids to women between 24+0 and 34+6 weeks of gestation at risk of PTB.
- In women presenting with spotting, where the most likely cause is lower genital tract bleeding, where imminent delivery is unlikely, corticosteroids are unlikely to be of benefit, but one can still consider it.

Tocolysis

- Do not use tocolysis to delay delivery in a woman presenting with a major APH who is haemodynamically unstable, or if there is fetal compromise.
- Tocolysis is contraindicated in placental abruption and is 'relatively contraindicated' in 'mild haemorrhage' due to placenta praevia.
- Women most likely to benefit from use of a tocolytic drug are those who are very preterm, those needing in utero transfer, and those who have not yet completed a full course of corticosteroids.
- If tocolysis is used, choose a drug which has minimal maternal cardiovascular side effects. Avoid calcium antagonist (nifedipine) as it has risk of maternal hypotension.

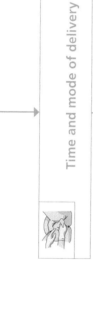

Ongoing antenatal care of following APH

- Following single or recurrent episodes of APH from a cervical ectropion, continue with routine ANC.
- Following APH from placental abruption or unexplained APH, reclassify pregnancy as 'high risk' and provide consultant-led ANC.
- Due to the increased risk of adverse perinatal outcomes including SGA fetus and FGR, arrange serial USS for fetal growth.
- Give anti-D Ig to all non-sensitized RhD-negative women, independent of whether routine antenatal prophylactic anti-D has been given. In the event of recurrent vaginal bleeding after 20 weeks, give anti-D Ig at a minimum of 6-weekly intervals, at least 500 IU anti-D Ig followed by a test to identify FMH > 4 ml red blood cells to give additional anti-D Ig if required.

Time and mode of delivery

Maternal or fetal compromise
- Obstetric emergency – resuscitate mother and deliver to control the bleeding. Delivery will usually be by CS, unless the woman is in established labour.

No maternal and/or fetal compromise
- Optimum timing of delivery of women presenting with unexplained APH and no associated maternal and/or fetal compromise is not established. Review by a senior obstetrician.

Fetal death
- Vaginal birth for most women (provided the maternal condition is satisfactory), but CS may be necessary in some.

Before 37 weeks
- Where there is no maternal or fetal compromise and bleeding has settled, there is no evidence to support elective premature delivery of the fetus; therefore can delay delivery.

After 37 weeks
- Differentiate between APH and blood-stained 'show'. If the APH is spotting or the blood is streaked through mucus it is unlikely to require active intervention.
- However, in the event of a minor or major APH, consider IOL for vaginal delivery.

Extremely preterm pregnancy (24 to 26 weeks)
- A senior paediatrician/neonatologist for counselling of women.
- Conservative management is usually appropriate when the mother's condition is stable.
- When the bleeding is considered life-threatening for the woman or there is evidence of cardiovascular compromise that fails to respond to resuscitation – consider delivery.
- Refer to The British Association of Perinatal Medicine framework for the management of babies born extremely preterm (less than 26+0 weeks of gestation).

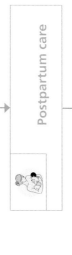

Intrapartum care

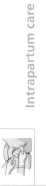

Intrapartum fetal monitoring

- Women in labour with active vaginal bleeding require continuous EFM. Provide continuous EFM in women who are in PTL whose pregnancies have been complicated by major APH or recurrent minor APH, or if there has been any clinical suspicion of an abruption.
- There is a lack of evidence to support continuous intrapartum fetal monitoring after APH. In women who have experienced one episode of minor APH, in which there have been no subsequent concerns regarding maternal or fetal wellbeing, intermittent auscultation is appropriate.
- Provide continuous EFM in women with minor APH with evidence of placental insufficiency (such as FGR or oligohydramnios).

Mode of anaesthesia

- Involve a consultant anaesthetist; the choice of anaesthesia is based on individual assessment. If the woman is haemodynamically stable, the magnitude of active bleeding will determine the appropriateness of regional anaesthesia.
- Regional anaesthetic is recommended for operative delivery unless there is a specific contraindication. Specific contraindications to regional anaesthesia relevant to APH include maternal cardiovascular instability and coagulopathy.
- In a case of APH where maternal or fetal condition is compromised and CS is required, consider a general anaesthetic to facilitate control of maternal resuscitation and to expedite delivery.
- In the case of severe fetal compromise but with a stable mother, it is reasonable to perform a general anaesthesia in the fetal interest to expedite rapid delivery.
- The optimal mode of anaesthesia will depend on the skill, expertise, and experience of the individual anaesthetist.

Management of the third stage of labour

- Anticipate PPH and provide active management of the third stage of labour.
- Consider ergometrine–oxytocin (Syntometrine) in the absence of hypertension.

Postpartum care

Postnatal issues

- Haemorrhage and blood transfusion are risk factors for VTE therefore commence thromboprophylaxis or reinstitute it as soon as the immediate risk of haemorrhage is reduced.
- Women at high risk of further haemorrhage (for example women with a coagulopathy) or women with continuing haemorrhage and in whom thromboprophylaxis is indicated may be more appropriately managed with unfractionated heparin and/or graduated compression stockings.
- Debriefing by an experienced obstetrician at the earliest possible time following delivery when the woman is able to comprehend and communicate.
- Provide a follow-up appointment at 4 to 6 weeks and contact numbers for access to medical and psychological support.

Neonate

- Major or massive APH (abruption and vasa praevia) may result in fetal anaemia and fetal compromise, therefore needs senior neonatologist review. Inform the neonatal staff of the likely diagnosis and extent of the blood loss so that arrangements for early neonatal blood transfusion can be made if necessary.
- In minor APH and continuing haemorrhage, it would be appropriate to request paediatric support at the time of delivery.
- In cases of vasa praevia, clamp the umbilical cord as soon as possible after delivery, and leave the longer part attached to the neonate so that umbilical artery catheterization is facilitated if required.

CHAPTER 30 Antepartum haemorrhage (APH)

Placental abruption

Prevention

- There is limited evidence to support interventions to prevent abruption.
- In view of the known associations between placental abruption and tobacco use, and cocaine and amphetamine misuse, advise and encourage women to modify these risk factors.
- Folic acid supplements:
  * Systematic review – no conclusive evidence of benefit in women who took folic acid supplements. An observational study reported that women who use folic acid and multivitamins during pregnancy are significantly less likely to develop placental abruption (OR 0.7).
- Antithrombotic therapy – there are no good data to support their role (low dose aspirin ± LMWH) in the prevention of abruption in women with thrombophilia. A pilot study of antithrombotic therapy in women with a previous placental abruption reported that women who received enoxaparin in the subsequent pregnancy experienced fewer placental vascular complications (including abruption, PET or LBW).

Risk factors

- Abruption is more likely to be related to conditions occurring during pregnancy and placenta praevia is more likely to be related to conditions existing prior to pregnancy.
- APH has a heterogeneous pathophysiology and cannot reliably be predicted. It is usually a sudden and unexpected obstetric emergency, not predictable by known reproductive risk factors.
- Approximately 70% of cases of placental abruption occur in low-risk pregnancies.

- Abruption in a previous pregnancy – 4.4% risk of recurrence after one previous pregnancy with abruption (OR 7.8) and 19–25% after previous pregnancies complicated by abruption.
- Risk of abruption later in the pregnancy increases with first trimester bleeding (OR 1.6) and when an intrauterine haematoma is identified on USS in the first trimester (RR 5.6).
- Threatened miscarriage increases the risk of placental abruption from 1% to 1.4% (OR 1.5).

- Other risk factors for placental abruption: PET, FGR, non-vertex presentations, polyhydramnios, advanced maternal age, multiparity, low BMI, pregnancy following ART, intrauterine infection, PROM, abdominal trauma (both accidental and from domestic violence), smoking, and drug misuse (cocaine and amphetamines) during pregnancy.

- Maternal thrombophilias – overall, thrombophilias are associated with an increased risk of placental abruption, but significant association is only observed with factor V Leiden (OR 4.7) and prothrombin 20210A (OR 7.7).
- Assess women for these and this information may be used to assign women to high-risk or low-risk antenatal care.

Placenta praevia

Definition and background

- **Placenta praevia** – when the placenta is inserted wholly or in part into the lower segment of the uterus.
- Ultrasound classification according to what is relevant clinically: if the placenta lies over the internal cervical os, it is considered a major praevia; if the leading edge of the placenta is in the lower uterine segment but not covering the cervical os, it is considered a minor or partial praevia.
- A morbidly adherent placenta includes placenta accreta, increta, and percreta as it penetrates through the decidua basalis into and then through the myometrium.

History

- Clinical suspicion – history of vaginal bleeding after 20 weeks of gestation (painless bleeding, or bleeding provoked by sexual intercourse).
- A high presenting part, an abnormal lie are suggestive of a low-lying placenta (LLP).
- The definitive diagnosis relies on USS.

Diagnosis

- **Offer routine USS (transabdominal scan) at 20 weeks to include placental localization.**
- TVS – improves the accuracy of placental localization and is safe. Confirm the suspected diagnosis of placenta praevia at 20 weeks by TVS. A second trimester TVS will reclassify 26–60% of cases where the abdominal scan diagnosed a low-lying placenta (sensitivity 87.5%, specificity 98.8%, PPV 93.3%, NPV 97.6%, and false negative rate 2.3%).

Risk factors

- Previous placenta praevia (OR 9.7).
- Previous CSs (RR 2.6; background rate 0.5%): 1 previous CS – OR 2.2; 2 previous CSs – OR 4; 3 previous CSs – OR 22.
- Previous termination of pregnancy.
- Multiparity; advanced maternal age (> 40 years).
- Multiple pregnancy; smoking; assisted conception.
- Deficient endometrium due to presence or history of: uterine scar, endometritis, manual removal of placenta, curettage, submucous fibroid.

Prevention

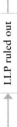

- There is limited evidence to support interventions to prevent placenta praevia.
- Avoid vaginal and rectal examinations in women with placenta praevia, and advise these women to avoid penetrative sexual intercourse.
- Cervical cerclage to prevent or reduce bleeding and prolong pregnancy is not supported by sufficient evidence.
- There is no place for the use of prophylactic tocolytics in women with placenta praevia to prevent bleeding.

LLP ruled out → **Routine care**

LLP

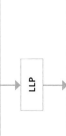

- Provide follow-up imaging. Placental 'apparent' migration, owing to the development of the lower uterine segment, occurs during the second and third trimesters, but is less likely to occur if the placenta is posterior or if there has been a previous CS. Although significant migration to allow vaginal delivery is unlikely if the placenta substantially overlaps the internal os, such migration is still possible.
- Women with a previous CS require a higher index of suspicion to exclude: placenta praevia and placenta accreta. Even with a partial 'praevia' at 20–23 weeks, the chance of persistence of the placenta praevia requiring abdominal delivery was 50% in women with a previous CS compared with 11% in those with no uterine scar.

Repeat TVS

- Asymptomatic women without a previous CS whose placenta has just reached but not covered the cervical os and in whom pregnancy is progressing normally – offer further imaging at 36 weeks.

- **Placenta accreta and major placenta praevia** – asymptomatic suspected major placenta praevia or if the placenta is anteriorly placed and reaching the os in a woman with a previous CS, making placenta accreta more likely – offer TVS at 32 weeks for earlier diagnosis to enable planning.
  - Of those women in whom the placenta is still low at 32 weeks of gestation, 73% will remain so at term, and up to 90% of major praevias at this gestation will persist.

- Symptomatic –women who bleed.

Arrange appropriate cervical management.

Diagnosis of morbidly adherent placenta

- Women who had a previous CS who also have an anterior placenta underlying the old CS scar at 32 weeks of gestation are at increased risk of placenta accreta. Manage as if they have placenta accreta, with appropriate preparations for surgery.
- Techniques to help diagnosis – USS and MRI.
- Consider MRI in equivocal cases to distinguish those women at special risk of placenta accreta.

USS

Greyscale:

- Loss of the retroplacental sonolucent zone.
- Irregular retroplacental sonolucent zone.
- Thinning or disruption of the hyperechoic serosa–bladder interface.
- Presence of focal exophytic masses invading the urinary bladder.
- Abnormal placental lacunae.

Colour Doppler:

- Diffuse or focal lacunar flow.
- Vascular lakes with turbulent flow (peak systolic velocity over 15 cm/s).
- Hypervascularity of serosa–bladder interface.
- Markedly dilated vessels over peripheral subplacental zone.

Three-dimensional power Doppler:

- Numerous coherent vessels involving the whole uterine serosa–bladder junction (basal view).
- Hypervascularity (lateral view).
- Inseparable cotyledonal and intervillous circulations, chaotic branching, detour vessels (lateral view).

MRI

- The role of MRI in diagnosing placenta accreta is still debated.
- Many authors recommend MRI for women in whom ultrasound findings are inconclusive. The main MRI features of placenta accreta include.
  * Uterine bulging.
  * Heterogeneous signal intensity within the placenta.
  * Dark intraplacental bands on T2-weighted imaging.

NICE – If LLP is confirmed at 32–34 weeks in women who have had a previous CS, offer colour-flow Doppler ultrasound as the first diagnostic test for morbidly adherent placenta. If it suggests morbidly adherent placenta:
- **MRI may help to diagnose morbidly adherent placenta and clarify the degree of invasion.**
- **MRI is safe, but there is a lack of evidence on long-term risks to the baby.**
- **Offer MRI if acceptable to the woman.**

Management of placenta praevia

Antenatal care

- Prevention and treatment of anaemia during the antenatal period.
- Counsel women in the third trimester about the risks of PTD, obstetric haemorrhage, and their care.

Place of care

- Encourage all women with major APH to remain close to the hospital for the duration of the third trimester of pregnancy.
- Conduct home-based care only within a research context.
- Provide outpatient care only after careful counselling, ensure close proximity with the hospital, and constant presence of a companion. Advise to attend hospital immediately if any bleeding, contractions or any pain (including vague suprapubic period-like aches).

Cervical cerclage

- Do not offer cervical cerclage to reduce bleeding and prolong pregnancy outside clinical trial.
- Cochrane Review – only one trial showed a possible benefit, with a reduction in the number of babies born before 34 weeks of gestation or weighing < 2 kg.

Tocolysis

- Tocolysis for treatment of bleeding due to placenta praevia may be useful in selected cases. Tocolysis was associated with prolongation of pregnancy and an increased birth weight. No adverse effects to mother or baby were shown, and particularly no increased risk of bleeding was found.
- Prophylactic terbutaline to prevent bleeding is not found to benefit women with placenta praevia.

Thromboembolism

- Prolonged inpatient care can be associated with an increased risk of VTE; encourage mobility, thromboembolic deterrent stockings, and adequate hydration.
- Prophylactic anticoagulation in women at high risk of bleeding can be hazardous; individualize the decision based on risk factors for VTE. Limiting anticoagulant thromboprophylaxis to those at high risk of VTE is reasonable.

Preparations before surgery

- Place of CS – unit with a blood bank and high-dependency care facilities.

Consent:

- Explain the risks associated with CS in general and the specific risks of placenta praevia in terms of MOH, the need for blood transfusion, and the chance of hysterectomy.
- Risk of MOH is approximately 12 times more likely with placenta praevia.
- The risk of hysterectomy is increased and rises when associated with previous CS.

- **Blood products** – make sure blood is readily available for the peripartum period.
  - If women have atypical antibodies, liaise with the local blood bank.
  - Do not offer autologous blood transfusion.
  - Consider cell salvage in women at high risk of MOH and women who refuse donor blood.
- **Interventional radiology** – consider uterine artery embolization in cases of uncontrolled MOH as it can be life saving and uterus sparing. The place of prophylactic catheter placement for balloon occlusion or in readiness for embolization if bleeding ensues requires further evaluation.

Delivery

Anaesthetic technique – The choice of anaesthesia for CS for placenta praevia and suspected placenta accreta must be made by the anaesthetist conducting the procedure. There is insufficient evidence to support one technique over another.

Mode of delivery

- Decide mode of delivery based on clinical judgement and USS information.
- As the lower uterine segment continues to develop beyond 36 weeks, there is a place for TVS to check if the fetal head is engaged prior to planned CS.
- USS – a woman with a placental edge < 2 cm from the internal os in the third trimester is likely to need delivery by CS, especially if the placenta is thick.

Time of delivery

- Do not offer elective CS in asymptomatic women before 38 weeks for placenta praevia, or before 36–37 weeks for suspected placenta accreta.
- Placenta praevia and placenta accreta are associated with 40% PTD before 38 weeks which results in neonatal morbidity, but equally waiting too long can increase the risk of perinatal mortality secondary to APH.

Care bundle

- For cases where there is a placenta praevia and a previous CS or an anterior placenta underlying the old CS scar. The 6 elements of care bundle are:
  * Consultant obstetrician to plan and directly supervise delivery.
  * Consultant obstetric anaesthetist to plan and directly supervise anaesthesia at delivery.
  * Blood and blood products available on-site.
  * Multidisciplinary involvement in pre-operative planning.
  * Discussion and consent includes possible interventions (such as hysterectomy, leaving the placenta in place, cell salvage, and intervention radiology).
  * Local availability of a level 2 critical care bed.

Grade of obstetrician

- A junior doctor should not be left unsupervised and a senior experienced obstetrician should be scrubbed in theatre. As a minimum, a consultant obstetrician and anaesthetist should be present within the delivery suite.
- Any woman going to theatre electively with suspected placenta praevia accreta should be attended by a consultant obstetrician and anaesthetist. When an emergency arises, consultant staff should be alerted and attend ASAP.

What not to do

- Vaginal examination – if placenta praevia is suspected.
- Kleihauer test for diagnosis of abruption.
- Continuous EFM if active obstetric intervention in the interests of the fetus is not planned, for example at gestations <26 + 0 weeks.
- Tocolysis in a woman presenting with a major APH, or who is haemodynamically unstable, or if there is evidence of fetal compromise.
- Tocolysis in placental abruption (it is also 'relatively contraindicated' in 'mild haemorrhage' due to placenta praevia).
- The calcium antagonist nifedipine for tocolysis.
- Folic acid supplements for prevention of APH.
- Antithrombotic therapy (low dose aspirin ± LMWH) for the prevention of abruption in women with thrombophilia.
- Cervical cerclage to prevent or reduce bleeding and prolong pregnancy.
- Prophylactic tocolytics in women with placenta praevia to prevent bleeding.
- Routine home-based care.
- Elective delivery by CS in asymptomatic women before 38 weeks for placenta praevia, or before 36–37 weeks for suspected placenta accreta.
- Use of autologous blood transfusion.
- The outcomes of prophylactic arterial occlusion require further evaluation.
- Routine methotrexate or arterial embolization.
- National screening programme for vasa praevia.
- Various tests to differentiate between fetal and maternal blood, as they are not applicable in the clinical situation.

Placenta accreta, increta, and percreta

Surgical approach

- Avoid going straight through the placenta to achieve delivery as it is associated with more bleeding and a high chance of hysterectomy.
- Consider opening the uterus at a site distant from the placenta, and delivering the baby without disturbing the placenta, in order to enable conservative management of the placenta or elective hysterectomy.
- The choice of skin and uterine incision needed to avoid the placenta will depend on the location of the placenta. It is therefore useful for the surgeon to perform an ultrasound scan before surgery to plot out the extent of placenta before starting. The antenatal diagnosis and surgical avoidance of the placenta, and its separation, may be associated with reduced maternal morbidity.
- Conservative management of placenta accreta when the woman is already bleeding is unlikely to be successful.

Placenta separates, or partially separates

- If the placenta separates, deliver it and deal with any PPH in the standard way.
- If the placenta partially separates, deliver the separated portion(s) and deal with any PPH in the normal way.
- Leave adherent portions attached as trying to separate them can cause severe bleeding.

Massive haemorrhage – See Chapter 54 Prevention and management of postpartum haemorrhage (PPH)

- Uterotonic agents and bimanual compression or aortic compression can buy time for extra help to arrive.
- Uterine and vaginal packing with gauze, balloon tamponade, the B-Lynch suture, vertical compression sutures, and suturing an inverted lip of cervix over the bleeding placenta bed.
- Uterine and internal iliac artery ligation have been reported but it makes subsequent access for intervention radiology techniques and embolization extremely difficult or impossible.
- Available evidence on prophylactic occlusion or embolization of pelvic arteries in the management of women with placenta accreta is equivocal. **Prophylactic arterial catheterization (with a view to embolization) could be considered where facilities permit.**

If placenta does not separate after delivery of the baby

- The placenta can be left in place and uterus closed with or without hysterectomy. Both options are associated with less blood loss than trying to separate it.
- Significantly reduced short-term morbidity (ICU admission, massive blood transfusion, coagulopathy, urological injury, re-laparotomy) if the placenta is left in place and hysterectomy performed electively compared with attempting to remove the placenta (36% vs 67%).
- Women desiring uterine preservation – leaving the placenta in place is an option.

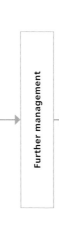

Further management

Management after placental retention

- Warn the woman of the risks of bleeding and infection postoperatively; prophylactic antibiotics may be helpful in the immediate postpartum period to reduce this risk.
- Risks – infection 18%, bleeding 35%, and DIC in 7%. Bleeding can start a few hours after surgery up until 3 months post-delivery.
- Do not offer routine methotrexate or arterial embolization as they do not reduce these risks. Review of the case reports – the outcomes for the women who received no additional treatment was the same as those receiving either methotrexate or embolization.

Follow-up

- USS and serum beta-hCG measurements. Weekly serum beta-hCG to check if it falls continuously, but since low levels do not guarantee complete placental resolution supplement it with imaging.
- Due to the protracted nature of recovery with complications occurring months after delivery – ensure regular review and ready access if the woman experiences any problems.
- Chance of success for a future pregnancy – there are insufficient data to make any firm prognosis about future pregnancy.

Vasa praevia

Definition and incidence

- Fetal vessels coursing through the membranes over the internal cervical os and below the fetal presenting part, unprotected by placental tissue or the umbilical cord.
- This can be secondary to a velamentous cord insertion in a single or bilobed placenta (vasa praevia type 1), or from fetal vessels running between lobes of a placenta with one or more accessory lobes (vasa praevia type 2).
- Incidence – 1 in 2000 to 6000 pregnancies, but the condition may be under-reported.

Risks or complications

- When the fetal membranes are ruptured (spontaneously or artificially), the unprotected fetal vessels are at risk of disruption with consequent fetal haemorrhage.
- Because the fetal blood volume is around 80–100 ml/kg, the loss of relatively small amounts of blood can have major implications for the fetus.
- The mortality rate is around 60%, although significantly improved survival rates of up to 97% have been reported where the diagnosis has been made antenatally.

Screening

- Although vasa praevia is detectable by USS, there remains insufficient information on the case definition, natural history, and epidemiology of the condition. The accuracy and practical application of the screening test has not been elucidated in the general pregnant population. There is currently no agreed management pathway for those with confirmed vasa praevia. Taking all of this into account, there is uncertainty about the balance of benefit versus harm to be derived from screening all pregnant women with a view to offering CS to those at risk.
- **The UK National Screening Committee does not recommend a national screening programme for vasa praevia.**

Risk factors

- Placental anomalies such as a bilobed placenta or succenturiate lobes where the fetal vessels run through the membranes joining the separate lobes together.
- History of low-lying placenta in the second trimester.
- Multiple pregnancy and IVF where the incidence of vasa praevia has been reported to be as high as 1 in 300. The reasons for this association are not clear, but disturbed orientation of the blastocyst at implantation, vanishing embryos, and the increased frequency of placental morphological variations have been postulated.
- The incidence of velamentous cord insertion in an unselected population is around 1%, and that of bilobed or succenturiate placenta is around 1.7%, two-thirds of which have a velamentous cord insertion. The reported coexistence of velamentous cord insertion and vasa praevia has been reported to be between 2 and 6%. Adding the other groups thought to be at increased risk of vasa praevia, i.e., multiple pregnancies, IVF conceptions, and those with a low-lying placenta, a significant minority of women will be identified as being at increased risk of vasa praevia.

Clinical features

In the absence of vaginal bleeding:

- Antenatal period – there is no method to diagnose vasa praevia clinically.
- Intrapartum period – vasa praevia can occasionally be diagnosed by palpation of fetal vessels in the membranes at the time of vaginal examination. However, high index of suspicion is necessary if one feels something unusual and to confirm the diagnosis prior to membrane rupture.
- Direct visualization using an amnioscope has some use, but this only gives visual access to the area of membranes exposed by the dilated cervix.
- Very rarely, FHR abnormalities in the absence of bleeding may be present secondary to compression of the fetal vessels by the fetal presenting part.

In the presence of vaginal bleeding:

- Vasa praevia often presents with fresh vaginal bleeding at the time of membrane rupture and FHR abnormalities. More rarely, bleeding can occur in the absence of membrane rupture.

Tests to differentiate between fetal and maternal bleeding

- **Various tests exist that can differentiate between fetal and maternal blood, but they are often not applicable in the clinical situation.**
- The Kleihauer–Bekte test and haemoglobin electrophoresis accurately identify fetal cells in the maternal circulation and fetal haemoglobin. Both can detect the presence of fetal haemoglobin in concentrations as low as 0.01%, and both can be used to identify fetal cells in vaginal blood loss. The disadvantage – they are laboratory-based tests that take a significant amount of time before a result is obtained, thus rendering them of little use in this clinical situation.
- The resistance of fetal haemoglobin to denaturation with alkali has been used by various methods to identify fetal bleeding. Lindqvist and Gren described a simpler bedside test using 0.14 M sodium hydroxide solution, which denatures adult haemoglobin, turning it a brownish-green colour, while fetal haemoglobin is resistant to denaturation and retains its red colour. This method may have some applicability in the clinical situation but requires further validation.

Ultrasound scan

- Vasa praevia can be accurately diagnosed with colour Doppler TVS. The ultrasound appearance of vasa praevia is of linear echolucent structures overlying the cervix. The use of colour Doppler improves the diagnostic accuracy.
- Factors such as maternal obesity, scarring, and fetal position can influence accuracy, and care must be taken not to mistake cord presentation for vasa praevia. Using both the abdominal and vaginal routes of scanning and changing maternal position can improve diagnostic accuracy.
- In cases with the diagnosis made antenatally, the perinatal outcome is significantly better than those diagnosed acutely.

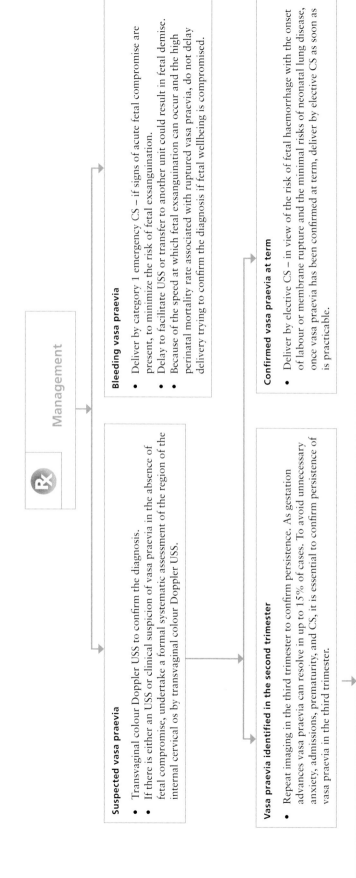

Management

Suspected vasa praevia

- Transvaginal colour Doppler USS to confirm the diagnosis.
- If there is either an USS or clinical suspicion of vasa praevia in the absence of fetal compromise, undertake a formal systematic assessment of the region of the internal cervical os by transvaginal colour Doppler USS.

Vasa praevia identified in the second trimester

- Repeat imaging in the third trimester to confirm persistence. As gestation advances vasa praevia can resolve in up to 15% of cases. To avoid unnecessary anxiety, admissions, prematurity, and CS, it is essential to confirm persistence of vasa praevia in the third trimester.

Confirmed vasa praevia in the third trimester

- Antenatal admission from 28 to 32 weeks of gestation to a unit with appropriate neonatal facilities will facilitate quicker intervention in the event of bleeding or labour.
- In view of the increased risk of PTD, consider corticosteroids for fetal lung maturity.
- Outpatient management may be possible if there is no evidence of cervical shortening on TVS and there are no symptoms of bleeding or preterm uterine activity.
- Laser ablation in utero may have a role in the treatment of vasa praevia.

Bleeding vasa praevia

- Deliver by category 1 emergency CS – if signs of acute fetal compromise are present, to minimize the risk of fetal exsanguination.
- Delay to facilitate USS or transfer to another unit could result in fetal demise.
- Because of the speed at which fetal exsanguination can occur and the high perinatal mortality rate associated with ruptured vasa praevia, do not delay delivery trying to confirm the diagnosis if fetal wellbeing is compromised.

Confirmed vasa praevia at term

- Deliver by elective CS – in view of the risk of fetal haemorrhage with the onset of labour or membrane rupture and the minimal risks of neonatal lung disease, once vasa praevia has been confirmed at term, deliver by elective CS as soon as is practicable.

- Deliver by elective CS prior to the onset of labour, between 35 and 37 weeks of gestation, when the risks of prematurity have significantly decreased.

Consent – caesarean section for placenta praevia

Discuss

- Explain the procedure.
- **Intended benefits** – the aim of the procedure is to secure the safest route of delivery to avoid the anticipated risks to the mother and/or baby of the heavy bleeding that would occur during labour and attempted vaginal delivery owing to the position of the placenta. These would be much greater than the risks of routine elective CS.
- **Procedure – the benefits and risks of any available alternative treatments, including no treatment.**
- The procedure involves delivery of the baby and placenta through an open approach using an abdominal incision and an incision into the uterus. Both incisions are usually transverse. Inform the woman of the reasons and the added risks if either a midline abdominal incision or a classic uterine incision is being considered.
- Discuss the reason for the CS and the great risk to mother and baby of not performing the CS. An informed, competent woman may choose the no-treatment option, i.e., she may refuse CS even when this would be detrimental to her own health or the wellbeing of her fetus. In such a situation every attempt must be taken to ensure the woman and her birth partner realize the critical importance of the CS in this specific situation.
- Other procedures, which may be appropriate but not essential at the time, such as ovarian cystectomy/oophorectomy – discuss and record woman's wishes.
- Form of anaesthesia planned.

Complications –differ from those of a CS performed in the presence of a normally sited placenta

- **Serious risks:**

Maternal –

In all women with placenta praevia:
  * Emergency hysterectomy – up to 11/100.
  * Need for further laparotomy during recovery – 75/1000.
  * Thromboembolic disease – up to 3/100.
  * Bladder or ureteric injury – up to 6/100.
  * Future placenta praevia – 23/1000.
  * MOH – 21/100.

In women with placenta praevia and previous CS:
  * emergency hysterectomy – up to 27/100.

In women with an abnormally adherent placenta:
  * Hysterectomy is highly likely; it may be safer to leave the placenta inside the uterus or to perform a planned caesarean hysterectomy to avoid heavy bleeding than to attempt removal.

- **Frequent risks:**

Maternal
  * Admission to intensive care.
  * Infection.
  * Blood transfusion.

Fetal
  * Admission to NICU.
  * Surgical and anaesthetic risks are increased in those with obesity, who have significant pathology, who have had previous surgery or who have pre-existing medical conditions.

Extra procedures

- Any extra procedures which may become necessary – repair of damage to bowel, bladder or blood vessels.
- Where placenta accreta is suspected owing to the combination of placenta praevia and previous CS and/ or imaging information, discuss the following (where available):
  * Cell salvage: reduces the small risk of transmission of infection and transfusion reactions associated with the use of donated blood; however, there is a theoretical risk of maternal sensitization to the baby's blood and rarely amniotic fluid embolism.
  * Interventional radiology: occludes the uterine blood vessels by cannulation of the femoral artery under X-ray screening. Foam plugs, balloons or coils are passed through these cannulas to block the vessels and control bleeding, either temporarily or permanently. The risks of it should be discussed by the radiologist in advance.

Risks

Very common	1/1 to 1/10
Common	1/10 to 1/100
Uncommon	1/100 to 1/1000
Rare	1/1000 to 1/10000
Very rare	Less than 1/10000

Placenta Praevia, Placenta Praevia Accreta and Vasa Praevia: Diagnosis and Management. RCOG Green-top Guideline No. 27; January 2011.
Caesarean section. NICE CGN 132, 2011.
Caesarean Section for Placenta Praevia. RCOG Consent Advice No. 12; December 2010.

CHAPTER 31 Preterm prelabour rupture of membranes (PPROM)

Prevalence and background

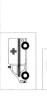

- PPROM complicates 2% of pregnancies but is associated with 40% of preterm deliveries.
- Women with intrauterine infection deliver earlier than non-infected women.
- There is an association between ascending infection from the lower genital tract and PPROM.
- In patients with PPROM, about one-third of pregnancies have positive amniotic fluid cultures, and studies have shown that bacteria have the ability to cross intact membranes.

Risks

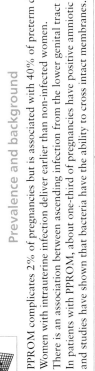

Neonatal –
- Prematurity, sepsis, and pulmonary hypoplasia leading to neonatal morbidity and mortality.
- Infants born with sepsis have a mortality rate 4 times higher than those without sepsis.

Maternal –
- Preterm delivery.
- Chorioamnionitis.

History and examination

- **History** of rapid passage of fluid from the vagina.
- **Sterile speculum** – pooling of fluid in the posterior vaginal fornix.
- **Avoid V/E** – micro-organisms may be transported from vagina into the cervix, leading to intrauterine infection, prostaglandin release, and PTL.
- History with speculum examination has similar accuracy to the other tests, therefore sufficient to make a diagnosis.

Investigations

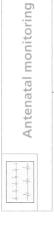

- USS in some cases confirms the diagnosis by oligohydramnios.
- Nitrazine test – detects pH change – sensitivity of 90% and a false positive rate 17%.
- Ferning test – sensitivity of 90%, false positive rate 6%.
- AmniSure – rapid immunoassay, sensitivity, and specificity of 99% and 100%, respectively.
- FBC, CRP, and HVS are commonly performed by many clinicians.

Antenatal monitoring

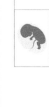

Maternal

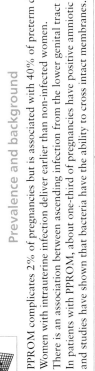

- Observe for **signs** of clinical chorioamnionitis – maternal pyrexia (>37.8°C), tachycardia, leucocytosis, uterine tenderness, offensive vaginal discharge, and fetal tachycardia (rate > 160) – **monitor maternal temperature, pulse, and FHR every 4 to 8 hours.**
- It is not necessary to carry out weekly maternal FBC or CRP because the sensitivity of these tests in the detection of intrauterine infection is low.
- Leucocytosis – the sensitivity and FPR range from 29 to 47% and 5 to 18%, respectively.
- CRP – the specificity is 38–55%.

Fetal

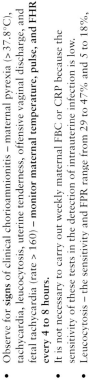

- **Non-invasive tests** to differentiate fetuses that are not infected and will benefit from remaining in utero from those who are infected and need to be delivered – overall the tests are of limited value.
- CTG – fetal tachycardia predicts 20–40% of cases of intrauterine infection with a FPR of about 3%. Fetal tachycardia, if present, may represent a late sign of infection.
- **Do not offer** BPP scoring or Dopplers (raised systolic/diastolic ratio in **umbilical artery**) as first-line surveillance or diagnostic tests for fetal infection, since they are of limited value in differentiating between fetuses with and without infection.

Management

Prophylactic routine antibiotics

- Reduces maternal and neonatal morbidity, delays delivery, allowing sufficient time for prophylactic prenatal corticosteroids to take effect.
- Systematic review – use of antibiotics is associated with a significant reduction in chorioamnionitis, neonatal infection, numbers of babies born within 48 hours and 7 days, and the number of babies with an abnormal cerebral USS prior to discharge from hospital. There is no significant reduction in PNM although there is a trend for reduction.
- Avoid co-amoxiclav as it increases the risk of neonatal necrotizing enterocolitis.
- Erythromycin is the antibiotic of choice.
- If GBS is isolated – give antibiotics in line with GBS intrapartum prophylaxis guidelines.

Antenatal corticosteroids

- Give to women with PPROM between 24 and 34 weeks of gestation.
- Systematic review – antenatal corticosteroids reduce the risks of RDS, IVH, and necrotizing enterocolitis and may also reduce the risk of neonatal death.
- They do not appear to increase the risk of infection in either mother or baby.

Tocolysis

- Do not offer prophylactic tocolysis if there is no uterine activity.
- Therapeutic tocolysis – consider in women with PPROM and uterine activity who require intrauterine transfer or antenatal steroids.
- In the absence of clear evidence that tocolysis improves neonatal outcome following PPROM it is reasonable not to use it. It is possible that tocolysis could have adverse effects, such as delaying delivery from an infected environment.

Fibrin sealants

- Do not offer as routine treatment for second-trimester oligohydramnios caused by PPROM.
- The 'amniopatch' resulted in an increase in amniotic fluid volume in some cases. Larger studies are needed to examine neonatal outcome before this treatment can be recommended.

Transabdominal amnioinfusion

- Do not offer as a method of preventing pulmonary hypoplasia in very preterm PPROM outside the research context.
- There are no significant differences between amnioinfusion and no amnioinfusion for CS, low Apgar scores, and neonatal death.

Outpatient monitoring

- Only after a period of 48–72 hours of inpatient observation.
- Advise women to take their temperature twice daily and inform them of the symptoms associated with infection.
- There are insufficient data to make recommendations of home, day care, and outpatient monitoring rather than continued hospital admission.

Time of delivery

- **To deliver vs expectant management** – assess the risks related to the development of intrauterine infection compared with the gestational age-related risks of prematurity.

Immediate delivery

If any signs of chorioamnionitis or fetal distress.

Conservative management

- Studies have demonstrated benefits in conservative management for gestations of < 34/40, whereas the management of pregnancy complicated by PPROM between 34 and 37/40 continues to be debated.

PPROM before 34 weeks

- Conservative management.
- Consider delivery at 34 weeks.

PPROM between 34 and 37 weeks

- Further research is needed to elucidate the optimal gestational age at delivery for women with PPROM between 34 and 37/40.
- Current data question the benefit of continued expectant management beyond 34 weeks of gestation. There is little evidence that intentional delivery after 34 weeks adversely affects neonatal outcome, whereas the expectant management beyond 34 weeks is associated with an increased risk of chorioamnionitis. Therefore consider delivery.

What not to do

- VE in suspected PPROM.
- Rely on any single test to diagnose or rule out chorioamnionitis.
- Prophylactic amoxicillin (risk of necrotizing enterocolitis).
- Amniocentesis.
- Fibrin sealants as routine treatment for second-trimester oligohydramnios caused by PPROM.
- Transabdominal amnioinfusion as a method of preventing pulmonary hypoplasia in very preterm PPROM.

Preterm Prelabour Rupture of Membranes. RCOG Green-top Guideline No. 44; November 2006 (minor amendment October 2010).

CHAPTER 32 Preterm labour (PTL)

Prevalence and background

- Birth at less than 37+0 weeks of gestation and more than 23 completed weeks of gestation. It is the most important single determinant of adverse infant outcome in terms of both survival and quality of life.
- 30–40% of all cases of preterm births (PTB) are the result of elective delivery for a maternal or a fetal complication. The remaining 60–70% of PTBs occur due to spontaneous PTL and/or PPROM.
- PTB complicates about 3% of pregnancies before 34 weeks and 7–12% before 37 weeks.
- In the UK, infant mortality among PTBs is 42/1000 live births, compared with 5/1000 live births overall. For very PTBs (< 32+0 weeks of gestation), mortality in the first year is 144/1000 live births, compared with 1.8/1000 live births for babies born at term (38+0 to 41+6 weeks).
- Very PTB accounts for 1.4% of UK births but 51% of infant deaths.

Risks

- Leading cause of perinatal death and disability.
- Risk of death or neurosensory disability increases with decreasing gestational age.
- Mortality increases from about 2% for infants born at 32 weeks to more than 90% for those born at 23 weeks. Although birth at 32 to 37 weeks is associated with less risk than very PTB, even this moderately PTB is associated with increased risk of infant death.
- Psychosocial and emotional effects on the family, and increased cost for health services.

Risk factors

- History – previous history of PTB.
- Symptomatic UTI.
- Smoking.
- Uterine developmental anomalies.
- History of cervical trauma.
- Asymptomatic bacteriuria.
- Bacterial vaginosis.
- Multiple pregnancy.

Prevention

- High-risk women identified in early pregnancy can be targeted for more intensive antenatal surveillance and prophylactic interventions.
- When women present with symptoms of threatened PTL, if the likelihood of having a spontaneous PTB can be determined, interventions can be deployed to prevent or delay birth and to improve subsequent neonatal mortality/morbidity.
- Unfortunately, few tests offer useful predictive value.
- Fetal fibronectin is promising, however has limited accuracy in predicting PTB within 7 days for women with symptoms of PTL.
- USS assessment of cervical length is promising for symptomatic women.
- It is unclear whether any predictive test, or combination of tests, is sufficiently accurate to be cost effective.

Health Technology Assessment – screening for PTL

Test accuracy reviews – for the prediction of spontaneous preterm birth (SPTB)

History –
- Previous history of SPTB for predicting SPTB before 34 weeks' gestation – LR for a positive test result (LR+) of 4.62 and a LR for a negative test result (LR−) of 0.68.

In asymptomatic antenatal women:
- For predicting SPTB before 34 weeks' gestation – only a few tests reach LR+ estimates > 5 putting them in the useful tests category:
  - * Ultrasonographic cervical length (USCL) and funnelling measurement.
  - * Cervicovaginal fetal fibronectin screening.
- Tests with LR− estimates of < 0.2 were:
  - * Detection of uterine contraction (home uterine monitoring device).
  - * Amniotic fluid CRP.

In symptomatic women with threatened PTL, tests with LR+ point estimate > 5 and LR− point estimate < 0.2 were:
- For predicting SPTB within 2–7 days:
  - * Absence of fetal breathing movements.
  - * USCL and funnelling.
  - * Amniotic fluid interleukin-6 (IL-6).
  - * Serum CRP.
- For predicting SPTB before 34 or 37 weeks' gestation:
  - * Cervicovaginal fetal fibronectin.

Cervicovaginal fetal fibronectin (fFN)

- A glycoprotein, which is usually undetectable in the cervicovaginal secretion; a higher quantity is purported to be an indication of imminent labour onset. The test is available as a commercial rapid test kit. A cotton swab is used to collect samples of cervicovaginal secretions during a speculum examination. The result is either positive or negative, obtained within 10–15 minutes.
  - * **Asymptomatic women –** > before 34 weeks – LR+ of 7.65, and LR− of 0.80.
    > before 37 weeks – LR+ of 3.17 and LR− of 0.87.
  - * **Symptomatic women –** > within 7–10 days – LR+ of 4.10 and LR− of 0.35.
    > before 34 weeks – LR+ 3.58 and LR− of 0.34.
    > before 37 weeks – LR+ 3.62 and LR− of 0.50.

Antenatal USCL and cervical funnelling

- **USCL –** there is a wide variation in the gestation at which USCL measurement was carried out and the definition for thresholds of abnormality. The most common gestation at which USCL measurement was carried out was in the late second trimester, between 20 and 24 weeks and the most common threshold used in asymptomatic women was 25 mm; and 15 mm in symptomatic women to predict SPTB within 7 days.
- **Cervical funnelling screening** has variable LRs depending on the chosen threshold.

Asymptomatic women
- **Ultrasound cervical length (USCL)**
  - * Predicting SPTB before 34 weeks – performed before 20 weeks using a threshold of 25 mm – LR+ of 13.38 and LR− of 0.80.
  - * Predicting SPTB before 37 weeks – measured between 20 and 24 weeks using a threshold of 32.5 mm, it had LR+ of 3.99 and LR− 0.33.
- **Cervical funnelling –** performed between 20 and 24 weeks, using a threshold of 25 mm – LR+ 4 and LR− 0.68.

Symptomatic women
- **Ultrasound cervical length (USCL)**
  - * Within 7 days – for the most commonly used threshold (<15 mm) – LR+ 8.61 and LR− 0.026.
  - * Before 34 weeks – for the most commonly used threshold (<30 mm) – LR+ 1 and LR− 0.30.
  - * Before 37 weeks –
    > Using a threshold < 18 mm – LR+ 3.36 and LR− 0.35.
    > With a threshold < 30 mm – LR+ 2.29 and LR− 0.29.
- **Cervical funnelling –**
  - * For predicting SPTB before 34 weeks – LR+ 4.70 and LR− 0.61.
  - * For predicting SPTB before 37 weeks – LR+ 2.53 and LR− 0.86.

Health Technology Assessment – screening for PTL – conclusion

- In preventing SPTB, it may be difficult from a clinical and patient perspective to distinguish between false-positive and false-negative results and so the optimal screening or testing modality will be one which minimizes both false-positive (high LR+) and false-negative (low LR−) results.
- Given the quality, level, and precision of the accuracy evidence, no single test emerged as a front runner in predicting SPTBs when the test result was positive, nor to exclude it when the test result was negative.
- Currently, considering cost-effectiveness, there are no practical recommendations for prevention of SPTB with testing performed before preventative treatment.

Risk factors and interventions for women at risk of PTL – Health Technology Assessment

Antibiotics

Others

Asymptomatic bacteriuria

- Occurs in 5–10% of pregnancies and is associated with an increased risk of SPTB and a LBW infant.
- Antibiotic therapy is effective in preventing PTB at <37 weeks and in reducing the incidence of pyelonephritis.
- Effectiveness of different duration of antibiotics is unclear.

Symptomatic UTI

- UTIs, including pyelonephritis, occur in up to 8% of pregnancies. UTIs are associated with an increased risk of SPTB and neonatal infection.
- Because of the lack of placebo/no treatment comparators, summary RRs are not available for the decision analysis for the use of antibiotics.
- There is no significant differences between different antibiotic regimens in incidence of SPTB <37 weeks, admission to NICU or other perinatal and maternal outcomes.
- Overall, ampicillin and gentamicin appear to be the most promising treatment combination but the evidence to support this is limited.

Bacterial vaginosis (BV)

- Asymptomatic BV is present in up to 35% of pregnancies. It has been linked to an increased risk of poor pregnancy outcome including PTD.
- Antibiotic therapy does not significantly affect the incidence of SPTB birth before 34 weeks, perinatal mortality or admission to NICU.
- SPTB before 37 weeks is significantly reduced in the subgroup of women with intermediate vaginal flora as well as BV.

Periodontal care

- One trial – when compared with no treatment, periodontal therapy reduced the incidence of SPTB before 37 weeks.

- Prophylactic antibiotics
- Infections, such as maternal genital tract infection or colonization by some infectious organisms, have been implicated in the aetiology of PTB, and associated with maternal and perinatal mortality and morbidity.
- A strategy of routine antibiotic prophylaxis has been suggested as an alternative to routine antenatal detection and treatment of infections.
- No beneficial effect of antibiotic prophylaxis was reported for incidence of SPTB <37 weeks or the risk of perinatal mortality in high-risk women.
- No data were reported for PTB <34 weeks or requirement of NICU admissions.

Antioxidants – supplementation with vitamin C or zinc does not significantly reduce the risk of SPTB <37 weeks, admission to NICU or perinatal mortality. These results do not support the prophylactic use of antioxidants for the prevention of SPTB.

Energy and protein intake – there is insufficient evidence to support the use of energy and protein intake interventions.

Fish oil supplements – compared to placebo/no treatment, marine oil supplementation was shown to reduce the incidence of SPTB before 34 and 37 weeks but no statistically significant differences were seen on the incidence of neonatal mortality or admission to NICU.

Smoking cessation programmes in pregnancy – smoking cessation programmes significantly reduce the incidence of SPTB <37 weeks and LBW (<2500 g) infants but there is no difference in the perinatal mortality.

Antenatal educational programmes – SPTB prevention educational programmes do not reduce the incidence of SPTB or neonatal mortality compared to no intervention.

Home uterine monitoring – no statistically significant difference is shown for the incidence of SPTB <34 weeks or 37 weeks or admission to NICU in women who received home uterine activity monitoring compared to controls.

Home visits – the results do not support a beneficial effect of home visits for the inhibition of SPTB.

Bed rest – no difference was shown between women prescribed bed rest and women who received no treatment for risk of SPTB <37 weeks.

Elective cervical cerclage

- 2 RCTs demonstrated a small but significant reduction in the incidence of SPTB <34 weeks in women receiving cerclage. No differences were found for incidence of SPTB <37 weeks gestation, or perinatal mortality.

Progestational agents

- Studies reported a reduction in risk of SPTB <34 and 37 weeks. No statistically significant difference was found for incidence of perinatal mortality. Further research is needed regarding the use of vaginal progesterone in the prevention of SPTB. (RCOG)

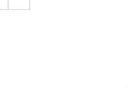

Guideline comparator – the use of progesterone for prevention of preterm birth

SOGC – recommendations

- Inform women about the lack of data for many neonatal outcome variables and about the lack of comparative data on dosing and route of administration. Inform women with short cervix of the single large RCT showing the benefit of progesterone in preventing PTL.
- A previous PTL and/or short cervix (<15 mm at 22–26 weeks) on TVS could be used as an indication for progesterone therapy. Start the therapy after 20 weeks and stop when the risk of prematurity is low.
- Use the dosage:
  * For prevention of PTL in women with history of previous PTL – 17 alpha-hydroxyprogesterone 250 mg IM weekly or progesterone 100 mg daily vaginally.
  * For prevention of PTL in women with short cervix of <15 mm detected on TVS at 22–26 weeks – progesterone 200 mg daily vaginally.

ACOG committee opinion

- Offer progesterone supplementation for the prevention of recurrent PTB to women with a singleton pregnancy and a prior SPTB or PROM.
- Current evidence does not suggest routine use of progesterone in women with multiple gestation.
- Consider progesterone supplementation for asymptomatic women with incidentally identified very short cervical length (<15 mm); however do not offer routine cervical length assessment.
- Progesterone has not been studied as a supplemental treatment to cervical cerclage for suspected cervical insufficiency, as a preventive agent for asymptomatic women with a positive cervico-vaginal fetal fibronectin screen result and it should not be used at this time for this indication alone.
- The optimum formulation for progesterone is not known.

Cervical cerclage (RCOG)

Background

- Cervical cerclage is performed in women with a history of mid-trimester loss or SPTB suggestive of cervical 'incompetence', with the aim of preventing recurrent loss.
- Cervical incompetence (CI) is an imprecise clinical diagnosis applied to women with a history where it is assumed that the cervix is weak and unable to remain closed during the pregnancy.
- CI is likely to be a continuum influenced by factors related not solely to the intrinsic structure of the cervix but also to processes driving premature effacement and dilatation.
- While cerclage may provide a degree of structural support to a 'weak' cervix, its role in maintaining the cervical length and the endocervical mucus plug as a mechanical barrier to ascending infection may be more important.

Time of procedure

Asymptomatic women/elective

- **A. History-indicated cerclage:**
  * Insertion of a cerclage as a result of factors in a woman's obstetric or gynaecological history that increase the risk of spontaneous second-trimester loss (STL) or PTB – performed as a prophylactic measure in asymptomatic women and normally inserted electively at 12–14 weeks of gestation.
- **B. Ultrasound-indicated cerclage:**
  * Insertion of a cerclage as a therapeutic measure in cases of cervical length shortening seen on TVS.
  * Performed on asymptomatic women who do not have exposed fetal membranes in the vagina.
  * Sonographic assessment of the cervix is usually performed between 14 and 24 weeks of gestation.

Symptomatic women/emergency

- **C. Rescue cerclage** – insertion of cerclage as a salvage measure in the case of premature cervical dilatation with exposed fetal membranes in the vagina. This may be discovered by USS of the cervix or as a result of a speculum/physical examination performed for symptoms such as vaginal discharge, bleeding or 'sensation of pressure'.

Prepregnancy diagnosis of cervical weakness

Prepregnancy techniques (e.g., hysterography, cervical resistance indices, insertion of cervical dilators) to assess cervical weakness:
- Studies are all observational.
- The largest study of cervical resistance indices (force required to dilate the cervix to 8 mm) reported that women with a history of STL had a lower cervical resistance index than parous women with no such history ($P < 0.001$). In this study all women with a history of low cervical resistance index had a suture inserted, with a successful pregnancy outcome in 75%. This rate is no higher than that expected with expectant management and the absence of a control group makes it inappropriate to draw any evidence-based conclusions on its usefulness.
- **Insufficient evidence to recommend the use of prepregnancy diagnostic techniques aimed at diagnosing 'cervical weakness' in women with a history of PTB/STL in the decision to place a history-indicated cerclage.**

Procedures

- Transvaginal cerclage (McDonald) – a transvaginal purse-string suture placed at the cervicovaginal junction, without bladder mobilization.
- High transvaginal cerclage (Shirodkar) – a transvaginal purse-string suture placed following bladder mobilization, to allow insertion above the level of the cardinal ligaments.
- Transabdominal cerclage – a suture performed via a laparotomy or laparoscopy, placing the suture at the cervicoisthmic junction.
- Occlusion cerclage – occlusion of the external os by placement of continuous non-absorbable suture to help retention of the mucus plug.

Cervical cerclage

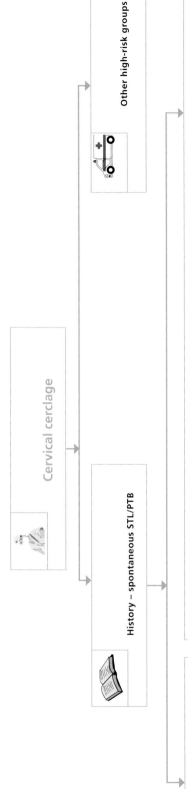

Other high-risk groups

History – spontaneous STL/PTB

Singleton pregnancy with no history of STL/PTB

- Meta-analysis (4 RCTs) of cerclage versus expectant management in women with a short cervix – no evidence of benefit of cerclage in women with cervical length <25 mm who had no other risk factors for SPTB.
- The insertion of an ultrasound-indicated cerclage is not recommended in women without a history of STL/PTB who have an incidentally identified short cervix of 25 mm or less.

A. Women with a history of spontaneous STL/PTB

- 3 RCTs compared history-indicated cerclage with expectant management.
- Largest trial MRC/RCOG Trial –
  * Fewer deliveries < 33 weeks in the cerclage group compared with the controls (13% vs 17%; RR 0.75) – NNT 25. No significant difference in fetal/neonatal outcome. Insufficient data to allow any conclusions to be drawn as to whether women were more likely to benefit if the previous loss had features suggestive of cervical incompetence (e.g., painless cervical dilatation or PPROM).
  * Subgroup analyses – only women with a history of ≥ 3 pregnancies ending < 37 weeks benefitted from cerclage, which halved the incidence of PTB < 33 weeks of gestation (15% vs 32%).
  * No effect was observed in those with:
    > 1 previous delivery < 33 weeks (14% vs 17%).
    > 2 previous deliveries < 33 weeks (12% vs 14%).
    > Previous cervical surgery or first-trimester loss/uterine anomaly.
- Offer history-indicated cerclage to women with ≥ 3 previous PTB/STL.
- Do not offer it routinely to women with ≤ 2 previous PTB/STL.
- Characteristics of the previous adverse event, such as painless dilatation of the cervix or rupture of the membranes before the onset of contractions, or additional risk factors, such as cervical surgery, are not helpful in the decision to place a history-indicated cerclage.

Women (singleton pregnancy) with a history of spontaneous STL/PTB who have not undergone a history-indicated cerclage

Serial sonographic surveillance

- Where serial sonographic surveillance of cervical length is carried out – 40–70% of women maintain a cervical length of > 25 mm before 24 weeks of gestation; > 90% of these women delivered after 34 weeks of gestation. This suggests that serial sonographic surveillance may differentiate between women with a prior STL/PTB who might benefit from cerclage and women who do not need intervention.
- Offer these women serial sonographic surveillance, as there is evidence to suggest that those who experience cervical shortening are at an increased risk of subsequent STL/PTB and may benefit from ultrasound-indicated cerclage, while those whose cervix remains long have a low risk of STL/PTB.

Expectant management

- In the MRC/RCOG study, women with a history of 1, 2, or 3 or more previous STLs or SPTBs had an 83%, 86%, and 68% chance of delivery after 33 weeks when managed expectantly, respectively.
- Expectant management is a reasonable alternative since there is a lack of direct evidence to support serial sonographic surveillance over expectant management. Furthermore, the majority of women with a history of STL/PTB will deliver after 33 weeks of gestation.

B. Ultrasound-indicated cerclage

- Meta-analysis (4 RCTs) – in the subgroup of women with singleton pregnancies with a history of STL (16–23 weeks) or birth <36 weeks; when compared with expectant management, cerclage resulted in a significant reduction in delivery before 35 weeks of gestation.

- There are no studies evaluating ultrasound-indicated cerclage performed solely on the presence of funnelling. However, studies have demonstrated that funnelling is a function of cervical shortening and does not appear to independently add to the risk of PTB associated with cervical length.

- Offer women with a history of one or more spontaneous STL or PTBs who are undergoing TVS surveillance of cervical length an ultrasound-indicated cerclage if the cervix is ≤25 mm before 24 weeks of gestation.

- Do not offer ultrasound-indicated cerclage for funnelling of the cervix (dilatation of the internal os on USS) in the absence of cervical shortening to ≤25 mm.

Cervical cerclage in other groups considered at increased risk of SPTB

Multiple pregnancies

- Ultrasound-indicated cerclage – subgroup analysis from meta-analysis of twin pregnancies demonstrated a doubling in delivery rates before 35 weeks of gestation with the ultrasound-indicated cerclage compared with expectant management in women with a cervical length < 25 mm. It may also be associated with increased perinatal mortality.

- History-indicated cerclage in twin pregnancies – one study demonstrated that cerclage was not effective in prolonging gestation or improving fetal outcome.

- Do not offer the insertion of a history- or ultrasound-indicated cerclage in women with multiple pregnancies as there is some evidence to suggest it may be detrimental and associated with an increase in PTB and pregnancy loss.

Uterine anomalies and cervical trauma

- Ultrasound-indicated cerclage – subgroup analysis from meta-analysis of women with a history of cone biopsy or more than one dilatation and evacuation showed no difference in PTB before 35 weeks. There were insufficient women with müllerian anomalies to perform subgroup analyses.

- History-indicated cerclage – the MRC/RCOG study subgroup analysis of women with a history of cone biopsy or cervical amputation showed no significant difference in delivery before 33 weeks of gestation in the cerclage group compared with the expectant group (19% vs 22%).

- Do not offer history- or ultrasound-indicated cerclage in other high-risk groups such as women with müllerian anomalies, previous cervical surgery (cone biopsy, LLETZ, laser ablation or diathermy) or multiple dilatation and evacuation.

- Individualize the decision to place a concomitant cerclage at radical trachelectomy.

C. Rescue cerclage

Indications

- Individualize decision taking into account the gestation as even with rescue cerclage the risks of severe PTD and neonatal mortality and morbidity remain high.
- Insertion of a rescue cerclage may delay delivery by a further 5 weeks on average compared with expectant management.
- It may be associated with a 2-fold reduction in the chance of delivery before 34 weeks of gestation.
- However, there are limited data to support an associated improvement in neonatal mortality or morbidity.
- Advanced dilatation of the cervix (> 4 cm) or membrane prolapse beyond the external os is associated with a high chance of cerclage failure.

Gestation at which cerclage can be offered

- There is no clear evidence that the gestation at which the cerclage is inserted affects the magnitude of prolongation in gestation; however, in cases presenting before 20 weeks of gestation, insertion of a rescue cerclage is highly likely to result in a PTD before 28 weeks.
- Individualize the decision to place a rescue cerclage beyond 24 weeks of gestation and take into account the local gestational age of viability.
- Improvements in neonatal intensive care have advanced the gestational age of viability to 24 weeks of gestation in most developed countries and, given the potential risk of iatrogenic membrane rupture and subsequent PTD, rescue cerclage can rarely be justified after this gestation.

Contraindications

- Active preterm labour.
- Clinical evidence of chorioamnionitis.
- Continuing vaginal bleeding.
- PPROM.
- Evidence of fetal compromise.
- Lethal fetal defect.
- Fetal death.

Transabdominal cerclage

Transabdominal vs transvaginal cerclage

- A transabdominal cerclage is usually inserted following a failed vaginal cerclage or extensive cervical surgery.
- Systematic review of transabdominal versus transvaginal cerclage in women with a prior failed transvaginal cerclage:
  * A lower risk of perinatal death/delivery before 24 weeks of gestation (6% vs 12.5%) in women who had undergone transabdominal cerclage compared with those who had a repeat insertion of transvaginal cerclage.
  * However, there is a higher incidence (3.4% vs 0%) of serious operative complications (bleeding requiring transfusion, injury to bladder/bowel/uterine artery, anaesthesia problems).
- Consider insertion of a transabdominal cerclage in women with a previous failed transvaginal cerclage, but this may be associated with increased maternal morbidity.
- There is no evidence to support a laparoscopic approach over laparotomy in the insertion of an abdominal cerclage.

Preconceptual transabdominal cerclage

- There are no studies directly comparing the insertion of a preconceptual transabdominal cerclage with insertion in early pregnancy.
- However, consider preconceptual insertion when possible because of the technical advantage of operating on the uterus of a woman who is not pregnant.
- There is no evidence that preconceptual transabdominal cerclage has any detrimental impact on fertility or management of early miscarriage.
- Abdominal cerclage can be safely left in place if a further pregnancy is desired.
- Transabdominal cerclage can be performed preconceptually or in early pregnancy.

Delayed miscarriage/fetal death in women with an abdominal cerclage

- Successful evacuation through the stitch by suction curettage or by dilatation and evacuation (up to 18 weeks of gestation) has been described; alternatively, the suture may be cut, usually via a posterior colpotomy.
- Failing this, a hysterotomy may be required or caesarean section may be necessary.

Cervical cerclage – procedure

Preoperative investigations

- Before a history-indicated cerclage – arrange a first-trimester USS and screen for aneuploidy to ensure both viability and the absence of lethal/major fetal abnormality. Arrange an anomaly scan prior to ultrasound-indicated/rescue cerclage.
- Do not routinely use maternal white cell count and CRP to detect subclinical chorioamnionitis. Decide to perform these tests based on the overall clinical picture. Do not delay rescue cerclage in the absence of clinical signs of chorioamnionitis.
- **Amniocentesis** – there is insufficient evidence to recommend routine amniocentesis before rescue or ultrasound-indicated cerclage. In selected cases where there is suspicion of intra-amniotic infection, amniocentesis may be performed to aid the decision, as the presence of infection is associated with a poor prognosis. Amniocentesis before rescue cerclage does not appear to increase the risk of PTD before 28 weeks of gestation.
- **Routine genital tract screening for infection** – there is an absence of data to support routine genital tract screening. Give a complete course of antimicrobial eradication therapy before cerclage insertion in the presence of a positive culture from a genital swab.

Potential complications

- A doubling in risk of maternal pyrexia but no apparent increase in chorioamnionitis.
- Not associated with an increased risk of PPROM, IOL or CS.
- Not associated with an increased risk of PTD or STL.
- A small risk of intraoperative bladder damage, cervical trauma, membrane rupture, and bleeding is reported but these are rare (<1%).
- Shirodkar cerclage usually requires anaesthesia for removal and therefore carries the risk of an additional anaesthetic.
- May be associated with a risk of cervical laceration/trauma if there is spontaneous labour with the suture in place. Cervical laceration requiring suturing at the time of delivery was reported in 11% of Shirodkar and 14% of McDonald procedures, which was higher than that reported in other deliveries (2%).
- Several case series have reported high risks of membrane rupture and infection associated with rescue cerclage; however, the lack of a control group makes it difficult to separate the procedure-related risk from that inherent to the underlying condition.

Operative issues

- Perioperative tocolysis – do not offer routine perioperative tocolysis.
- Perioperative antibiotics at the discretion of the operating team.
- Mode of anaesthesia at the discretion of the operating team.
- Hospital stay elective transvaginal cerclage can be safely performed as a day-case procedure. Women undergoing ultrasound-indicated or rescue cerclage, given the higher risk of complications such as PPROM, early PTD, miscarriage and infection, may benefit from at least a 24-hour postoperative period of observation in hospital. In women undergoing insertion of transabdominal cerclage via laparotomy, offer an inpatient stay of at least 48 hours.
- Choice of suture material and the choice of transvaginal cerclage technique (Shirodkar vs McDonald) at the discretion of the surgeon.
- There is no evidence to support the placement of two purse-string sutures over a single suture and to support the placement of a cervical occlusion suture in addition to the primary cerclage.

Postoperative management

- Do not advise bed rest routinely; individualize the decision based on clinical circumstances and the potential adverse effects of bed rest.
- Do not advice abstinence from sexual intercourse routinely. There are no studies on this issue; there is no evidence that sexual intercourse in early pregnancy increases the risk of PTD in women with a PTB.
- Do not offer routine serial sonographic measurement of the cervix; it may be useful in individual cases following ultrasound-indicated cerclage to offer timely administration of steroids or in utero transfer. A postoperative upper cervical length (closed cervix above the cerclage) of <10 mm before 28 weeks of gestation provides the best prediction of subsequent PTD before 36 weeks following the placement of an ultrasound-indicated cerclage.
- Do not routinely offer repeat cerclage when cervical shortening is seen postcerclage. It may be associated with an increase in both pregnancy loss and delivery before 35 weeks of gestation.
- Do not offer routine fetal fibronectin testing postcerclage. High NPV of fetal fibronectin testing for subsequent delivery at <30 weeks of gestation in asymptomatic high-risk women with a cerclage in place may provide reassurance to women and clinicians in individual cases. However, the increased false-positive rate of fetal fibronectin testing in such women makes the finding of a positive result less useful.
- Do not offer routine progesterone supplementation following cerclage.

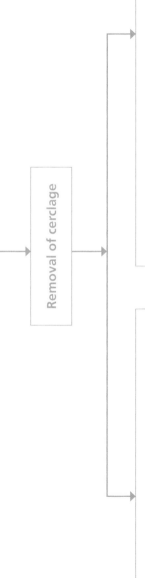

Removal of cerclage

Time of removal

- Remove transvaginal cervical cerclage before labour, usually between 36 and 37 weeks of gestation (owing to the potential risk of cervical injury in labour and the minimal risk to a neonate born at this gestation), unless delivery is by elective CS, in which case suture removal could be delayed until this time.
- In women presenting in established PTL, remove the cerclage to minimize potential trauma to the cervix.
- A Shirodkar suture will usually require anaesthesia for removal.
- All women with a transabdominal cerclage require delivery by CS, and the abdominal suture may be left in place following delivery.

PPROM

- PPROM between 24 and 34 weeks and without evidence of infection or PTL:
  * Consider delaying removal of the cerclage for 48 hours, to provide a course of prophylactic steroids for fetal lung maturation and/or arrange in utero.
  * Delayed removal (> 24 hours) is associated with significantly more women delivering >48 hours after presentation (96% vs 54%) compared with immediate removal, accompanied by a trend towards lower neonatal mortality (4% vs 11%). There is no higher rate of maternal infection (44% vs 22%) and neonatal sepsis (16% vs 5%).
- Do not delay suture removal until labour ensues or delivery, as it is associated with an increased risk of maternal/fetal sepsis.
- PPROM before 23 weeks and after 34 weeks given the risk of neonatal and/or maternal sepsis and the minimal benefit of 48 hours of latency in pregnancies with PPROM before 23 and after 34 weeks; delayed suture removal is unlikely to be advantageous in this situation.

H Honest, CA Forbes, KH Durée, G Norman, SB Duffy, A Tsourapas, TE Roberts, PM Barton, SM Jowett, CJ Hyde, and KS Khan. Screening to prevent spontaneous preterm birth: systematic reviews of accuracy and effectiveness literature with economic modelling.; Health Technology Assessment 2009;13: No. 43

Clinical Practice Guideline; Ultrasonographic Cervical Length Assessment in Predicting Preterm Birth in Singleton Pregnancies: SOGC No. 257. J Obstet Gynaecol Can 2011;33(5):486–499.

Assessment of Risk Factors for Preterm Birth: Practise Bulletin. Clinical Guidelines for Obstetrician and Gynaecologists; ACOG No. 31; Oct 2011.

Committee Opinion – Use of Progesterone in Reducing Preterm Birth. ACOG No. 419; Oct 2008.

Cervical Cerclage. Green-top Guideline RCOG No. 60; May 2011.

CHAPTER 33 Preterm labour: tocolysis and antenatal corticosteroids

Background – tocolysis compared with no treatment or placebo

Tocolysis for prevention of preterm labour

- Systematic review – tocolytic drugs – ritodrine, isoxuprine, terbutaline, magnesium sulphate, indomethacin, and atosiban.
  * Tocolytics were associated with a reduction in the odds of birth within 24 hours (OR 0.47), 48 hours (OR 0.57), and 7 days (OR 0.60). These effects were statistically significant for beta-agonists, indomethacin, and atosiban but not for magnesium sulphate.
  * However, use of any tocolytic drug was not associated with a statistically significant reduction in births <30 weeks (OR 1.33), <32 weeks (OR 0.81) or <37 weeks of gestation (OR 0.17).

Tocolytic drugs reduce the proportion of births occurring up to 7 days but with no significant effect on PTB.

Tocolytic drug to prevent perinatal or neonatal death and neonatal morbidity

- Tocolysis is not associated with a statistically significant reduction in perinatal mortality nor in neonatal morbidity, such as RDS or IVH.
- Plausible explanations for the lack of effect of tocolytic drugs on substantive perinatal outcomes:
  * Trials may have included too many women who were so advanced in gestation that any further prolongation of pregnancy would have little potential to benefit the baby.
  * Trials may have included too many women who were not genuinely in PTL.
  * Time gained by tocolytic treatment may not have been used to implement potentially beneficial measures, such as corticosteroids or transfer to a unit with better neonatal health services.
  * There may be direct or indirect adverse effects of tocolytic drugs (including prolongation of pregnancy when this is detrimental to the baby), which counteract their potential gain.

There is no clear evidence that tocolytic drugs improve outcome and therefore it is reasonable not to use them. However, consider tocolysis if the few days gained would be put to good use, such as completing a course of corticosteroids or in utero transfer.

Tocolytic drug

- Beta-agonists (ritodrine) reduce risk of giving birth within 48 hours compared with placebo, but there is no evidence that they are more effective than other tocolytic drugs at preventing PTB.
- Calcium channel blockers (nifedipine) compared with other tocolytic drugs are associated with a reduction in the number of women giving birth within 7 days of treatment and before 34 weeks of gestation (Cochrane review). Compared with beta-agonists, nifedipine is associated with improvement in neonatal outcome, although there are no long-term data.
- Oxytocin receptor agonist (atosiban) compared with beta-agonists – no difference between the groups either in birth within 48 hours or birth within 7 days.
- COX inhibitors (indomethacin) – reduce birth before 37 weeks of gestation (Cochrane review). Short-term use of NSAIDs in the third trimester of pregnancy is associated with a significant increase in the risk of premature ductal closure.
- No evidence that COX-2 inhibitors (rofecoxib) reduce the risk of PTB.
- Nitric oxide donor (nitroglycerine – although there was a reduction in births before 37 weeks of gestation, there was no clear impact on birth before 32–34 weeks of gestation.
- Magnesium sulphate – no clear evidence that it reduces the risk of PTB. However, it reduces the risk of cerebral palsy.
- Nifedipine and atosiban have comparable effectiveness in delaying birth for up to 7 days.

Multiple pregnancy

- Insufficient evidence about whether or not tocolysis leads to any benefit in PTL in multiple pregnancy.
- Case reports – an association between nifedipine use in multiple pregnancy and pulmonary oedema, suggesting that atosiban may be preferable to nifedipine in this context, although not confirmed in a prospective cohort study.

Indications for tocolysis

- Consider tocolysis for women with suspected PTL with otherwise uncomplicated pregnancy.
- In the absence of clear evidence that tocolytic drugs improve outcome following PTL, it is reasonable not to use them.
- Any contraindication to prolonging pregnancy is a contraindication to tocolytic therapy – known lethal congenital or chromosomal malformation, intrauterine infection, severe PET, placental abruption, advanced cervical dilatation, and evidence of fetal compromise or placental insufficiency.
- Relative contraindications – mild haemorrhage due to placenta praevia, non-reassuring CTG or FGR.
- Choose the drug which is most effective with the fewest adverse effects, both immediate and long-term.
- Women most likely to benefit from use of a tocolytic drug are those who are in very preterm labour, those needing transfer to a hospital with NICU, and those who need a full course of corticosteroids.

Tocolytics – adverse effects

Maternal

- Ritodrine has a high frequency of unpleasant and sometimes severe or potentially life-threatening adverse effects. Women allocated beta-agonists were far more likely to stop treatment because of adverse effects than those allocated placebo.
  - Common side effects – palpitations, tremor, nausea, vomiting, headache, chest pain, dyspnoea.
  - Rare but serious and life-threatening adverse effects – reports of a small number of maternal deaths. Pulmonary oedema usually associated with aggressive intravenous hydration.
- Calcium channel blockers – fewer side effects and less need to stop treatment.
- Nifedipine – flushing, palpitations, nausea and vomiting, and HT. Contraindicated in women with cardiac disease; use with caution in diabetes or multiple pregnancy due to the risk of pulmonary oedema.
- Atosiban – nausea, vomiting, headache, chest pain, dyspnoea, and injection site reactions. Women are more likely to stop treatment because of adverse effects. Diabetes and cardiac disease are not contraindications to atosiban.
- COX inhibitors are well tolerated by women.
- Avoid using more than one tocolytic in combination as it increase the risk of adverse effects.
- Nifedipine, atosiban, and COX inhibitors have fewer adverse effects compared with beta-agonists.

Recommended dose regimens

- No clear consensus on the ideal dose regimen for nifedipine.
- Nifedipine – initial oral dose of 20 mg followed by 10–20 mg 3–4 times daily, adjust according to uterine activity for up to 48 hours. A total dose above 60 mg appears to be associated with a 3- to 4-fold increase in side effects, such as headache and hypotension.
- Atosiban – initial bolus dose of 6.75 mg over 1 minute, followed by an infusion of 18 mg/hour for 3 hours, then 6 mg/hour for up to 45 hours (to a maximum of 330 mg).
- For both, duration of treatment is 48 hours.

Maintenance tocolytic therapy

- Insufficient evidence on whether or not maintenance tocolytic therapy following threatened PTL is worthwhile. Do not offer maintenance therapy.

Fetal/neonatal

- Calcium channel blockers:
  * Associated with less neonatal RDS, less necrotizing enterocolitis and less IVH than other tocolytic drugs. No difference in SBs or neonatal deaths.
  * Nifedipine – no specific congenital defects have been associated with its use.
  * Atosiban – no difference in neonatal deaths or neonatal morbidity.
- COX inhibitors – premature closure of the ductus arteriosus with consequent pulmonary HT, persistent patent ductus arteriosus, necrotizing enterocolitis, and IVH.
- Magnesium sulphate – increases risk of fetal, neonatal or infant death.
- Insufficient data on long-term follow-up for reliable conclusions about the effects on the baby for any of these tocolytic drugs.

- Nifedipine and atosiban have comparable effectiveness, with fewer maternal side effects and less risk of rare serious adverse events than alternatives such as ritodrine or indomethacin.
- Limited evidence that use of nifedipine, rather than a beta-agonist, is associated with improved short-term neonatal outcome.
- Little information on the long-term growth and development of the children for any of the drugs.
- Although the use of nifedipine for PTL is an unlicensed indication, it has the advantages of oral administration and a low purchase price.

Antenatal corticosteroids (ANCS) to reduce neonatal morbidity and mortality

Safety

- Use of a single course of ANCS does not appear to be associated with any significant short-term maternal or fetal adverse effects. Evidence on the longer-term benefits and risks shows no difference in adverse neurological or cognitive effects.
- Insufficient evidence on the longer-term benefits and risks of multiple courses of ANCS. Increasing the number of glucocorticoid exposures, for the purpose of enhancing lung maturation prior to PTB, is associated with reduced birth weight and behavioural disorders at 3 years of age. There was a non-significant higher risk of cerebral palsy among children who had been exposed to repeat doses of ANCS.

Contraindications

- In a woman with systemic infection, they may theoretically suppress the immune response to infection. There is no evidence to suggest that a single course of ANCS would have a profound effect in women with systemic infection, but be cautious in women with systemic infection including tuberculosis or sepsis.
- Clinical chorioamnionitis is significantly associated with both cystic periventricular leucomalacia and cerebral palsy. With chorioamnionitis, a course of ANCS may be started, but do not delay delivery if indicated by maternal or fetal condition.

Benefits

- Cochrane review – in women at risk of PTB, a single course of ANCS reduces the risk of neonatal death by 31%, RDS by 44%, and intraventricular haemorrhage (IVH) by 46%.
- ANCS use is also associated with a reduction in necrotizing enterocolitis, respiratory support, NICU, and systemic infections in the first 48 hours of life.
- ANCS enhance the efficacy of neonatal surfactant therapy and reduce the cost and duration of NICU.

Timing of the effect of the drug

- ANCS are most effective in reducing RDS in pregnancies that deliver 24 hours and up to 7 days after administration of the second dose. No reduction in neonatal death, RDS or IVH is seen in infants delivered >7 days after treatment with ANCS. ANCS use reduces neonatal death even when infants are born <24 hours after the first dose has been given.
- ANCS use reduces neonatal death within the first 24 hours; therefore give if delivery is expected within this time.

Dose and route of administration

- Betamethasone 12 mg IM two doses or dexamethasone 6 mg IM four doses. As long as 24 mg of either drug is given within a 24- to 48-hour period, any dosing regimen can be used.
- Cochrane review – betamethasone causes a larger reduction in RDS than dexamethasone. Dexamethasone may decrease the incidence of IVH compared with betamethasone.
- Comparison of oral vs IM administration of dexamethasone – oral administration increased the incidence of neonatal sepsis.

Repeat courses of ANCS

- Multiple courses of steroids may lead to possible harmful effects including growth delay, brain developmental delay, lung development problems, necrotizing enterocolitis, maternal and neonatal sepsis, adrenal gland insufficiency, and placental infarction. Weekly repeat courses of ANCS reduce the occurrence and severity of neonatal respiratory disease, but the short-term benefits are associated with a reduction in weight and head circumference. Do not offer weekly repeat courses. Consider a repeat rescue course with caution in pregnancies where the first course was given at <26 weeks and another obstetric indication arises later in pregnancy. This would be justified by the paucity of data on the efficacy of the current dosing regimens on babies <26 weeks.

Indications – gestational age

34+6 and 38+6 weeks – give ANCS to all women in whom an elective CS is planned prior to 38+6 weeks of gestation.

24+0 and 34+6 weeks
- Offer a single course of ANCS to women between 24+0 and 34+6 weeks of gestation who are at risk of PTB (iatrogenic or spontaneous).
- Despite the paucity of data at earlier gestations, the reduction in outcomes other than RDS at 26+0 weeks of gestation would suggest that there is some benefit in corticosteroid prophylaxis at earlier gestations between 24+0 and 26+0 weeks.
- EPICure study – babies born at <26+0 weeks assessed at 2.5 years and assessed at 6 years – ANCS was associated with an increased mental development index.

<24+0 weeks
- Consider ANCS for women between 23+0 and 23+6 weeks of gestation who are at risk of PTB.

Indications – other groups

Prophylactic steroids
- There is no evidence to support a practice of prophylactic steroids in women with a previous history of PTD or multiple pregnancy who show no signs of PTB.

Women undergoing elective CS
- Compared with elective CS births at 39 weeks, births at 37 and at 38 weeks are associated with an increased risk of a composite outcome of neonatal death and/or respiratory complications, hypoglycaemia, newborn sepsis, and admission to the NICU. Give ANCS to reduce the risk of respiratory morbidity in babies delivered by elective CS prior to 38+6 weeks. This has been shown to reduce the need for admission to the NICU.

Multiple pregnancy
- Offer a single course of ANCS treatment to women with multiple pregnancy at risk of imminent PTD between 24+0 and 34+6 weeks.
- Although there are limited data to support the use of ANCS in multiple pregnancy, the overall improvement in outcomes in singleton fetuses would suggest that steroids could be beneficial in multiple pregnancy.

Diabetes mellitus
- It is not a contraindication to ANCS for fetal lung maturation.
- Provide women who have impaired glucose tolerance or diabetes and who are receiving ANCS with additional insulin and monitor closely.
- Maternal hyperglycaemia can adversely affect fetal lung maturity. It is possible that any benefit of ANCS could be offset by corticosteroid-induced hyperglycaemia.

Fetal growth restriction
- Offer a single course of ANCS to pregnancies affected by FGR between 24 and 35+6 weeks and at risk of delivery.
- Case–control study of infants between 26 and 32 weeks with FGR secondary to placental insufficiency – survival without disability or handicap at 2 years of age was better in the ANCS group than in the control group who did not receive ANCS.
- The benefits from ANCS for early preterm growth-restricted infants appear to outweigh the possible adverse effects.

Antenatal magnesium sulphate (AMS) to prevent cerebral palsy (CP) following preterm birth

Prevalence and background

- While the survival of infants born preterm has improved, the prevalence of CP has risen. Incidence of CP decreases significantly with increasing gestational age: 15% at 22–27 weeks, 6% at 28–31 weeks, 0.7% at 32–36 weeks, and 0.1% at term. 25% of all cases of CP are in infants born at < 34 weeks.
- In children born preterm the proportion whose CP is considered to have a perinatal origin (49%) is greater than in those born at term (35%).
- Infants born to mothers given magnesium sulphate to prevent eclamptic seizures or as tocolysis showed a reduction in rates of cystic periventricular leucomalacia (PVL) and CP (OR 0.14).
- The exact mechanism of action of magnesium as a neuroprotective agent is unknown.
- Cochrane review – AMS given to women at risk of PTB reduces the risk of CP in children (RR 0.68). There is also a significant reduction in the rate of substantial gross motor dysfunction (RR 0.61).
- Australian/SOGC guidelines – in women at risk of early PTB use AMS for neuroprotection of the fetus, infant, and child.

- **Maternal side effects** – 70% reported side effects such as flushing, nausea and vomiting, sweating, and injection site problems. 50% increase in hypotension and tachycardia is reported. Rarely in those with neuromuscular disorders it can result in muscle weakness and paralysis. There is no evidence of maternal death, cardiac respiratory arrest, pulmonary oedema, respiratory depression, severe PPH or increase in CS rates.
- When given in conjunction with calcium channel antagonists, cardiovascular and neuromuscular effects may be exaggerated.

RCOG opinion

- AMS given to mothers shortly before delivery reduces the risk of CP and protects gross motor function in preterm birth. The effect may be greatest at early gestations and is not associated with adverse long-term fetal or maternal outcome.
- There is an increase in minor side effects.
- Issues against its use – one study showed adverse neonatal outcomes following AMS; the lack of a statistically significant difference in primary outcome measures from all the RCTs; and a large NNT for benefit, compared with ANCS to improve neonatal lung function.
- Issues for its use – meta-analyses show that AMS reduces CP and motor deficits, no matter what the original indication for AMS administration. Unlike steroids that need to be administered up to 24 hours before PTB to have their optimal effect, AMS has a much more rapid neuroprotective effect, making it more widely relevant. Major maternal adverse effects are uncommon.

Dose and timing of administration

- Loading dose varied between 4 and 6 g. Some trials administered a maintenance infusion with varied doses: 1 g/hr, 2 g/hr or 2–3 g/hr. Meta-analysis confirmed that the beneficial effect of AMS on CP persisted in those studies using lower doses.
- Australian guideline – IV 4 g loading dose over 20–30 minutes followed by a 1 g/hr maintenance regime to continue for 24 hours or until birth, whichever occurs sooner.
- Discontinue therapy if birth was not achieved within 12 hours.
- The Australian guideline – commence infusion at least 4 hours before birth but agrees that there may still be a benefit if given less than 4 hours before delivery.
- In situations where delivery needs to be expedited for reasons of maternal or fetal wellbeing, it should not be delayed solely for AMS administration.
- **Gestation at administration** – The gestational age at which AMS has its greatest effect is debated. As perinatal and neonatal factors are more prominent in the aetiology of CP in less mature infants, an intervention is more likely to be effective at earlier gestations. The NNT increases significantly with advancing gestational age.
- Australian guidelines – consider AMS in women at <30 weeks of gestation.

SOGC recommendations

- Active labour with ≥ 4 cm of cervical dilatation, with or without PPROM or planned PTB for fetal or maternal indications – consider AMS for fetal neuroprotection for PTB (≤31+6 weeks).
- Consider AMS for fetal neuroprotection from viability to ≤31+6 weeks.
- Consider tocolysis, if AMS is started for fetal neuroprotection.
- Dose – 4 g IV loading dose, over 30 minutes, followed by a 1 g/hr maintenance infusion until birth. Discontinue AMS if delivery is no longer imminent or a maximum of 24 hours of therapy has been administered.
- For planned PTB, start AMS within 4 hours before birth.
- Insufficient data on repeat course of AMS.
- Provide continuous fetal heart surveillance. Be aware of hypotonia or apnoea since magnesium sulphate has the potential to alter the neonate's neurological evaluation.
- AMS may be administered before tocolytic drugs have been cleared from the maternal circulation. If nifedipine has been used for tocolysis or hypertension, there is NO contraindication to the use of AMS for fetal neuroprotection.
- Monitoring of serum Mg levels is NOT required.

Antibiotics, preterm labour, and cerebral palsy (CP)

Prevalence and background

- Cerebral palsy – a group of disorders that can involve brain and nervous system functions such as movement, learning, hearing, seeing, and thinking. Most common cause of motor disability in childhood, with a prevalence of 1.5–3 cases per 1000 births.
- The risk of cerebral palsy is inversely proportional to gestational age; the prevalence of cerebral palsy is 80 times higher in infants born prior to 28 weeks compared to those born at term.
- PTB is the strongest known risk factor for cerebral palsy.
- Many children who were born preterm without disability develop significant behavioural and educational difficulties. There may be a link between fetal infections and other neurological and psychiatric conditions during childhood and in adults.

Link between infection and cerebral palsy

- Infection/inflammation is commonly associated with PTB (particularly with ruptured membranes) especially at less than 30 weeks of gestation.
- The high risk of brain injury in preterm infants could be directly related to the intrauterine hostile inflammatory environment. A higher risk of brain injury in infants born preterm with spontaneous onset of labour (high frequency of infection) compared with physician-initiated delivery (low frequency of infection) has been reported.
- Funisitis, high cytokines in amniotic fluid and fetal blood are associated with white matter injury and cerebral palsy.
- Systematic review – clinical chorioamnionitis is associated with white matter injury and cerebral and histological chorioamnionitis with periventricular leucomalacia.
- Infection/inflammation may not exert adverse effects alone but it may sensitize the immature brain to hypoxia–ischaemia and other insults.
- Although a causal link has been proposed between antibiotics and cerebral palsy, no direct association has been demonstrated.

Short-term effect of antenatal antibiotics

- Subclinical infection is implicated in a large proportion of PTB - antibiotics could eradicate the infection, prolong the pregnancy, and improve neonatal outcome; alternatively, antibiotics might suppress the infection, prolong the pregnancy, but leave the fetus in a hostile inflammatory environment.
- **Asymptomatic women at risk of PTL**
  * Meta-analysis of antibiotic treatment showed no reduction in PTB. Antibiotics may increase PTB and routine treatment is therefore not recommended.
  * Bacterial vaginosis has been confirmed as a risk factor for PTB, maternal infectious morbidity, and miscarriage; yet trials of antibiotic therapy during the antenatal period to reduce these complications have yielded conflicting results.
- **Symptomatic women in PTL**
  * Cochrane review – the use of antibiotics following PPROM is associated with statistically significant reductions in chorioamnionitis and the numbers of babies born within 48 hours and 7 days. The following markers of neonatal morbidity were reduced: neonatal infection, use of surfactant, oxygen therapy, and abnormal cerebral ultrasound scan, although no reduction in perinatal mortality was observed. Co-amoxiclav was associated with an increased risk of neonatal necrotizing enterocolitis.
  * Cochrane review – the use of antibiotics for women with spontaneous PTB (with intact membranes) was associated with a reduction in maternal infection but had no benefit on neonatal outcomes. There was a suggestion of harm with a near significant increase in neonatal mortality in the antibiotic group.

Longer term effects of antibiotics on childhood outcomes

- **For children whose mothers had PPROM** – antibiotics seemed to have little effect on health and educational attainment. It might be linked to the length of antibiotic exposure which was fairly short, since about 60% gave birth within a week.
- **For children whose mothers had spontaneous PTL with intact membranes** –
  * Erythromycin (with or without co-amoxiclav) was associated with an increase in the proportions of children with any level of functional impairment from 38% to 42% and proportion of children with CP increased from 1.7% to 3.3% associated with erythromycin and from 1.9% to 3.2% with co-amoxiclav. More children who developed CP had been born to mothers who had received both antibiotics.
  * Antibiotic-treated spontaneous PTL group – it may be related to an ongoing low-grade antenatal neurological insult. This is because despite later birth, the injury is consistent with a more preterm origin.

RCOG opinion

- **Women with clinical infection** – treat with antibiotics since clinical chorioamnionitis is an important cause of maternal, fetal, and neonatal death.

- **Women with spontaneous PTL with intact membranes and no evidence of overt infection** –
  * Do not routinely prescribe antibiotics because there is evidence that antibiotics given under these circumstances increase the risk of functional impairment and CP in children.
  * Women with spontaneous PTL and intact membranes may be at increased risk of GBS infection. However, the RCOG does not recommend routine prophylaxis in this situation.

- **Women with PPROM and without evidence of overt infection** –
  * Current guidance endorses the routine use of antibiotics for women with PPROM in the acute situation.
  * Balance the benefits in some short-term outcomes (prolongation of pregnancy, reductions in infection, need for surfactant, oxygen therapy, and fewer babies with abnormal cerebral ultrasound) against a lack of evidence of benefit in perinatal mortality and longer term outcomes.
  * Given the lack of any long-term demonstrable benefit, a decision not to prescribe antibiotics to women with PPROM without evidence of infection is also reasonable, especially in a high-income setting where support is available.
  * There may be a stronger argument for routine antibiotic treatment in low income settings, where access to other interventions (antenatal steroids, surfactant therapy, ventilation, and antibiotic therapy) may be low.
  * Erythromycin is the antibiotic of choice after being tested by the ORACLE.
  * Avoid co-amoxiclav in women at risk of PTL due to increased risk of neonatal necrotizing enterocolitis.
  * Do not prescribe antibiotics unless a definite diagnosis of PPROM is made.

What not to do

- Tocolysis to prolong pregnancy in known lethal congenital or chromosomal malformation, intrauterine infection, severe PET, placental abruption, advanced cervical dilatation and evidence of fetal compromise or placental insufficiency.
- Tocolysis is relatively contraindicated in mild haemorrhage due to placenta praevia, non-reassuring CTG, FGR.
- Routine use of tocolysis to prevent PTL in multiple pregnancy.
- Do not use Nifedipine in women with cardiac disease, use it with caution in diabetes or multiple pregnancy due to the risk of pulmonary oedema.
- Avoid using more than one tocolytic in combination as it increases the risk of adverse effects.
- Do not offer maintenance tocolytic therapy.
- Women with spontaneous PTL with intact membranes and no evidence of overt infection – do not routinely prescribe antibiotics; do not offer routine GBS prophylaxis.
- Avoid co-amoxiclav in women at risk of PTL.
- Do not prescribe antibiotics unless a definite diagnosis of PPROM is made.

Clinical Practice Guideline: Magnesium Sulphate for Fetal Neuroprotection; SOGC No. 258, May 2011.

Tocolysis for Women in Preterm Labour. RCOG Green-top Guideline No. 1b; February 2011.

Antenatal Corticosteroids to Reduce Neonatal Morbidity and Mortality. RCOG Green-top Guideline No. 7; October 2010.

Magnesium Sulphate to Prevent Cerebral Palsy Following Preterm Birth. RCOG Scientific Advisory Committee Opinion Paper 29; August 2011.

Preterm Labour, Antibiotics, and Cerebral Palsy. RCOG Scientific Impact Paper No. 33; February 2013.

SL Kenyon, DJ Taylor, W Tarnow-Mordi. Broad-spectrum antibiotics for preterm, prelabour rupture of fetal membranes: the ORACLE I randomised trial. ORACLE Collaborative Group. Lancet 2001 – europepmc.org

SL Kenyon, DJ Taylor, W Tarnow-Mordi. Broad-spectrum antibiotics for spontaneous preterm labour: the ORACLE II randomised trial. ORACLE Collaborative Group. Lancet 2001 - europepmc.org

CHAPTER 34 Chronic hypertension

Background and definition

- **Chronic hypertension** is hypertension that is present at the booking visit or before 20 weeks or if the woman is already taking antihypertensive medication prior to pregnancy.
- It can be primary or secondary in aetiology.
- Rates for chronic HT during pregnancy – 0.6% and 2.7%.
- Classification –
  Mild HT: DBP 90–99 mmHg, SBP 140–149 mmHg.
  Moderate HT: DBP 100–109 mmHg, SBP 150–159 mmHg.
  Severe HT: DBP 110 mmHg or greater, SBP 160 mmHg or greater.

Risks or complications

Pre-eclampsia (PET) and eclampsia – see Chapter 27

Prepregnancy advice

- Angiotensin-converting enzyme (ACE) inhibitors or angiotensin II receptor blockers (ARBs): increased risk of congenital abnormalities if taken during pregnancy.
- Chlorothiazide: there may be an increased risk of congenital abnormality and neonatal complications if taken during pregnancy; discuss and change to other antihypertensives.
- Antihypertensive treatments other than ACE inhibitors, ARBs or chlorothiazide: limited evidence has not shown an increased risk of congenital malformation.
- Diet: encourage women to keep their dietary sodium intake low, either by reducing or substituting sodium salt, because this can reduce BP.

Antenatal care – treatment of hypertension

- Antihypertensive treatment dependent on pre-existing treatment, side-effect profiles, and teratogenicity.
- Stop ACE inhibitors or ARBs and offer alternatives.
- Women with uncomplicated chronic HT – aim to keep BP <150/100 mmHg. Do not offer treatment to lower DBP <80 mmHg.
- Women with target-organ damage secondary to chronic HT (e.g., kidney disease) treat with the aim of keeping BP <140/90 mmHg.
- Women with secondary chronic HT – refer to a specialist in hypertensive disorders.

Antenatal care – monitoring

- **Antenatal consultations** – schedule additional antenatal consultations based on the individual needs of the woman and her baby.
- **Fetal monitoring:**
  * USS fetal growth and AFV, UmAD velocimetry between 28 and 30 weeks and between 32 and 34 weeks.
  * If results are normal, do not repeat at more than 34 weeks, unless otherwise clinically indicated.
  * Only carry out CTG if fetal activity is abnormal.

Timing of birth

- Do not offer delivery if BP is <160/110 mmHg with or without antihypertensive treatment before 37 weeks.
- Women with BP <160/110 mmHg after 37 weeks with or without antihypertensive treatment – individualize timing of delivery based on maternal and fetal indications for birth.
- Plan delivery in women with refractory severe chronic HT, after a course of corticosteroids (if required) has been completed.

Intrapartum care

Mild or moderate hypertension (BP ≤ 159/109 mmHg)

- Continue antenatal antihypertensive treatment.
- Measure BP hourly.
- Haematological and biochemical monitoring according to criteria from antenatal period even if regional analgesia being considered.
- If BP stable do not routinely limit duration of second stage.

Severe hypertension (BP ≥ 160/110 mmHg)

- Continue antenatal antihypertensive treatment.
- Measure BP continually.
- If BP controlled within target ranges do not routinely limit duration of second stage.
- If BP does not respond to initial treatment advise operative delivery.

Postnatal investigation, monitoring, and treatment

- Measure BP: ＊ daily for the first 2 days; ＊ at least once between day 3 and day 5; ＊ as clinically indicated if antihypertensive treatment is changed after birth.
- Aim to keep blood pressure <140/90 mmHg.
- Continue antenatal antihypertensive treatment. Review long-term antihypertensive treatment 2 weeks after birth.
- If a woman has taken methyldopa to treat chronic HT during pregnancy, stop within 2 days of birth and restart the antihypertensive treatment the woman was taking before the pregnancy.
- Offer a medical review at the postnatal review with the pre-pregnancy care team.
- **If the woman is breastfeeding:**
  - ＊ Avoid diuretic treatment for hypertension.
  - ＊ Assess clinical wellbeing of baby, especially adequacy of feeding, at least daily for first 2 days.

Follow-up care

- Review long-term treatment 2 weeks after birth.
- Medical review at 6–8 weeks postnatal review with pre-pregnancy care team.

What not to do

- Angiotensin-converting enzyme (ACE) inhibitors or angiotensin II receptor blockers (ARBs) and chlorothiazide in pregnancy.
- Routine repeat fetal growth scans after 34 weeks if previous growth scans were normal.
- Deliver if BP is < 160/110 mmHg (with or without antihypertensive treatment) before 37 weeks.
- Limit duration of second stage if BP is stable in mild to moderate HT or severe HT.
- Diuretic treatment if woman is breastfeeding.
- Methyldopa in postnatal period.

Hypertension in Pregnancy: The Management of Hypertensive Disorders During Pregnancy; NICE CGN 107, August 2010.

Introduction and prevalence

- A disorder of carbohydrate metabolism associated with long-term vascular complications, including retinopathy, nephropathy, neuropathy, and vascular disease.
- Incidence 2–5% of pregnancies; approximately 87.5% of pregnancies complicated by diabetes are due to GDM, 7.5% due to type 1 DM, and 5% being due to type 2 DM.
- The prevalence of type 1 and type 2 DM is increasing.
- Type 2 DM is increasing in ethnic groups such as African, black Caribbean, South Asian, Middle Eastern, and Chinese origin.
- Risks associated with pregnancies complicated by DM increase with the duration of diabetes.

Risks or complications

Maternal

- Miscarriage, PET, and PTL are more common.
- Increased likelihood of birth trauma, IOL, and CS.
- Diabetic retinopathy can worsen rapidly during pregnancy.

Fetus

- Stillbirth, congenital malformations, macrosomia, birth injury, perinatal mortality, and postnatal adaptation problems (such as hypoglycaemia) are more common.
- Newborn – transient morbidity in the neonatal period; may require admission to neonatal unit.
- Long term risk – the risk of the baby developing obesity and/or diabetes in later life.

Preconception care

Contraception, diet, body weight, and exercise

- Discuss the importance of avoiding unplanned pregnancy. Advise to use contraception until good glycaemic control (assessed by HbA1c) is achieved.
- Review glycaemic targets, glucose monitoring, medications for diabetes, and medications for complications of DM before and during pregnancy. Good glycaemic control before conception and throughout pregnancy will reduce the risk of miscarriage, congenital malformation, stillbirth, and neonatal death. Risks can be reduced but not eliminated.
- Advice on weight loss to women who have a BMI >27 kg/m².
- Give folic acid (5 mg/day) until 12 weeks to reduce the risk of baby with a neural tube defect.
- Nausea and vomiting in pregnancy can affect glycaemic control. Individualize dietary advice.

Retinal assessment – arrange retinal assessment (by digital imaging) at the first appointment (unless an annual retinal assessment has been done within previous 6 months) and annually thereafter if no diabetic retinopathy is found.

- Defer rapid optimization of glycaemic control until after retinal assessment and treatment have been completed.

Renal assessment – measure microalbuminuria before discontinuing contraception. If serum creatinine is abnormal (≥120 micromol/l) or the estimated glomerular filtration rate (eGFR) is <45 ml/minute/1.73 m², refer to a nephrologist.

Medications for DM before and during pregnancy

- Metformin may be used as an adjunct or alternative to insulin in the preconception period and during pregnancy, when the likely benefits from improved glycaemic control outweigh the potential for harm.
- Discontinue all other oral hypoglycaemic agents before pregnancy and substitute with insulin. Rapid-acting insulin analogues (aspart and lispro) are safe in pregnancy.
- Insufficient evidence on the use of long-acting insulin analogues during pregnancy. Isophane insulin (NPH insulin) is the first choice for long-acting insulin during pregnancy.
- Discontinue ACE inhibitors, angiotensin-II receptor antagonists, and statins before conception or as soon as pregnancy is confirmed. Substitute with alternative agents suitable for pregnancy.

Monitoring and target ranges BG and ketones

- Measure HbA1c monthly.
- Advise on self-monitoring of BG with individualized targets of BG levels.
- Women who require intensification of hypoglycaemic therapy should increase the frequency of self-monitoring of BG to include fasting and a mixture of pre- and PP levels.
- Offer ketone testing strips and advise to test for ketonuria or ketonaemia if they become hyperglycaemic or unwell.
- Aim to maintain the HbA1c <6.1%. Any reduction in HbA1c towards the target of 6.1% is likely to reduce the risk of congenital malformations.
- Advise strongly to avoid pregnancy in women whose HbA1c is >10%.
- Provide information on the risks of hypoglycaemia and hypoglycaemia unawareness.

Specific antenatal care – MDT care. Provide assessment with diabetes care team for glycaemic control every 1–2 weeks throughout pregnancy.

First appointment (joint diabetes and antenatal clinic)
- Information, advice, and support in relation to optimizing glycaemic control.
- Take a clinical history to establish the extent of diabetes-related complications.
- Review medications for diabetes and its complications.
- Retinal and/or renal assessment if these have not been undertaken in the previous 12 months.
- Folic acid 5 mg daily.

7–9 weeks
- Confirm viability of pregnancy and gestational age.

Booking appointment (ideally by 10 weeks)
- Education and advice about how diabetes will affect the pregnancy, birth, and early parenting (such as breastfeeding and initial care of the baby).

16 weeks
- Retinal assessment in women with pre-existing diabetes who showed signs of diabetic retinopathy at the first antenatal appointment

20 weeks
- Four-chamber view of the fetal heart and outflow tracts plus anomaly scans including assessment for NTD.

28 weeks
- USS – fetal growth and AFV.
- Retinal assessment in women with pre-existing diabetes who showed no diabetic retinopathy at their first antenatal clinic visit.

32 weeks
- USS – fetal growth and AFV; nulliparous women – all investigations as part of routine antenatal care.

36 weeks
- USS –fetal growth and AFV.
- Information and advice about: timing, mode, and management of birth; analgesia and anaesthesia; changes to hypoglycaemic therapy during and after birth; management of the baby after birth; initiation of breastfeeding and the effect of breastfeeding on glycaemic control; contraception and follow-up.

38 weeks
- IOL or CS if indicated, and start regular tests of fetal wellbeing for women with diabetes who are awaiting spontaneous labour.

39, 40, 41 weeks
- Tests of fetal wellbeing.

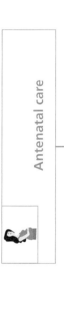

Antenatal care

Target ranges and monitoring for BG

- Individualize targets for self-monitoring of BG. Aim – FBG between 3.5 and 5.9 mmol/l and 1-hour PP BG <7.8 mmol/l. FBG levels and BG levels 1 hour after every meal. Advise women with insulin-treated diabetes to test BG levels before going to bed at night (additional).
- Do not use HbA1c routinely for assessing glycaemic control in the second and third trimesters.
- Offer women with type 1 diabetes ketone testing strips and to test for ketonuria or ketonaemia if they become hyperglycaemic or unwell.

Retinal assessment

- Retinal assessment at first antenatal appointment and at 28 weeks if the first assessment is normal. If retinal assessment has not been performed in the preceding 12 months, offer it ASAP in pregnancy.
- If any diabetic retinopathy is present, offer an additional retinal assessment at 16–20 weeks.
- Diabetic retinopathy is a contraindication to rapid optimization of glycaemic control in women who present with a high HbA1c in early pregnancy.
- Women with preproliferative diabetic retinopathy diagnosed during pregnancy – refer for ophthalmological follow-up following delivery.
- Diabetic retinopathy is not a contraindication to vaginal birth.

Renal assessment

- If renal assessment has not been done in the preceding 12 months, arrange it at the first contact in pregnancy.
- If serum creatinine is abnormal (≥120 micromol/l) or if total protein excretion > 2 g/day – refer to a nephrologist.
- Do not use eGFR during pregnancy.
- Consider thromboprophylaxis in women with proteinuria > 5 g/day (macroalbuminuria).

Management of diabetes

- Consider rapid-acting insulin analogues (aspart and lispro) during pregnancy as they have advantages over soluble human insulin.
- Women with insulin-treated diabetes (ITDM):
  * Inform regarding risks of hypoglycaemia and hypoglycaemia unawareness in pregnancy, particularly in the first trimester.
  * Provide a concentrated glucose solution and glucagon to women with type 1 diabetes.
  * Offer continuous SC insulin infusion if adequate glycaemic control is not obtained by multiple daily injections of insulin without significant disabling hypoglycaemia.
- If women with type 1 diabetes become unwell, exclude DKA urgently and admit for medical and obstetric care.

Fetal monitoring

- Offer first trimester nuchal translucency (possibly with first trimester biochemical screening with PAPP-A and β-hCG) (Australian).
- Screen for congenital malformations along with four-chamber view of the fetal heart and outflow tracts at 18–20 weeks.
- Monitor fetal growth and wellbeing – USS of fetal growth and AFV every 4 weeks from 28 to 36 weeks.
- Routine monitoring of fetal wellbeing before 38 weeks is not recommended, unless there is a risk of IUGR.
- Women at risk of IUGR (macrovascular disease and/or nephropathy) – individualize care to monitor fetal growth and wellbeing.

Intrapartum care

Timing and mode of birth

- Women with a normally grown fetus – offer IOL or elective CS if indicated, after 38 completed weeks.
- Diabetes in itself is not a contraindication to VBAC.
- Women with an USS diagnosed macrosomic fetus (>4.5kg) – inform of the risks and benefits of vaginal birth, IOL, and CS.
- Place of birth – units with advanced neonatal resuscitation care available 24 hours a day.

Analgesia and anaesthesia

- Offer anaesthetic assessment in the third trimester of pregnancy for women with comorbidities such as obesity or autonomic neuropathy.
- If GA is used, monitor BG regularly (every 30 minutes) from induction of general anaesthesia until after the baby is born and the woman is fully conscious.

Glycaemic control

- Monitor capillary BG hourly to maintain it between 4 and 7 mmol/l.
- Consider IV dextrose and insulin infusion from the onset of established labour in women with type 1 diabetes.
- Use IV dextrose and insulin infusion during labour in women whose BG is not maintained at between 4 and 7 mmol/l.

Preterm labour

- Diabetes is not a contraindication to antenatal steroids for fetal lung maturation or to tocolysis. Provide additional insulin and closely monitor women with insulin-treated DM who are receiving steroids for fetal lung maturation.
- Do not use betamimetic drugs for tocolysis.

Postnatal care

Breastfeeding and effects on glycaemic control

- Insulin requirements fall rapidly during labour and in the puerperium.
- Women with insulin-treated DM:
  * Reduce insulin immediately after birth and monitor BG levels to establish the appropriate dose.
  * Are at increased risk of hypoglycaemia, especially when breastfeeding.
- Women with type 2 diabetes who are breastfeeding can resume or continue to take metformin and glibenclamide immediately following birth but avoid other oral hypoglycaemic agents while breastfeeding.
- Women who are breastfeeding – avoid any drugs for the treatment of diabetic complications that were discontinued for safety reasons in the pre-conception period.
- Refer back women to their routine diabetes care arrangements.

Neonatal care

- Keep babies with their mothers unless there is a clinical complication or there are abnormal clinical signs that warrant admission for special care.
- Test BG 2–4 hours after birth.
- Test for polycythaemia, hyperbilirubinaemia, hypocalcaemia, and hypomagnesaemia in babies with clinical signs.
- ECG if any signs of congenital heart disease or cardiomyopathy, including heart murmur.
- Admit to NICU if: hypoglycaemia associated with abnormal clinical signs; respiratory distress; signs of cardiac decompensation; neonatal encephalopathy; polycythaemia; need for IV fluids or tube feeding; jaundice requiring intense phototherapy and frequent monitoring of bilirubinaemia; born before 34 weeks (or between 34 and 36 weeks if dictated clinically).
- Do not transfer babies to community care until they are at least 24 hours old, maintaining BG levels, and are feeding well.

Prevention and assessment of neonatal hypoglycaemia

- Feed babies ASAP after birth (within 30 minutes) and then at frequent intervals (every 2–3 hours) until feeding maintains prefeed BG levels at a minimum of 2.0 mmol/l.
- Give tube feeding or IV dextrose if BG values are <2.0 mmol/l on 2 consecutive readings despite maximal support for feeding; if there are abnormal clinical signs or if the baby does not feed orally effectively.
- If clinical signs of hypoglycaemia – test BG and treat with IV dextrose ASAP.

What not to do

- Routine HbA1c for assessing glycaemic control in the second and third trimesters.
- eGFR use during pregnancy.
- Routine monitoring of fetal wellbeing before 38 weeks.
- Betamimetic drugs for tocolysis.

Diabetes in Pregnancy: Management of Diabetes and its Complications from Pre-conception to the Postnatal Period; NICE CGN 63, March 2008.

CHAPTER 36 Cardiac disease and pregnancy

Background and prevalence

- Cardiac disease is a leading cause of maternal death in pregnancy in many developed countries, including the UK.
- UK – overall rate of mortality from cardiac disease 22.7/million births.
- The major part of this increase is due to acquired heart disease.
- One-third of these deaths are a result of myocardial infarction (MI)/ ischaemic heart disease (IHD) and a similar number of late deaths are associated with peripartum cardiomyopathy (CMP).
- Other significant contributors (5–10% each) are rheumatic heart disease, congenital heart disease, and pulmonary hypertension.
- The majority of pregnant women who die of heart disease have not previously been identified as 'at risk'.

Risks or complications

Fetal –

- FGR, PTB.
- 3–5% risk of congenital heart disease (risk varies, depending on the precise condition); about five times the average risk. If the partner has a heart problem, the risk is even higher.

Maternal –

- Prolonged hospitalization.
- Reduced life span of patient herself.
- There is a small risk of dying as a result of the pregnancy – in the UK it is currently about 1 in 8000. In cases of very severe heart disease (Eisenmenger's syndrome or primary pulmonary HT), the risk of death is as high as 25–40%. It is often difficult to give a precise estimate of risk for the more unusual forms of heart defect.

Cardiac conditions in pregnancy

MI, IHD

- Pregnancy itself raises the risk of acute MI by 3- to 4-fold, with the risk being 30 times higher for women over the age of 40 years compared with women aged < 20 years.
- The rate of maternal death from IHD in the UK – 1/132 000 pregnancies. Up to 1/13 women with an MI in pregnancy will die.
- Risk factors include chronic HT, PET, DM, smoking, obesity, and hyperlipidaemia. Many of these risk factors are becoming increasingly common, and most women affected will be asymptomatic before pregnancy with no history of heart disease.
- Keep a high index of suspicion for MI in any pregnant woman presenting with chest pain. Perform an ECG in women with chest pain in pregnancy and get someone who is skilled at detecting signs of cardiac ischaemia and infarction to interpret it. If the pain is severe, arrange a CT or MRI of the chest. A serum troponin I measurement can also be useful.

Peripartum cardiomyopathy (CMP)

- Cause of peripartum CMP is unknown in most cases. It usually presents in late pregnancy or early in the puerperium up to 6 months after delivery.
- Consider it in any pregnant or puerperal woman who complains of increasing shortness of breath, especially on lying flat or at night. Arrange an ECG, chest X-ray, and an echocardiogram. As 25% of affected women will be hypertensive, it can be confused with PET.
- If any pregnant or postpartum woman has unexpected and persistent dyspnoea or is noted to be unusually tachypnoeic or tachycardic, and PE has been excluded, she may have peripartum CMP. Investigate it further by echocardiography and refer to a cardiologist.

Aortic dissection

- Systolic HT is a key factor in most of the deaths from aortic dissection. Monitor BP during pregnancy and treat with antihypertensives promptly. CT scan/MRI will provide the diagnosis.
- Aortic dissection is the most common serious complication of Marfan syndrome.

Rheumatic heart disease

- Almost 25% of women currently giving birth in the UK are migrants; the figure is >50% in London. Many of these women have never undergone medical screening and some will be unaware that they have valvular heart disease.
- Undertake a careful cardiovascular assessment at the beginning of pregnancy of all women not born in a country where there is effective medical screening in childhood.
- Mitral valve stenosis (the most common lesion and the one that carries the highest risk) is a difficult clinical diagnosis. Keep a low threshold for echocardiography.

Congenital heart disease (CHD)

- Although deaths from CHD are uncommon, the prevalence of this condition in pregnancy is about 0.8%.
- CHD is one of the most common congenital abnormalities and the majority of those affected will survive to adulthood because of the development of effective corrective surgery.

Preconception

- Refer girls with CHD to a joint cardiac/obstetric clinic for advice about contraception and preconception counselling at the age of 12–15 years. Provide preconception counselling to older women with a new diagnosis. Give an estimate of the risks as accurately as possible, and reassess this risk every 5 years (or more often if their condition deteriorates significantly).
- Discuss and offer contraception to prevent unwanted pregnancy because pregnancy carries substantially increased risks for women with CHD. Provide this information at the appropriate age and do not delay until transfer to the adult cardiac services.
- Review all women with significant heart disease regularly to ensure that there has been a recent assessment prior to pregnancy.
- Women with heart disease are often at increased risk with assisted conception. Seek MDT advice before any such treatment is commenced.

- Preconception assessment and risk stratification for women with pre-existing heart disease can be refined by cardiopulmonary exercise testing.
- Inform the issues relating to pregnancy with CHD – increased risk of mortality, CHD in the offspring, and the need for increased medical surveillance during pregnancy.
- Immigrants to the UK (or to other developed countries) are a high-risk group for undiagnosed heart disease. Undertake a careful clinical and echocardiographic assessment if any cardiovascular or respiratory symptoms and consider any additional imaging as appropriate.
- Any cardiac surgical interventions in women of childbearing age should take into account the effect they may have on pregnancy. For example, because of the risks associated with prosthetic mechanical valves in pregnancy, consider using tissue valves for valve replacement.

Symptoms

- At each visit – ask about SOB (especially at night), exercise tolerance, palpitations.
- Be aware of prepregnancy symptoms, to detect any deterioration in symptomatic status ASAP. Many pregnant women will experience deterioration of one class as pregnancy progresses. These women may need to take more rest than usual during pregnancy, although it is also important for them to maintain their fitness as much as possible.
- Refer to cardiologist – any woman who complains of feeling suddenly less well, who develops any loss of consciousness, a sudden increase in SOB or new palpitations associated with other symptoms.

Examination

- Measure BP manually.
- Pulse rate and rhythm – a rising pulse rate can be the first signs of cardiac decompensation.
- Auscultate heart sounds at each visit to check if there is any substantial change. It is usual for a murmur to increase by one grade as pregnancy progresses because of the increase in cardiac output. A sudden increase in the loudness of a heart murmur can suggest the development of vegetations from endocarditis. The appearance of a new murmur is always significant.
- Auscultate lung bases posteriorly at each visit to check for crackles, which can indicate developing pulmonary oedema (incipient heart failure).
- Women with cyanotic heart disease – check oxygen saturations periodically (each trimester or more often if there are any clinical signs of deterioration).

Fetal monitoring

- Women with CHD are at a relatively increased risk of having a baby affected with CHD.
- Fetal NT scan – a significant indicator of recurrent cardiac disease in the fetus.
- Standard fetal anomaly scan at 20 weeks of gestation.
- Fetal cardiac scan at 22 weeks by fetal cardiologist.
- Up to 80% of heart abnormalities can be detected using USS between 11 and 24 weeks of pregnancy (the later the scan, the bigger the baby and the more detailed the scan can be).
- Screening efficiency will improve if fetal cardiac ultrasound screening is offered on the basis of an NT being > 3.5 cm, as well as on the basis of family or personal history.
- If a fetal cardiac anomaly is identified, it carries a 4–5% risk of an associated chromosomal abnormality – offer amniocentesis. SOGC
- In women on beta blockers (for treatment of HT or to reduce the risk of arrhythmia) there is a small increased risk of IUGR. Monitor fetal growth regularly if there is any clinical suspicion of poor growth.

Investigation

- Baseline ECG and echocardiogram.
- Symptomatic women – ECG, emergency echocardiogram, arterial blood gases, and a chest X-ray with screening of the fetus.
- Chest pain – measure troponin I levels and repeat it 24 hours later to assess whether there has been any significant myocardial damage. An exercise treadmill test is the first non-invasive test of choice to investigate the possibility of coronary artery disease, assuming the patient is well enough. A myocardial perfusion scan or coronary angiography can be considered if symptoms continue or worsen despite treatment.
- Consider and rule out PE – V/Q scan or CTPA.
- Doppler examination of the leg vessels to identify any DVT.
- Dissection of the aorta – echocardiography; MRI is more sensitive.
- CT scan can also be used but exposes the fetus to a considerable radiation dose.

Management

General care

- MDT – obstetricians, cardiologists, anaesthetists, midwives, neonatologists, and intensivists.
- Because there are so many types of cardiac disease, often with very different implications, carry out risk assessment of any woman with a heart murmur or a history of any cardiac defect early in pregnancy in a joint clinic by MDT. Risk stratification to determine the frequency and content of antenatal care.
- Women at low risk can be returned to routine care.
- Depending on cardiac status, see the woman every 2–4 weeks until 20 weeks of gestation; every 2 weeks until 24 weeks of gestation and then weekly thereafter.
- Continuity of carer is important, because this makes it much easier to detect any deterioration in the woman's condition.

Specific condition

- Mitral and aortic stenosis that are not problematic in non-pregnant women may be poorly tolerated in pregnancy. Reduction of heart rate with beta blockers is useful.
- Women with pulmonary arterial HT, irrespective of aetiology, carry a high risk to pregnancy (30–50% mortality). Discuss contraception. For some of these women, pulmonary arterial vasodilators during pregnancy and puerperium may improve the chances of maternal survival.
- Pregnant women with tachyarrhythmias and underlying heart disease – timely restoration of sinus rhythm is crucial. Direct current (DC) cardioversion is safe with careful fetal monitoring.

Antibiotics

- There is currently no evidence that prophylactic antibiotics are necessary to prevent endocarditis in an uncomplicated vaginal delivery.
- However, give prophylactic antibiotics in all cases of operative delivery and to women at increased risk such as those with mechanical valves or a history of previous endocarditis.
- Provide prophylactic antibiotic cover before any intervention which is likely to be associated with significant or recurrent bacteraemia.
- Consider the possibility of endocarditis in any woman with a cardiac defect who has positive blood cultures. It is important to minimize the strain on the heart by vigorous treatment of any infections (for example, chest, urinary).
- **SOGC** – the risk of bacteremia at the time of vaginal delivery or CS is low.
- **The American Heart Association guidelines** – antibiotic prophylaxis is not required at vaginal delivery or CS except in some high-risk patients.

Thromboprophylaxis

- Keep a lower threshold for starting thromboprophylaxis.
- There is currently no ideal regimen of anticoagulation in women with mechanical heart valves in pregnancy. Discuss the higher rate of fetal loss associated with warfarin vs higher risk of maternal valve thrombosis with subcutaneous heparin.
- Low-dose aspirin is a safe and possibly effective adjunct to LMWH in pregnant women with mechanical heart valves or an otherwise increased risk of intracardiac thrombosis.
- Thrombolysis may cause bleeding from the placental site but should be given in women with life-threatening thromboembolic disease or acute coronary insufficiency.

Cardiac surgery

- Acute coronary insufficiency or myocardial infarction – coronary angiography is appropriate. The radiation exposure of the fetus is not sufficient to contraindicate this essential diagnostic procedure. The first choice for treatment of acute coronary syndrome in pregnancy is percutaneous catheter intervention.
- Percutaneous catheter intervention is safe and effective in the treatment of coronary disease and mitral and pulmonary valve stenosis.
- Consider balloon dilatation for aortic valve disease for highly selected cases as it carries a higher risk and a lower success rate.
- Consider only for women who are refractory to medical treatment or when there is no catheter-based interventional alternative.
- If cardiac surgery requiring use of cardiopulmonary bypass does need to be performed, consider early delivery of the fetus if it is viable. If cardiopulmonary bypass is necessary, the deep hypothermia and low perfusion pressure associated with the standard techniques carries a 30% risk of fetal mortality. In the interests of the fetus, if possible, avoid hypothermia and keep perfusion pressures as high as possible. With these adjustments, fetal mortality can be as low as 10%.

Intrapartum care

- The main objective is to minimize any additional load on the cardiovascular system from delivery and puerperium. This is best achieved by aiming for spontaneous onset of labour, providing effective pain relief with low-dose regional analgesia, and if necessary, assisting vaginal delivery to limit or avoid active maternal efforts.
- Vaginal delivery is the preferred mode of delivery over CS for most women whether they have a congenital or acquired heart condition unless obstetric or specific cardiac considerations determine otherwise.
- IOL may be appropriate to optimize the timing of delivery in relation to anticoagulation and the availability of specific medical staff or because of deteriorating maternal cardiac function. However, IOL before 41 weeks, especially in nulliparous women with an unfavourable cervix, increases the likelihood of CS.

- Pregnancies progressing satisfactorily – MDT assessment at 32–34 weeks to plan care around the time of delivery and to establish optimum management.
- Advise woman to ring labour ward and to make herself known to the labour ward staff. Staff should inform consultants of the woman's admission.
- Involve senior anaesthetists who are familiar with the delivery plan and have experience of pregnant women with cardiac disease. Regional or general anaesthesia for CS should be used in such a way as to optimize cardiovascular stability.

- With any surgical intervention, pay meticulous attention to haemostasis. Excess bleeding can cause marked cardiovascular instability in pregnant women with reduced cardiac reserve.
- In the management of the third stage of labour, avoid bolus doses of oxytocin as it can cause severe hypotension. Low-dose oxytocin infusions are safer and may be equally effective.
- Avoid ergometrine as it can cause acute hypertension.
- Misoprostol may be safer but it can cause problems such as hyperthermia and data are still limited in this population. Use it only if the benefits outweigh any potential risks.
- At CS, uterine compression sutures may be effective in controlling uterine haemorrhage due to atony and may allow the avoidance of any uterotonic agent.

Postpartum care

- Transfer woman to a high-dependency unit where she can be monitored closely for 12 to 48 hours. High-level maternal surveillance is required until the main haemodynamic challenges following delivery have passed.
- For unstable cardiac conditions (such as pulmonary HT or CMP) surveillance may be required for up to 2 weeks.
- Do not transfer to a normal labour ward until she is reviewed by senior staff who can determine whether she will be safe in an area where monitoring will be less intensive.
- ACE inhibitors are safe in breastfeeding.
- DVTs are more common after birth, especially in women with CHD, and need anticoagulants until fully mobile.
- Because of the increased risk of PPH in women with heart disease who are anticoagulated, delay the introduction or reintroduction of warfarin until at least 2 days postpartum. Meticulous monitoring of anticoagulation is essential.

Postnatal check

- MDT follow-up assessment at 6 weeks after delivery (and in cases where there are continuing concerns, at 6 months), beyond which time the woman can return to her periodic cardiac outpatient care. Cardiac function should be checked by a cardiologist, and arrangements made for cardiological follow-up.
- Review contraceptive plans.

Contraception

Natural and barrier methods

- **Natural methods** – not reliable and depend very much on how carefully they are used. They do not have any adverse effects.
- **Barrier methods (condoms, diaphragm)** – have few adverse effects but have a high failure rate even when used with spermicidal creams.

Intrauterine contraceptive devices (IUCDs)

- 1:100 failure rate over a period of 5 years.
- Copper (e.g., TT380).
- Mirena – advantage of less bleeding and less infection than copper coils, and can be used more safely in women who have never had children (who are more at risk of infection).
- About 1 in 1000 women have a fainting reaction at the time the coil is inserted. This can be dangerous for women with severe heart disease; therefore it should be inserted in hospital, with cardiac anaesthetic expertise on standby in case of this rare complication.

Sterilization

- Vasectomy is more reliable and safer.
- In women – laparoscopic sterilizations under anaesthetic with clips applied to the tubes. Failure rate – 1 in 500.
- A mini-laparotomy under a regional anaesthetic may be safer for some women (laparoscopy with gas insufflation at high pressure into the abdomen can affect the heart).
- Hysteroscopic sterilization – can be done under local anaesthetic or IV sedation in a centre fully equipped to deal with women with heart problems.

Hormonal

The combined pill

- Failure rates of <1/300 women per year if taken correctly.
- It has many advantages, especially regulating the periods.
- Also available as a patch or vaginal ring.
- Complication – DVT (3- to 4-fold increased risk). Certain heart conditions are associated with an increased risk of clotting and therefore this form of contraception is contraindicated.
- Emergency contraception:
  * Levonorgestrel – it may upset warfarin control.
  * Ulipristal acetate (ellaOne).

Low dose of progestogen

- Low-dose POP has almost no dangerous adverse effects and does not cause thrombosis. However, it has a higher failure rate than the combined pill.
- Cerazette (desogestrel) stops ovulation. There is a longer window of time for the woman to take her pill, so the occasional missed pill is less likely to result in pregnancy. Cerazette is related to the drug in Implanon and can be used as a test before the implant is inserted.

Progestogen depot and implant

- Depot injections – failure rate is 1 in 300 women per year. Injections might be a problem if woman is on warfarin or has a needle phobia.
- Implant – it is one of the safest and most effective forms of contraception, effective for 3 years. Failure rate is < 1 in 1000 per year.
- Nexplanon has replaced Implanon, which was sometimes difficult to insert correctly.

Progestogen implants (Implanon) and Mirena are the most efficacious and are also the safest methods for most women with significant heart disease.

Cardiac Disease and Pregnancy, RCOG. Good Practice RCOG No.13, June 2011.

Heart Disease and Pregnancy: RCOG Study Group Statement Consensus Views Arising from the 51st Study Group; 2006.

Heart Disease in Pregnancy 1: SOGC. Assessment and Management of Cardiac Disease in Pregnancy. J Obstet Gynaecol Can 2007;29(4):331–336.

Heart Disease in Pregnancy 2: SOGC. Congenital Heart Disease in Pregnancy. J Obstet Gynaecol Can 2007;29(5):409–414.

Heart Disease in Pregnancy 3: SOGC. Acquired Heart Disease in Pregnancy. J Obstet Gynaecol Can 2007;29(6):507–509.

Heart Disease in Pregnancy 4: SOGC. Ischemic Heart Disease and Cardiomyopathy in Pregnancy. J Obstet Gynaecol Can 2007;29(7):575–579.

Heart Disease in Pregnancy 5: SOGC. Prosthetic Heart Valves and Arrhythmias in Pregnancy. J Obstet Gynaecol Can 2007;29(8):635–639.

Guidelines on the management of cardiovascular diseases during pregnancy. European Society of Cardiologists. Eur Heart J 2011;32:3147–3197. doi:10.1093/eurheartj/ehr218.

Background – iodine nutrition during pregnancy

- Average iodine requirement in women of childbearing age is 150 μg per day.
- During pregnancy and breastfeeding daily iodine requirement is 250 μg.
- Iodine intake during pregnancy and breastfeeding should not exceed twice the daily recommended intake, i.e., 500 μg iodine per day.
- To assess the adequacy of the iodine intake during pregnancy in a population, urinary iodine concentration (UIC) should ideally range between 150 and 250 μg/l.

Screening for thyroid dysfunction during pregnancy

- The benefits of universal screening for thyroid dysfunction (primarily hypothyroidism) are not justified by current evidence. Undertake a high-risk screening for thyroid disease by measurement of TSH in women with:
  * History of hyperthyroid or hypothyroid disease, PPT, or thyroid lobectomy.
  * Symptoms or clinical signs suggestive of thyroid under-function or over-function including anaemia, elevated cholesterol, and hyponatraemia.
  * Family history of thyroid disease.
  * Thyroid antibodies (when known).
  * Other autoimmune disorders.
  * Previous therapeutic head or neck irradiation.
  * Goitre.
  * Type 1 diabetes.
  * History of recurrent miscarriage or PTD.

Thyroid hormones in pregnancy

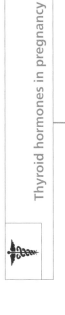

- Serum total T4 – The range of normal serum total T4 is modified due to the rapid increase in T4-binding globulin (TBG) levels and changes in serum albumin. Total thyroid hormone levels increase and therefore measurements of total T4 and total T3 are not reliable.
- Free T4 (fT4) and free T3 (fT3) **remain relatively constant and are the tests of choice in pregnancy; interpret them in relation to pregnancy-trimester specific reference ranges.** As up to 28% of singleton pregnancies with a serum TSH > 2 SD above the mean would not have been identified by using the non-pregnant serum TSH range, each laboratory should establish trimester-specific reference ranges for pregnant women.
- For practical purposes, keep the fT4 in the upper non-pregnant normal range.
- Alternatively, as the changes in total T4 levels during gestation are predictable, adjust the non-pregnant reference limits by a factor of 1.5 to determine the normal range for pregnancy.

- Serum TSH values are influenced by the thyrotropic activity of elevated circulating hCG concentrations, particularly (but not only) near the end of the first trimester. hCG and TSH have similar alpha subunits and receptors. In the first trimester hCG stimulates the TSH receptor and gives a biochemical picture of hyperthyroidism.
- In the normal pregnant woman, TSH levels typically fall in the mid to late first trimester coincident with rising hCG levels. Therefore, do not interpret subnormal serum TSH levels in the first half of pregnancy as diagnostic of hyperthyroidism.

- Thyroid hormone is an important contributory factor to normal fetal brain development.
- At early gestational stages the presence of thyroid hormones in fetal structures can only be explained by transfer of maternal thyroid hormones to the fetal compartment because fetal production of thyroid hormones does not become efficient until mid-gestation.
- Prior to 12 weeks' gestation, maternal thyroxine (but not fT3) crosses the placenta. From 12 weeks onwards, fetal thyroid function is controlled independently of the mother, provided that her iodine intake is adequate.
- The fetal thyroid begins concentrating iodine at 10–12 weeks and is under control of fetal pituitary TSH by approximately 20 weeks.
- TSH does not cross the placenta. However, clinically significant amounts of maternal T4 do cross the placenta. In addition, TSH-releasing hormone (TRH), iodine, TSH receptor (TSH-R) antibodies, and antithyroid drugs (ATDs) cross the placenta readily.

Hypothyroidism

Prevalence

- Prevalence of hypothyroidism during pregnancy is estimated to be 0.3–0.5% for overt hypothyroidism (OH) and 2–3% for subclinical hypothyroidism (SCH).
- Subclinical hypothyroidism – serum TSH concentration above the upper limit of the reference range with a normal free T4.
- Thyroid autoantibodies are found in 5–15% of women of childbearing age, and chronic autoimmune thyroiditis is the main cause of hypothyroidism during pregnancy. Other causes of thyroid insufficiency – treatment of hyperthyroidism (radioiodine ablation or surgery) or surgery for thyroid tumours. A hypothalamic–hypophyseal origin of hypothyroidism is rare and can include lymphocytic hypophysitis occurring during pregnancy or postpartum.
- Worldwide the most important cause of thyroid insufficiency remains iodine deficiency, known to affect over 1.2 billion individuals.

Clinical features

- Weight gain, sensitivity to cold, dry skin; asthenia, drowsiness, constipation.
- Many women may remain asymptomatic. Only thyroid function tests (TFTs) confirm the diagnosis.

Investigations

- Raised TSH suggests primary hypothyroidism.
- Serum fT4 levels distinguish between SCH and OH, depending on whether fT4 is normal or below normal for gestational age.
- Thyroid autoantibodies titers – thyroid peroxidase (TPO) and thyroglobulin (TG) antibodies (TPO-Ab and TG-Ab) to confirm the autoimmune origin of the disorder.

Risks or complications

Maternal

- Decreased fertility.
- Increased miscarriage, anaemia, gestational HT, placental abruption, and PPH.
- Risks are more frequent with OH than with SCH; adequate thyroxine treatment greatly decreases the risk of a poorer obstetrical outcome.
- Systematic review – SCH in early pregnancy compared with normal thyroid function is associated with an increased risk of PET (OR 1.7) and perinatal mortality (OR 2.7).
- The presence of thyroid antibodies is associated with an increased risk of unexplained subfertility (OR 1.5), miscarriage (OR 3.73), recurrent miscarriage (OR 2.3), PTB (OR 1.9), and maternal postpartum thyroiditis (OR 11.5).

Fetal

- Untreated maternal OH is associated with PTB, LBW, neonatal respiratory distress, and increased fetal and perinatal mortality.
- Though less frequent than with OH, complications are described in newborns from mothers with SCH with a doubling of the PTD rate. Women with very PTDs (<32 weeks) have a 3-fold increase in SCH.
- A significant decrease in the rate of PTD among thyroid antibody-positive women who are treated with thyroxine, compared with thyroid antibody-positive women who were not treated with thyroxine has been reported.

Fetal brain development

- Psychoneurological outcome – significantly increased risk of impairment in neuropsychological developmental indices, IQ scores, and school learning abilities in the offspring of hypothyroid mothers.
- There are 3 times as many children with IQs that were 2 SD scores below the mean IQ of controls in the children born to untreated hypothyroid women. A 3-fold increased predisposition for having learning disabilities is reported.

Treatment and monitoring

- Levothyroxine is the treatment of choice, if the iodine nutrition status is adequate.
- Hypothyroid pregnant women require larger thyroxine replacement doses than non-pregnant patients. Women who already take thyroxine before pregnancy usually need to increase their daily dosage by on average 30–50% above preconception dose. The thyroxine dose usually needs to be incremented by 4–6 weeks of gestation.
- The reasons for the increased thyroid hormone requirements: the rapid rise in TBG levels, the increased distribution volume of thyroid hormones, and increased placental transport and metabolism of maternal T4.
- Start thyroxine treatment with a dose of 100–150 μg thyroxine/day or titrate according to body weight. In non-pregnant women, the full replacement thyroxine dose is 1.7–2.0 μg/kg/day. During pregnancy increase the dose to 2.0–2.4 μg/kg/day.
- As a simple rule of thumb, the increment in thyroxine dose can be based on the initial degree of TSH elevation. For women with a serum TSH between 5 and 10 mIU/l, the average increment in thyroxine dosage is 25–50 μg/day; for those with a serum TSH between 10 and 20 mIU/l is 50–75 μg/day; and for those with a serum TSH >20 mIU/l is 75–100 μg/day.

Subclinical hypothyroidism

- T4 treatment improves obstetric outcome but has not been proved to modify long-term neurological development in the offspring.
- **Given that the potential benefits outweigh the potential risks, provide T4 replacement in women with subclinical hypothyroidism.**

- Maintain serum TSH concentrations of <2.5 μU/ml in the first trimester (or 3 μU/ml in the second and third trimester) or to trimester-specific normal TSH ranges.
- Measure serum fT4 and TSH levels within 1 month after the initiation of treatment and any change in the dose. Aim to achieve and maintain normal fT4 and TSH levels normal for pregnancy throughout gestation.
- Once the TFTs have been normalized by treatment, monitor every 6–8 weeks.
- Measuring the fT4 or FTI every 2–4 weeks can be helpful (ACOG).

Overt hypothyroidism

- If diagnosed before pregnancy – adjust preconception thyroxine dose to reach a TSH level not higher than 2.5 μU/ml prior to pregnancy.

- If diagnosed during pregnancy – normalize TFTs as rapidly as possible.
- In women in whom hypothyroidism has not been diagnosed until after the first trimester, the offspring may suffer from impairment in final intellectual and cognitive abilities. The present consensus is to maintain the ongoing pregnancy, while rapidly normalizing maternal thyroid function by the administration of thyroxine. However, despite thyroxine treatment, it is not possible to fully reassure patients that there will not be any neurological effect of longstanding untreated hypothyroidism.

Antenatal care

- Hypothyroidism itself does not influence pregnancy outcome or complications.
- The majority of their antenatal care can be midwifery-led unless risk factors dictate otherwise.

Postnatal

- After delivery, reduce the levothyroxine dose over 4 weeks.
- Women with evidence of thyroid autoimmunity are at risk of developing postpartum thyroiditis (PPT). Therefore continue monitoring TFTs for at least 6 months after delivery.

Hyperthyroidism in pregnancy

Prevalence and background

- Prevalence is 0.1% to 0.4%, with Graves' disease accounting for 85% of cases.
- Graves' disease is 5- to 10-fold more common in women, with a peak incidence during the reproductive age.
- Other causes – single toxic adenoma, multinodular toxic goitre, and thyroiditis, gestational thyrotoxicosis, factitious thyrotoxicosis, and hydatidiform mole.
- The activity level of Graves' disease fluctuates during gestation, with exacerbation during the first trimester and gradual improvement during the latter half; with an exacerbation shortly after delivery. Rarely, labour, CS, and infections may aggravate hyperthyroidism and trigger a thyroid storm.
- Autoimmune thyroiditis occurs in up to 10% of women in the reproductive age. Generally the result is hypothyroidism, although a hyperthyroid phase of Hashimoto's thyroiditis and silent thyroiditis may both occur.
- Postpartum thyroiditis (PPT) occurs after up to 10% of all pregnancies and may have a hyperthyroid phase, usually within the first month or two. The hyperthyroid phase of PPT is often followed by a hypothyroid phase, an important risk for fetal development. Therefore, careful sequential monitoring is necessary.

- **Inhibitory TRAbs may** cause transient neonatal hypothyroidism in neonates.

Risks or complications

- The risks are related to the duration and control of maternal hyperthyroidism.
- **Maternal –**
  - ∗ PET, congestive heart failure, thyroid storm. Untreated women are twice as likely to develop PET, compared to women receiving antithyroid drugs (ATDs).
  - ∗ Limited data suggest that untreated maternal hyperthyroidism is associated with miscarriage.
- **Fetal –** fetal and neonatal risks are related to the disease itself and/or to the medical treatment of the disease.
  - ∗ Inadequately treated maternal thyrotoxicosis is associated with an increased risk of PTD, IUGR, LBW, and IUD.
  - ∗ Overtreatment of the mother with thioamides can result in iatrogenic fetal hypothyroidism.

Effect on fetal thyroid function

- Women with Graves' disease have thyroid receptor antibodies (TRAbs) that can stimulate or inhibit the fetal thyroid.
- Because TRAbs can cross the placenta (Graves' disease and chronic autoimmune thyroiditis), there is risk of immune-mediated **hypothyroidism or hyperthyroidism in the neonate.**

- Stimulatory TRAbs can cause hyperthyroidism. 1–5% of neonates of mothers with Graves' disease have hyperthyroidism or neonatal Graves'.
- Signs of thyrotoxicosis: Fetus – hydrops fetalis, IUD, polyhydramnios related to oesophageal pressure, obstructed labour from neck extension related to goitre. Neonate – tachycardia, excessive movements, fetal goitre, IUGR, fetal cardiac failure, craniosynostosis and associated intellectual impairment.
- Fetal goitre associated with treatment of Graves' disease with thioamides can be due to either fetal hypothyroidism from maternal ATD treatment or fetal hyperthyroidism from maternal antibody transfer. The risk factors for significant fetal and neonatal thyroid disease – fetal signs, maternal history of a prior affected baby or prior treatment with ^{131}I, and elevated maternal thyroid-stimulating antibodies (TSAb).
- Maternal antibodies are cleared less rapidly than thioamides in the neonate, sometimes resulting in delayed presentation of neonatal Graves' disease.

- The incidence of neonatal Graves' disease is not directly related to maternal thyroid function.
- Women who have been treated surgically or with ^{131}I before pregnancy and require no thioamide treatment are at higher risk for neonatal Graves' disease, due to the lack of the suppressive thioamide and the potential persistence of TRAb.
- Measure these antibodies before pregnancy or by the end of the first/second trimester in mothers – with current Graves' disease, with a history of Graves' disease and treatment with ^{131}I or thyroidectomy, or with a previous neonate with Graves' disease.

- Women who have a negative TRAb and do not require ATD have a very low risk of fetal or neonatal thyroid dysfunction.

- Women with elevated TRAb or treated with ATD – monitor with monthly fetal USS after 20 weeks.
- **Fetal USS** for evidence of fetal thyroid dysfunction – FGR, hydrops, goitre, or cardiac failure.

- Umbilical cord blood sampling – when non-invasive studies do not distinguish fetal hypothyroid from hyperthyroid disease in the presence of fetal goitre.
- Consider if the diagnosis of fetal thyroid disease is not certain from the clinical data and if the information gained from cord blood sampling would change the treatment. It carries a risk of fetal loss of 1–2%.

Clinical features

- Non-specific symptoms of hyperthyroidism such as tachycardia, warm moist skin, tremor, and systolic murmur may be mimicked by normal pregnancy.
- Rarely, the presence of classic thyroid ophthalmopathy, a significant goitre, or pretibial myxoedema (while rare) may point to Graves' disease.
- Thyroid storm – a rare condition affecting 1% of pregnant women with hyperthyroidism characterized by severe, acute exacerbation of the signs and symptoms of hyperthyroidism which is a medical emergency.

Investigations

- Measurement of serum TSH, fT4, fT3 levels, and TRAb.
- If in doubt – measure serum total T3 concentration as only 12% of women with hyperemesis gravidarum have an elevated fT3 index.
- Most patients with Graves' disease have detectable TRAb. Measurement of TRAb may also help to distinguish Graves' disease from gestational thyrotoxicosis in the first trimester as TRAb is negative in gestational hyperthyroidism. Because Graves' disease tends to undergo immunological remission after the late second trimester, detection of TRAb may depend upon gestational age at measurement.

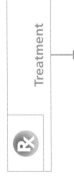

Treatment

1. Maternal antithyroid drug (ATD) therapy

- ATDs are the main treatment (propylthiouracil [PTU] and methimazole [MMI] and carbimazole) as they inhibit thyroid hormone synthesis.
- Pregnancy itself does not alter the maternal pharmacokinetics of MMI, although serum PTU levels may be lower in the latter part of gestation than in the first and second trimesters.
- Theoretically, there is increased transplacental passage of MMI relative to PTU. However recent evidence suggests that the differential placental transfer of PTU and MMI appears unlikely, and by itself does not support the preferential use of PTU vs MMI. Moreover, the effect on fetal/neonatal thyroid function appears to be similar for the two.
- For overt hyperthyroidism due to Graves' disease or hyper-functioning thyroid nodules – start or adjust ATD therapy to maintain the maternal free T4 in the upper non-pregnant reference range.
- Because MMI may be associated with congenital anomalies PTU is the first line drug, especially during first trimester organogenesis. MMI may be prescribed if PTU is not available or if a patient cannot tolerate it.
- Measure TFTs monthly when control is good and more frequently when the diagnosis is new or there is a relapse: titrate the ADT against the results.
- Clinical disease activity follows the titre of TRAb, which rises in the first trimester and puerperium and falls in the second and third trimesters. Most women can, therefore, reduce their dose and almost one-third of women can stop treatment during pregnancy, which helps prevent fetal hypothyroidism. Most women will need to restart or increase their dose in the puerperium to avoid a relapse.

Differential diagnosis

DDx

- **Gestational thyrotoxicosis** presents in the mid to late first trimester, often with hyperemesis. Usually classic hyperthyroid symptoms are absent or minimal, except for weight loss, which may be a result of vomiting and poor nutrition. Differentiate Graves' disease from gestation thyrotoxicosis to decide about ATD therapy.
- **Subnormal serum TSH concentration** – it is important to differentiate hyperthyroidism from normal physiology during pregnancy and hyperemesis gravidarum because of the adverse effects of overt hyperthyroidism on the mother and fetus. Differentiation of Graves' disease from gestational thyrotoxicosis is supported by evidence of autoimmunity, a goitre, and presence of TRAb.
- **Subclinical hyperthyroidism** (TSH below normal limits with free T4 and total T4 in the normal pregnancy range, and unaccompanied by specific clinical evidence of hyperthyroidism) – there is no evidence that treatment improves pregnancy outcome, and treatment can potentially adversely affect fetal outcome.

- **Effects on the fetal thyroid: hypothyroidism** – aim to restore normal maternal thyroid function while ensuring that fetal thyroid function is minimally affected.
- The lack of correlation between maternal dosage and fetal thyroid function reflects maternal factors, as there is individual variability in serum PTU levels after a standard oral dose as well as the transplacental passage of maternal TRAbs that stimulate the fetal thyroid.
- Current maternal thyroid status is the most reliable marker for titration of ATD therapy to avoid fetal hypothyroidism. If the maternal serum free T4 concentration is either elevated or maintained in the upper third of the normal non-pregnant reference range, serum free T4 levels are normal in more than 90% of neonates.

Teratogenicity – MMI and carbimazole – aplasia cutis and choanal/oesophageal atresia – controversial data.

- There may be a higher incidence of choanal and oesophageal atresia in fetuses exposed to MMI and carbimazole in the first trimester than expected. There are no data to support an association between congenital anomalies and PTU.
- MMI and carbimazole are the only medications available in many countries, and therefore these drugs must be employed despite the potential complications. However, where available, PTU is preferred as the initial therapy for maternal hyperthyroidism.
- Both drugs cause agranulocytosis. Advise women to report any sore throat immediately. This is unpredictable and is a reason not to change agent routinely during pregnancy.

Lactation – historically, women treated with ATDs were advised against breastfeeding due to the presumption that the ATD was present in breast milk in concentrations sufficient to affect the infant's thyroid. Recent studies reported no alteration in thyroid function in newborns breastfed by mothers treated with daily PTU, MMI, or carbimazole. Therefore, consider ATD therapy (PTU < 300 mg/day, MMI < 20 mg/day) during lactation. Advise to take the drug after feeding. Until more studies are available, consider monitoring the infant's thyroid function.

Rx **Treatment contd – other agents**

2. Propranolol

- May be used to treat symptoms of acute hyperthyroid disease and for preoperative preparation. It can also be used until ATD therapy reduces thyroid hormone levels to reduce symptoms.
- Use of propranolol in late pregnancy is associated with mild and transitory neonatal hypoglycaemia, apnoea, and bradycardia (resolve within 48 hr). IUGR – remains controversial. If a patient requires long-term propranolol treatment, monitor fetal growth.
- Propranolol is safe in breastfeeding women.

3. Iodides

- Chronic use of iodides during pregnancy is associated with hypothyroidism and goitre in neonates, sometimes resulting in asphyxiation because of tracheal obstruction.
- As the experience with iodides is limited, do not use iodides as a first-line therapy for women with Graves' disease. They can be used transiently if needed in preparation for thyroidectomy.

4. Radioactive iodine (RAI)

- RAI diagnostic tests and therapy are contraindicated during pregnancy. All women who could potentially be pregnant should have a pregnancy test before RAI administration.
- The fetus is exposed to the radiation from the ^{131}I circulating in the mother's blood. Because fetal thyroid uptake of RAI commences after 12 weeks, exposure to maternal ^{131}I before the 12th week of pregnancy is not associated with fetal thyroid dysfunction. However, treatment after 12 weeks leads to significant radiation to the fetal thyroid causing fetal thyroid destruction and hypothyroidism; the woman should consider whether pregnancy should continue. There are no data for or against recommending TOP after ^{131}I exposure.
- [131]I is contraindicated in breastfeeding.
- Men – advise to avoid pregnancy for 4 months after RAI treatment to ensure that one cycle of spermatogenesis has occurred.

5. Surgery

- Thyroidectomy is for women who do not respond to ATD therapy.
- MDT – endocrinologist, surgeons, neonatologist, and anaesthetist.
- Subtotal thyroidectomy may be indicated during pregnancy for maternal Graves' disease if:
  * severe adverse reaction to ATD therapy;
  * persistently high doses of ATD are required; or
  * non-compliance with ATD therapy with uncontrolled hyperthyroidism.
- The optimal timing of surgery is the second trimester.
- If a woman experiences severe ATD-related side effects such as agranulocytosis, give transient therapy with potassium iodide solution (50–100 mg/day) for 10–14 days before surgery to reduce vascularity of the thyroid gland.
- Propranolol can also be administered preoperatively.

Fetus management – fetal hyperthyroidism or hypothyroidism associated with maternal antithyroid treatment for Graves' disease

Rx

Hypothyroid

Case reports –
- Intra-amniotic thyroxine treatment of a fetus with a goitre, or fetal hypothyroidism diagnosed by cord blood sampling.
- Simply stop or reduce maternal antithyroid treatment, if the patient is euthyroid.

- Consider delivery depending on the gestational age at diagnosis and the severity of fetal symptoms.

Fetal thyrotoxicosis

- Modulation of maternal antithyroid medication; PTU in a euthyroid mother and modulate the dose by repeated cord blood sampling to determine fetal thyroid functions.
- If this is not appropriate, give high doses of PTU or carbimazole to the mother and titrate her response against the FHR; the pregnant woman can take thyroxine if she becomes clinically hypothyroid as this will not cross the placenta.

- At delivery, measure TFTs on cord blood. Evaluate all newborns of mothers with Graves' disease for thyroid dysfunction and treat if necessary.
- Hypothyroidism is usually self-limiting.
- Hyperthyroidism typically presents 7–10 days postnatally, since the half-life of maternally derived antithyroid drugs is shorter than that of TRAb.
- Warn parents to look for changes in their baby, such as weight loss or deteriorating/poor feeding.
- Neonatal treatment rarely lasts for more than a few months.

Gestational hyperemesis and hyperthyroidism

- Measure TFTs in all patients with hyperemesis gravidarum. Few women with hyperemesis gravidarum will require ATD treatment.
- Treat overt hyperthyroidism believed to be due to Graves' disease with ATD.
- Gestational hyperthyroidism with clearly elevated thyroid hormone levels (free T4 above the reference range or total T4 > 150% of top normal pregnancy value and TSH < 0.1 μU/ml) and evidence of hyperthyroidism may require treatment.

Autoimmune thyroid disease and miscarriage

- Systematic review – association between thyroid autoantibodies and miscarriage:
  * Cohort studies – OR for miscarriage was 3.90.
  * Case–control studies the OR for miscarriage was 1.80.
- PTB – the OR for PTB is 2.
- With levothyroxine – a significant (52%) relative risk reduction in miscarriages (RR 0.48) and PTB (69%) are reported but the trials on this subject were small.
- Although a positive association exists between the presence of thyroid antibodies and pregnancy loss, universal screening for antithyroid antibodies is not currently recommended.

Postpartum thyroiditis (PPT)

- Insufficient data to recommend screening all women for PPT.
- Women known to be thyroid peroxidase antibody positive – test TSH at 3 and 6 months postpartum.
- The prevalence of PPT in women with type 1 diabetes is 3 times higher than in the general population. Postpartum screening (TSH) is recommended for women with type 1 diabetes mellitus at 3 and 6 months postpartum.
- Women with a history of PPT have a markedly increased risk of developing permanent primary hypothyroidism in the 5- to 10-year period following the episode of PPT. Perform an annual TSH level in these women.
- Asymptomatic women with PPT who have a TSH above the reference range but <10 μU/ml and who are not planning a subsequent pregnancy do not necessarily require intervention, but if untreated reassess in 4–8 weeks.
- Treat symptomatic women and women with a TSH above normal who are attempting pregnancy with levothyroxine.
- As hypothyroidism is a potentially reversible cause of depression, screen women with postpartum depression for hypothyroidism and treat appropriately.

Thyroid nodules and cancer

- Perform fine needle aspiration cytology (FNAC) for thyroid nodules > 1 cm discovered in pregnancy. Ultrasound-guided FNAC may have an advantage for minimizing inadequate sampling.
- Malignant nodules diagnosed in the first or early second trimester or exhibit rapid growth – offer surgery in the second trimester.
- Cytology indicative of papillary or follicular neoplasm without evidence of advanced disease – if women prefer to wait until the postpartum period for definitive surgery, reassure that most well-differentiated thyroid cancers are slow growing and that surgical treatment soon after delivery is unlikely to adversely affect prognosis.
- It is appropriate to administer thyroid hormone to achieve a suppressed but detectable TSH in pregnant women with a previously treated thyroid cancer or a FNA positive for cancer in those who elect to delay surgical treatment until postpartum. High-risk patients may benefit from a greater degree of TSH suppression compared to low-risk patients. The fT4 or total T4 levels should not be increased above the normal range for pregnancy.
- Advise women to avoid pregnancy for 6 months to 1 year if they have suffered thyroid cancer and received therapeutic RAI doses to ensure stability of thyroid function and confirm remission of thyroid cancer.

Management of thyroid dysfunction during pregnancy and postpartum: An Endocrine Society Clinical Practice Guideline. Journal of Clinical Endocrinology and Metabolism 2007 Aug;92(8) (Suppl):S1–S47.

van den Boogaard E, Vissenberg R, Land JA, van Wely M, van der Post JA, Goddijn M, Bisschop PH. Significance of (sub)clinical thyroid dysfunction and thyroid autoimmunity before conception and in early pregnancy: a systematic review. Human Reproduction Update. 2011 Sep-Oct;17(5):605–619.

Thangaratinam S, Tan A, Knox E, Kilby MD, Franklyn J, Coomarasamy A. Association between thyroid autoantibodies and miscarriage and preterm birth: meta-analysis of evidence. British Medical Journal 2011;342:d2616.

Girling J. Thyroid disease in pregnancy. The Obstetrician & Gynaecologist 2008;10:237–243.

Thyroid disease in pregnancy. ACOG Practice Bulletin No. 37, August 2002. International Journal of Gynaecology and Obstetrics 2002 Nov;79(2):171–180.

CHAPTER 38 Renal condition in pregnancy

Prevalence and background

- Prevalence rates vary from 2/10 000 to 12/10 000 women. This low incidence may be due to the fact that many women with significant renal insufficiency are beyond childbearing age or infertile.
- National Kidney Foundation classification of chronic kidney disease is based on eGFR. eGFR is calculated using serum creatinine values and is affected by age, sex, and race. Although this value is useful in non-pregnant women, the use of eGFR is not valid in pregnancy:

Stage	Description	eGFR
1	• Kidney damage and normal/raised GFR	>90
2	• Kidney damage and mildly reduced GFR	60–90
3	• Moderately reduced GFR	30–59
4	• Severely reduced GFR	15–29
5	• Kidney failure	<15 (or dialysis)

- The outcome of pregnancy depends on the degree of renal impairment, presence of proteinuria, and underlying renal pathology.
- Women with mild renal impairment do well in pregnancy with few problems.
- Women with moderate to severe kidney dysfunction face significant pregnancy-related complications as well as long -term renal deterioration.
- **Degree of renal impairment**
  * Mild: serum creatinine <125 μmol/l
  * Moderate: serum creatinine – 125–220 μmol/l
  * Severe: serum creatinine >220 μmol/l

Risks or complications

Pregnancy complications

- Depend on the severity of the renal dysfunction with progressive increase of these complications with the severity of the dysfunction:
  * Chronic HT, PET, anaemia.
  * FGR, PTD.
  * LBR falls from 98% in mild to 64% in severe dysfunction.
- UTI, bacteriuria, multiorgan failure, acute respiratory distress syndrome.
- Periarteritis nodosa – fetal prognosis is poor and maternal death often occurs.
- Consider therapeutic termination in this group of women.

Effect of pregnancy on renal condition

- Depends on the severity of the renal dysfunction – with progressive increase in these complications with the severity of the dysfunction:
  * Loss of renal function from 5% in mild cases to 75% in severe.
  * Postpartum deterioration 0% in mild to 60% in severe.
  * End-stage renal disease 0% in mild to 40% in severe dysfunction.

Prepregnancy counselling

- Offer to all women considering pregnancy or assisted reproduction.
- MDT counselling – fertility and pregnancy outcome, depends on the degree of renal insufficiency.
- Recommend single-embryo transfer with IVF.
- Women with normal or only mildly decreased prepregnancy renal function (serum creatinine <125 μmol/l) – obstetric outcome is favourable without adverse effects on the long-term course of their disease, although there is an increased risk of antenatal complications including PET.
- **Discuss:**
  * The risks of PET, FGR, and PTD.
  * Long-term risks to their own health.
  * The risk of deterioration in renal function following pregnancy.
- Consider modification of remediable risk factors, including optimization of medications.
- Establish baseline renal function and achieve optimal control of HT.
- ACE inhibitors and angiotensin receptor blockers are contraindicated in pregnancy. Change to safer drugs after the woman becomes pregnant.

Proteinuria alone

- Proteinuria can be an indicator of renal impairment in pregnancy.
- Asymptomatic women with significant proteinuria (>500 mg/24 hours) and no pre-existing renal disease or diabetes:
  * Renal insufficiency coexists in 62% of women and 40% of them have chronic HT.
  * PTD rate of 50% and a FGR of 25%.
  * 20% of these women progressed to end-stage renal disease within 5 years.
- In women with positive proteinuria >1+dipstick (in the absence of infection), quantify proteinuria either with 24-hour urine or urine PCR on a random sample of urine and follow up with urine PCR.
- Persistent proteinuria (>500 mg/24 hours) before 20 weeks of gestation – refer to nephrologist.
- Lesser degrees of proteinuria may constitute a risk for VTE.

Antenatal care

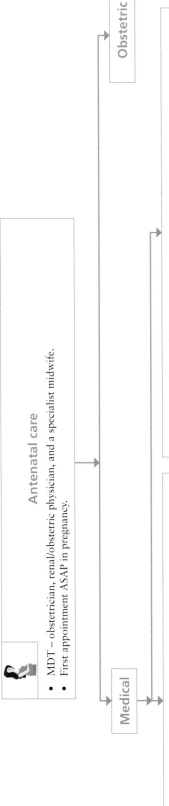

- MDT – obstetrician, renal/obstetric physician, and a specialist midwife.
- First appointment ASAP in pregnancy.

Obstetric

- Monitor and control BP.
- There is controversy over 'tight' vs 'non-tight' BP control, as every 10mmHg fall in MAP is associated with a 145 g reduction in mean birth weight. The current consensus is to maintain BP to less than 140/90 mmHg.
- Drugs – methyldopa, calcium channel blockers, hydralazine, and labetalol.
- Maternal anaemia occurs due to decreased erythropoietin production and shortened red cell survival. Manage with oral/IV iron therapy. Offer recombinant erythropoietin if the haematocrit falls <19%. Erythropoietin can cause HT, or aggravate pre-existing HT. BT may be required in rare cases where erythropoiesis-stimulating agents are safe to use.

- Regular scans every 4 weeks from 28 weeks of gestation onwards to check growth and liquor volume.
- PTL is common. There is no evidence to suggest safety of the oxytocin receptor antagonist atosiban in women with renal insufficiency.
- Treat UTIs promptly, including asymptomatic bacteriuria, as it can be helpful in prevention of PTL. Provide antibiotic prophylaxis to women with recurrent bacteriuria/UTIs and kidney disease throughout pregnancy.

Medical

- Get a baseline:
  * Renal profile – serum urea, creatinine, electrolytes, albumin, and FBC.
  * Urinalysis and urine culture, assessment of proteinuria (either by 24-hour collection of urine or by urine PCR).
- Repeat every 4 weeks or more frequently, depending on the clinical situation.
- No data on renal biopsy during pregnancy. It can be associated with severe bleeding, which can require BT and further invasive procedures. Hence, most specialists prefer to deliver early and investigate postnatally. Renal biopsy is indicated only in cases of florid nephrotic syndrome early in pregnancy or suspected rapidly progressive glomerulonephritis.

- Women found or suspected to have kidney disease in pregnancy – refer to a nephrologist. May need more frequent hospital visits, depending on the clinical situation.
- Early dating scan to estimate gestational age accurately.
- Nuchal and anomaly scans. The anomaly scan must include a detailed scan of the urinary tract to look for evidence of inherited conditions such as obstructive uropathy. Serum screening for Down syndrome is not a reliable screening tool in these women.
- Commence low-dose aspirin as prophylaxis against PET within the first trimester.
- Nephrotic syndrome is an indication for thromboprophylaxis with heparin in pregnancy and the puerperium.
- Women known to have lupus nephritis or suspected lupus flare – refer to the MDT.

Renal dialysis and renal transplant patients

- All renal units, in conjunction with obstetric units, should have a protocol for management of women receiving or starting dialysis in pregnancy.
- The indications for acute dialysis during pregnancy are similar to those in non-pregnant women. They include: severe refractory metabolic acidosis, electrolyte imbalance, especially severe refractory hyperkalaemia, volume overload leading to congestive heart failure, pulmonary oedema that is unresponsive to diuretics.
- Dialysis may be initiated earlier in pregnancy if there is an acute deterioration in renal function because of the increased risk of fetal demise.
- Prednisolone, azathioprine, cyclosporine or tacrolimus alone or in combination do not appear to be associated with fetal abnormality; do not discontinue in pregnancy. Safety of mycophenolate mofetil/enteric-coated mycophenolic acid, sirolimus/everolimus or rituximab is not determined.
- Women who have undergone renal transplantation and/or lower urological surgery – involve the appropriate surgical team, as part of the delivery plan where necessary.

Time and mode of delivery

- In the absence of maternal or fetal deterioration, plan delivery at or near term.
- Early delivery is usually necessary for obstetric indications such as PET and FGR or for rapidly deteriorating maternal renal function.
- CS for obstetric indications.

Postnatal

- Women with nephrotic syndrome – thromboprophylaxis with heparin in pregnancy as well as for 6 weeks postpartum.
- Follow-up in a combined clinic. Continue woman's established care with her nephrology team.
- Give appropriate contraceptive advice.
- Evaluate women with early-onset (necessitating delivery before 32 weeks) PET to identify women with underlying renal disease.
- Isolated microscopic haematuria with structurally normal kidneys does not need to be investigated during pregnancy but evaluate if it persists postpartum.

Consensus views arising from the 54th Study Group: Renal Disease in Pregnancy; RCOG: John M Davison, Catherine Nelson-Piercy, Sean Kehoe and Philip Baker. Kapoor N, Makanjuola D, Shehata H. Management of women with chronic renal disease in pregnancy. The Obstetrician & Gynaecologist 2009;11:185–191.

Prevalence and background

- Anaemia affects 1.62 billion people globally. Iron deficiency is the most common cause. Even in the developed world 30–40% of pregnant women have iron depletion.
- **Definition –**
  * Hb <2 standard deviations below the mean for a healthy matched population.
  * Hb or haematocrit value <5th centile of healthy reference population (US – CDC).
  * WHO – Hb concentration of <110 g/l. In view of the relative plasma expansion being particularly marked in the second trimester, take 105 g/l as the cut-off from 12 weeks (US – CDC).
- **There is variation in definition of normal Hb levels in pregnancy. A level of ≥ 110 g/l appears adequate in the first trimester and ≥ 105 g/l in the second and third trimesters. Postpartum anaemia is defined as Hb < 100 g/l.**
- There is a racial difference in normal Hb levels and the optimum Hb may be lower in those of African origin than in Europeans.
- It is a spectrum ranging from iron depletion to iron deficiency anaemia:
- **Iron depletion** – the amount of stored iron (serum ferritin concentration) is reduced but the amount of transport and functional iron may not be affected. Those with iron depletion have no iron stores to mobilize if the body requires additional iron.
- **Iron-deficient** – stored iron is depleted and transport iron (transferrin saturation) is reduced further; the amount of iron absorbed is not sufficient to replace the amount lost or to provide the amount needed for growth and function. In this stage, the shortage of iron limits red blood cell (RBC) production and results in increased erythrocyte protoporphyrin concentration.
- **Iron-deficiency anaemia** – there is a shortage of iron stores, transport and functional iron, resulting in reduced Hb in addition to low serum ferritin, low transferring saturation, and increased erythrocyte protoporphyrin concentration.

Risks or complications

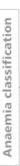

Maternal morbidity and mortality

- Iron deficiency may contribute to maternal morbidity through effects on immune function with increased susceptibility or severity of infections, poor work capacity and performance, and disturbances of postpartum cognition and emotion.
- There is little information regarding the Hb thresholds below which mortality increases, although this may be as high as 8.9 g/dl, which was associated with a doubling of the maternal death risk. However severe anaemia is likely to have multiple causes and the direct effect of the anaemia itself is unclear.
- **Effects on pregnancy outcome** – there is some evidence for the association between maternal iron deficiency and PTD, LBW, possibly placental abruption, and increased peripartum blood loss.

Effects on the fetus and infant

- The fetus is relatively protected from the effects of iron deficiency by up-regulation of placental iron transport proteins but maternal iron depletion increases the risk of iron deficiency in the first 3 months of life.
- Impaired psychomotor and/or mental development are described in infants with iron deficiency anaemia and may also negatively contribute to infant and social emotional behaviour and have an association with adult onset diseases, although controversial.

Anaemia classification

A. By inherited/acquired

Acquired

Deficiency anaemia – Fe, folic acid, B12
Haemorrhagic
Chronic disease
Acquired haemolytic
Aplastic

Inherited

Thalassaemia
Sickle cell
Other haemoglobinopathies
Inherited haemolytic

B. Anaemia by mechanism

Decreased red cell production

Fe deficiency, vitamin B12 deficiency, folic acid deficiency
Bone marrow disorders, bone marrow suppression
Low erythropoietin
Hypothyroidism
Deficiency – dietary deficiency, malabsorption or parasites

Increased red cell destruction

Inherited haemolytic anaemia – sickle cell, thalassaemia major, hereditary spherocytosis
Acquired haemolytic anaemia – autoimmune haemolytic, thrombotic thrombocytopenic purpura, haemolytic uraemic syndrome, malaria
Haemorrhagic anaemia - blood loss

C. By MCV

Microcytic (MCV <80 fl)

Fe deficiency, thalassaemia, sideroblastic anaemia
Chronic disease, copper deficiency, lead poisoning

Normocytic (MCV 80–100 fl)

Haemorrhagic anaemia, early Fe deficiency
Chronic disease, chronic renal insufficiency
Bone marrow suppression, endocrine dysfunction
Autoimmune haemolytic, hereditary spherocytosis
Paroxysmal nocturnal haemoglobinurea

Macrocytic (MCV >100 fl)

Vitamin B12 deficiency, folic acid deficiency
Drug-induced haemolytic anaemia (zidovudine)
Liver disease, alcohol abuse, acute myelodysplastic syndrome

Prevention of iron deficiency – universal supplementation

- The International Nutritional Anemia Consultative Group (INACG) and WHO recommend universal supplementation with 60 mg/day of elemental iron, from booking (WHO) or from the second trimester (INACG).
- Cochrane review – universal prenatal supplementation with iron or iron+folic acid has relative risk-reduction of anaemia at term by 30–50% for those receiving daily iron supplements. No evidence of significant reductions in substantive maternal and neonatal adverse clinical outcomes (low birth weight, delayed development, preterm birth, infection, postpartum haemorrhage).
- Iron ingestion has been the most common cause of paediatric poisoning deaths and doses as low as 60 mg/kg have proved fatal.

Issues with routine supplementation:

- Drug compliance is inconsistent and often poor.
- There is a risk of elevated Hb with the use of iron supplements in non-anaemic women and particularly those given daily regimes from an early gestational age < 20 weeks.
- A U-shaped association is observed between maternal Hb concentrations and birth weight.
- Higher rates of perinatal death, LBWs, and PTD in women with high (Hb > 132 g/l), compared to intermediate Hb levels, at 13–19 weeks of gestation is reported. A booking Hb of > 145 g/l is reported to be associated with a 42% risk of subsequent HT.
- Markers of oxidant stress have been found to be significantly elevated in the placentas of women with regular iron supplementation in pregnancy.
- The intestinal mucosa is also vulnerable to oxidative damage, caused by the continuous presence of a relatively small amount of excess iron intake and iron accumulation leading to intestinal abnormalities and injury which has been observed in patients receiving therapeutic iron.
- Associated side effects and particularly haemoconcentration during pregnancy may suggest the need for revising iron doses and schemes of supplementation during pregnancy.

- **Routine iron supplementation for all women in pregnancy is not recommended in the UK.**
- **An individual approach is preferable, based on results of blood count screening tests as well as identification of women at increased risk.**

Clinical symptoms and signs

- Nonspecific, unless the anaemia is severe. Fatigue is the most common symptom.
- Patients may complain of pallor, weakness, headache, palpitations, dizziness, dyspnoea, and irritability.
- Rarely pica develops, where there is a craving for non-food items such as ice and dirt.
- Iron deficiency anaemia may also impair temperature regulation and cause pregnant women to feel colder than normal.
- Storage iron is depleted before a fall in Hb and symptoms of iron deficiency may occur even without anaemia: fatigue, irritability, poor concentration, and hair loss.

- Hb and haematocrit levels are lower in African women compared with white women. For African women – it is recommended to lower the cut-off levels for Hb and Hct by 8 g/l, and 2% respectively. ACOG

Investigations

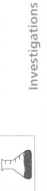

Full blood count, blood film, and red cell indices

- FBC – may show low Hb, mean cell volume (MCV), mean cell haemoglobin (MCH), and mean cell haemoglobin concentration (MCHC).
- Blood film may confirm presence of microcytic hypochromic red cells and characteristic 'pencil cells'.
- Microcytic, hypochromic indices may also occur in haemoglobinopathies. In milder cases of iron deficiency, the MCV may not have fallen below the normal range.
- Other tests to assess iron stores or the adequacy of iron supply to the tissues – low plasma iron levels, high total iron binding capacity, low serum ferritin levels, increased free erythrocyte protoporphyrin.

Serum ferritin

- Ferritin is a stable glycoprotein which accurately reflects iron stores in the absence of inflammatory change. It is the first test to become abnormal as iron stores decrease and it is not affected by recent iron ingestion. It is the best test to assess iron deficiency in pregnancy, although it is an acute phase reactant and levels will rise when there is active infection or inflammation. Concurrent measurement of the CRP may be helpful in interpreting higher levels.
- Even though the ferritin level may be influenced by the plasma dilution later in pregnancy, a concentration < 15 µg/l indicates iron depletion in all stages of pregnancy (specificity of 98% and sensitivity of 75%).
- Consider to treat when serum ferritin levels fall < 30 µg/l, as this indicates early iron depletion.

Serum iron (Fe) and total iron binding capacity (TIBC)

- Serum Fe and TIBC are unreliable indicators of availability of iron to the tissues because of wide fluctuation in levels due to recent ingestion of Fe, diurnal rhythm, and other factors such as infection. Transferrin saturation fluctuates due to a diurnal variation in serum iron and is affected by the nutritional status. This may lead to a lack of sensitivity and specificity.

Bone marrow iron – a bone marrow sample stained for iron is the gold standard for assessment of iron stores; however, this is too invasive. Only indicated in most complicated cases in pregnancy, where the underlying cause of anaemia is not identifiable by simpler means.

Others – zinc protoporphyrin, soluble transferrin receptor, reticulocyte haemoglobin content, and reticulocytes

Trial of iron therapy

- A trial of iron therapy is simultaneously diagnostic and therapeutic. Check ferritin first if the patient is known to have a haemoglobinopathy but otherwise microcytic or normocytic anaemia can be assumed to be caused by iron deficiency until proven otherwise. Assessment of response to iron is both cost and time effective. A rise in Hb by 2 weeks confirms iron deficiency.
- If haemoglobinopathy status is unknown, it is reasonable to start iron whilst screening. Screen immediately in accordance with the NHS sickle cell and thalassaemia screening programme guidelines.
- If there has been no improvement in Hb by 2 weeks, refer to secondary care to consider other causes of anaemia, such as folate deficiency.

Maternal – antenatal care

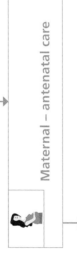

- FBC at booking and at 28 weeks.
- Women with a Hb < 110 g/l before 12 weeks or < 105 g/l beyond 12 weeks are anaemic. Offer a trial of therapeutic iron replacement unless they are known to have a haemoglobinopathy.
- Women with known haemoglobinopathy – check serum ferritin and offer therapeutic iron if the ferritin is < 30 µg/l.
- Anaemic women with unknown haemoglobinopathy status – offer a trial of iron and haemoglobinopathy screen without delay (iron deficiency can cause some lowering of the haemoglobin A2 percentage).
- The serum ferritin level < 30 µg/l – prompt treatment.
- Refer to secondary care – if there are significant symptoms and/or severe anaemia (Hb < 70 g/l) or advanced gestation (> 34 weeks) or if there is no rise in Hb at 2 weeks. In these cases commence 200 mg elemental iron daily.

- In non-anaemic women at increased risk of iron depletion such as those with previous anaemia, multiple pregnancy, consecutive pregnancies with less than a year's interval between, and vegetarians – consider a serum ferritin.
- Also consider in pregnant teenagers, women at high risk of bleeding, and Jehovah's witnesses.
- If the ferritin is < 30 µg/l – commence 65 mg elemental iron daily. Check FBC and ferritin 8 weeks later.
- Do not offer unselected screening with routine serum ferritin as this is an expensive use of resources and may cause delay in response to blood count results.

Management

A. Dietary advice

- The average daily iron intake in Great Britain is 10.5 mg. Approximately 15% of dietary iron is absorbed. Physiological iron requirements are 3 times higher in pregnancy, with increasing demand as pregnancy advances. The recommended daily intake (RDA) of iron for the latter half of pregnancy is 30 mg.
- There is an increased iron requirement during pregnancy because blood volume expands by approximately 50% and total red blood cell mass expands by 25%. Absorption of iron increases 3-fold by the third trimester, with iron requirements increasing from 1–2 mg to 6 mg per day. The amount of iron absorption depends upon the amount of iron in the diet, its bioavailability, and physiological requirements. The main sources of dietary haem iron are haemoglobin and myoglobin from red meats, fish, and poultry. Haem iron is absorbed 2- to 3-fold more readily than non-haem iron. Meat also contains organic compounds which promote the absorption of iron from other less bioavailable non-haem iron sources.
- However, approximately 95% of dietary iron intake is from non-haem iron sources. Vitamin C (ascorbic acid) significantly enhances iron absorption from non-haem foods, the size of this effect increasing with the quantity of vitamin C in the meal. Germination and fermentation of cereals and legumes improve the bioavailability of non-haem iron by reducing the content of phytate, a food substance that inhibits iron absorption. Tannins in tea and coffee inhibit iron absorption when consumed with a meal or shortly after.
- Education and counselling regarding diet may improve iron intake and enhance absorption but the degree of change achievable, especially in poorer individuals, remains in question.
- **Counsel all women regarding diet in pregnancy including details of iron-rich food sources and factors that may inhibit or promote iron absorption and why maintaining adequate iron stores is important in pregnancy.**

B. Oral iron supplements

- Once women become iron deficient in pregnancy dietary changes alone are insufficient to correct iron deficiency anaemia and iron supplements are necessary.
- Oral iron is an effective, cheap, and safe way to replace iron.
- Ferrous iron salts are the preparation of choice. Ferrous salts show only marginal differences between one another in efficiency of absorption of iron. Available ferrous salts include ferrous fumarate, ferrous sulphate, and ferrous gluconate.
- Ferric salts are much less well absorbed.
- Do not give higher doses as absorption is saturated and side effects are increased. The oral dose for iron deficiency anaemia is 100–200 mg of elemental iron daily.
- Advise women how to take oral iron supplements, i.e., on an empty stomach, 1 hour before meals, with a source of vitamin C (ascorbic acid) such as orange juice to maximize absorption. Advise not to take other medications or antacids at the same time.

Response to oral iron

- The Hb concentration should rise by approximately 20 g/l over 3–4 weeks. The degree of increase in Hb that can be achieved depends on the Hb and iron status at the start of supplementation, ongoing losses, iron absorption, and other factors contributing to anaemia, such as other micronutrient deficiencies, infections, and renal impairment.
- In anaemic women repeat Hb after 2 weeks of treatment to assess compliance, correct administration, and response to treatment.
- Once the Hb is in the normal range, continue for a further 3 months and at least until 6 weeks postpartum to replenish iron stores.
- **In non-anaemic women repeat Hb and serum ferritin after 8 weeks of treatment to confirm response.**
- Lack of compliance and intolerance can limit efficacy. Iron salts may cause gastric irritation and up to a third of patients may develop dose-limiting side effects, including nausea and epigastric discomfort.
- Titration of dose to a level where side effects are acceptable or a trial of an alternative preparation may be necessary. **For nausea and epigastric discomfort, try preparations with lower iron content.**
- Avoid enteric-coated or sustained release preparations as the majority of the iron is carried past the duodenum limiting absorption.

If response to oral iron replacement is poor, exclude concomitant causes which may contribute to anaemia, such as folate deficiency or anaemia of chronic diseases, and refer patient to secondary care.

C. Parenteral iron therapy

- Indicated if absolute non-compliance with, or intolerance to, oral iron therapy or proven malabsorption. Consider it from the 2nd trimester onwards and in postpartum period.
- It results in faster increase in Hb and better replenishment of iron stores in comparison with oral therapy. There is a paucity of trials that assess clinical outcomes and safety of these preparations.
- The dose of parenteral iron is calculated on the basis of pre-pregnancy weight, aiming for a target Hb of 110 g/l. The choice of parenteral iron preparation is based on local facilities, taking into consideration drug costs and facilities and staff required for administration.
- RCTs have shown non-inferiority and superiority to oral ferrous sulphate in the treatment of iron deficiency anaemia in the postpartum period with rapid and sustained increases in Hb.
- Iron sucrose has a higher availability for erythropoiesis than iron dextran and has a good safety profile in pregnancy. Its use is limited by the total dose that can be administered in one infusion, requiring multiple infusions. The preparations iron III carboxymaltose and iron III isomaltoside aim to overcome this problem, with single-dose administration in an hour or less.
- Anaphylactic reactions – 1%.

Fast-acting intravenous iron preparations

- Iron III carboxymaltose (Ferrinject) – ferric hydroxide carbohydrate complex, allows for controlled delivery of iron within the cells of the reticuloendothelial system (primarily bone marrow) and subsequent delivery to the iron-binding proteins ferritin and transferrin. IV as a single dose of 1000 mg over 15 minutes (maximum 15 mg/kg by injection or 20 mg/kg by infusion).
- Iron III isomaltoside (Monofer) – IV preparation with strongly bound iron in spheroid iron-carbohydrate particles, provide slow release of bioavailable iron to iron-binding proteins. There is rapid uptake by the reticuloendothelial system and little risk of release of free iron. An erythropoietic response is seen in a few days, with an increased reticulocyte count. Ferritin levels return to the normal range by 3 weeks as iron is incorporated into new erythrocytes. Doses > 1000 mg iron can be administered in a single infusion, although there are little data on its use in the obstetrics setting.

Intramuscular preparations

- Preparation available in the UK is low-molecular-weight iron dextran. Compared with oral iron it reduces the proportion of women with anaemia. However injections tend to be painful and there is significant risk of permanent skin staining. Its use is therefore generally discouraged but if given, use the Z-track injection technique to minimize risk of iron leakage into the skin.
- The advantage of IM iron dextran is that, following a test dose, it can be administered in primary care, although facilities for resuscitation should be available as there is a small risk of systemic reaction.

D. Blood transfusion

- Indications:
  * Unstable vital signs.
  * Severe anaemia with maternal Hb <60 g/l is associated with abnormal fetal oxygenation, resulting in non-reassuring FHR patterns, reduced AFV, fetal cerebral vasodilation, and fetal death. Therefore consider maternal transfusion for fetal indications in cases of severe anaemia.
- See Chapter 55 Blood transfusion (BT) in obstetrics

E. Erythropoietin

- Conflicting studies.
- Cochrane review – there is some evidence of favourable outcomes for treatment of postpartum anaemia with erythropoietin.

Management of delivery

- Consider delivery in hospital – a suggested cut-off would be Hb < 110 g/l for delivery in hospital, including hospital-based midwifery-led unit and <95 g/l for delivery in an obstetrician-led unit.
- IV access and blood group and save.
- Take active measures to minimize blood loss at delivery.
- Active management of the third stage of labour.

Postnatal anaemia

- Check FBC within 48 hours of delivery in all women with an estimated blood loss >500 ml and in women with uncorrected anaemia in the antenatal period or symptoms suggestive of postpartum anaemia.
- Women with Hb <110g/l who are haemodynamically stable, asymptomatic, or mildly symptomatic – offer elemental iron 100–200 mg daily for at least 3 months and repeat FBC and ferritin to ensure Hb and iron stores are replete.

Macrocytic anaemia (MCV > 100 fl)

Megaloblastic

- Folate and vitamin B12 deficiency; pernicious anaemia.
- MCV levels > 115 fl are almost exclusively seen in patients with folic acid or vitamin B12 deficiency.
- Folic acid deficiency – due to diet lacking fresh green vegetables, legumes or animal proteins.
- Measure serum folic acid and vitamin B12 levels; red cell folate levels.
- Treatment – nutritious diet and folic acid and iron supplements.
- Folic acid – 1 mg daily.
- Vitamin B12 deficiency – women with partial or total gastrectomy, Crohn's disease.
- Treatment – vitamin B12 injections.

Non-megaloblastic

- Alcoholism, liver disease, myelodysplasia, aplastic anaemia, hypothyroidism.

Peña-Rosas JP, Viteri FE. Effects and safety of preventive oral iron or iron+folic acid supplementation for women during pregnancy. Cochrane Database Syst Rev. 2009 Oct 7;(4):CD004736.

Reveiz L, Gyte GM, Cuervo LG. Treatments for iron-deficiency anaemia in pregnancy. Cochrane Database Syst Rev. 2007 Apr 18;(2):CD003094.

Dodd JM, Crowther CA, Dare MR, Middleton P. Oral betamimetics for maintenance therapy after threatened preterm labour. Cochrane Database Syst Rev. 2006 Jan 25;(1):CD003927.

UK Guidelines on the Management of Iron Deficiency in Pregnancy; British Committee for Standards in Haematology. July 2011.

Clinical Management Guidelines for Obstetrician and Gynaecologists. ACOG Practice Bulletin No. 95; 2008.

Prevalence and background

- Defined by the presence of recurrent, unprovoked seizures. Treatment is typically a daily, long-term antiepileptic drug (AED) regimen.
- UK – 0.5–1% of the population have epilepsy, one third of whom are women of childbearing age.
- There is exposure to AEDs in approximately 0.3–0.6% of pregnancies.
- USA – 3–5 births per 1000 are in woman with epilepsy (WWE).
- Norwegian cohort (365 107 singleton pregnancies) – 0.8% had a previous or present history of epilepsy; out of which about 30% were exposed to AED. The most commonly used AEDs were carbamazepine (46%), lamotrigine (25%), and sodium valproate (22%).
- The risks of uncontrolled convulsive seizures outweigh the potential teratogenic risk of medication, therefore advise women with active epilepsy to continue with medication during pregnancy.

Effects of pregnancy on AEDs

Pregnancy causes increased clearance of lamotrigine (LTG), phenytoin (PHT), active metabolite of oxcarbazepine, and levetiracetam. The decreased levels may be associated with an increase in seizure frequency.
Pregnancy causes a small decrease in concentration of carbamazepine (CBZ), Phenobarbital, valproate, primidone, and ethosuximide – evidence for a change in clearance or levels is inadequate.
- The physiological changes that occur in pregnancy influence the distribution, metabolism, clearance, and availability of AEDs – a reduction in total plasma concentration and the unbound fraction of AEDs occurs during pregnancy.
- Measurement of total plasma concentration for most AEDs is unreliable as it does not reflect the free (active) fraction of drug. Large inter-individual and intra-individual variations of drug levels limit interpretation of routine therapeutic drug monitoring.
- **Do not routinely monitor AED levels during pregnancy. If seizures increase or are likely to increase, monitoring AED levels (particularly levels of lamotrigine and phenytoin, which may be particularly affected in pregnancy) may be useful when making dose adjustments. NICE**

Maternal risks

- Maternal mortality (CESDI 2004) – there were 13 epilepsy-related deaths indirectly related to pregnancy. A review reported a 10-fold increase in mortality rate among pregnant WWE, compared to 2- to 3-fold mortality rate observed in people with epilepsy. Withdrawal of treatment may contribute to excess seizure-related deaths.
- Change in seizure frequency:
  * Increase in seizure frequency – 15–37% of pregnant women, possibly due to non-adherence to medication or sleep deprivation.
  * 1–2% of women experience a tonic–clonic seizure in labour and a further 1–2% within the first 24 hours after delivery.
  * Seizure freedom for at least 9 months prior to pregnancy is probably associated with a high likelihood (84–92%) of remaining seizure free during pregnancy.
- There is no increase in seizure rate or status epilepticus during pregnancy or an increased risk of seizure relapse during pregnancy for WWE who are seizure-free.
- Complications of pregnancy – Norwegian cohort:
  * Significantly increased risk of PET (OR 1.3; 1.4 for mild PET). No increased risks of placenta praevia, PPROM or eclampsia. However, the increased risk of PET was confined to women using AEDs (OR 1.5, mild PET 1.7). Risk was higher in the first pregnancy (OR 1.8).
  * Women using AEDs also have an increased risk of gestational HT (OR 1.5, 2.4 in the first pregnancy), PTD before the 34th week (OR 1.6), and an almost 2-fold increased risk of late vaginal bleeding (OR 1.9). Women who were not treated with AEDs had no increased risks of any of these complications. However 'the increased risks are small and the benefit of the drugs in preventing epilepsy is generally greater than the risks, although the balance of risk needs to be assessed on a case-by-case basis'.
  * IOL, instrumental deliveries, and CS may be more common.

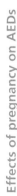

Fetal and neonatal risks

Major congenital malformations (MCMs)

- Major malformations – Structural defects that require medical or surgical intervention.
- A 2- to 3-fold increase in MCMs in children of mothers exposed to AEDs in utero, compared with the general population. The most common are: congenital heart defects, NTDs, urogenital defects (glandular hypospadias), and orofacial clefts. NTD – 1% risk with carbamazepine and 1–2% risk with VA.
- Absolute rates vary between 1 and 12% compared with 2–3% in the general population. The risk is highest in the first trimester during organogenesis.

AEDs taken during the first trimester of pregnancy compared to no AEDs in pregnancy:

- VA increases the risk of MCMs. CBZ does not substantially increase the risk of MCMs. There is insufficient evidence to determine if LTG or other specific AEDs increase the risk of MCMs. If possible, avoid VA as part of monotherapy or polytherapy during the first trimester of pregnancy.

  Specific AED during the first trimester of pregnancy – VA during the first trimester of pregnancy contributes to the development of MCMs compared to taking CBZ, PHT, and LTG. If possible avoid VA during the first trimester of pregnancy compared to the use of CBZ, PHT or LTG.

  Polytherapy compared to AED monotherapy – polytherapy contributes to the development of MCMs in the offspring of WWE as compared to monotherapy. Avoid AED polytherapy during the first trimester of pregnancy, if possible, compared to monotherapy.

  Dose of AEDs – there is a relationship between the dose of VA and LTG and the risk of development of MCMs. Limit the dosage of VA or LTG during the first trimester, if possible.

Specific MCMs associated with specific AEDs exposure in utero:

  * PHT – cleft palate, congenital heart defects.
  * CBZ – posterior cleft palate.
  * VA – neural tube defects and facial clefts and urogenital defects (hypospadias).
  * Phenobarbital and primidone – cardiac malformations.
- Animal data suggest a teratogenic risk for topiramate, but not for levetiracetam or gabapentin. Data in humans are very limited. The manufacturers recommend their avoidance in pregnancy.

Adverse perinatal outcomes

- Seizures – known association between tonic–clonic seizures and fetal hypoxia, fetal intracranial haemorrhage, and fetal loss. However, the absolute risk from convulsive seizures is unknown and may depend on seizure frequency. Although non-convulsive seizures are believed to be of little risk to the fetus, they have psychosocial and socioeconomic consequences for the mother.
- Fetal loss – 2-fold increased risk of spontaneous abortion, stillbirth, and perinatal loss.
- FGR – an association between LBW and AED exposure, ranging up to 200 g, has been reported. The risk of clinically significant LBW or SGA children is highly variable, representing up to a 2-fold risk compared with control groups. Much of this higher risk may be associated with the use of polytherapy.
- There is no substantially increased risk of perinatal death in neonates born to WWE.

- **Minor malformations** – anomalies are reported to occur in 6–20% of infants exposed to AEDs in utero, representing a 2-fold increase over the general population.
- The combination of characteristic facies with typical MCMs with or without developmental delay is referred to as the fetal anticonvulsant syndrome.

Long-term developmental effects

- Higher prevalence of developmental delay, especially in the first 2 years of life. Results from long-term follow-up are conflicting. Reported proportion of children with clinically significant cognitive impairment vary between 1.7 and 30%. A significantly lower mean verbal IQ has been reported among those exposed to valproate in utero compared with non-exposed children of mothers with epilepsy and those exposed to carbamazepine or phenytoin. Cognition is probably not reduced in children of WWE who are not exposed to AEDs in utero.
  * CBZ exposure probably does not produce cognitive impairment in offspring of WWE.
- Five or more tonic–clonic seizures during pregnancy were also independently associated with a lower verbal IQ.
- Polytherapy is more commonly associated with poorer developmental outcomes at an early age.

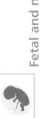

Fetal and neonatal risks contd

NTDs – Folic acid

- Alteration of folate metabolism due to AEDs may contribute to their teratogenicity. Lower folate levels in mothers taking AEDs are associated with a higher rate of malformation in their offspring. There is no direct evidence that folate supplementation reduces the risk of malformation among WWE. Nonetheless, 5 mg/day of folic acid is recommended before conception and up to at least the end of the first trimester in all women taking AEDs. Offer all women and girls on AEDs folic acid 5 mg/day before any possibility of pregnancy. (NICE CGN 137)

Haemorrhagic disease of the newborn

- Neonatal bleeding is reported in association with maternal use of enzyme-inducing AEDs, such as phenytoin, phenobarbital, and carbamazepine. There is insufficient evidence to support or refute a benefit of prenatal vitamin K supplementation for reducing the risk of haemorrhagic complications in the newborns of WWE. Give all women on enzyme-inducing AEDs oral vitamin K (20 mg/day) from 36 weeks of gestation to delivery.
- A study found no significant risk of neonatal haemorrhage despite lack of oral vitamin K supplementation in mothers taking AEDs, provided that neonates received the standard parenteral injection of 1 mg of parenteral vitamin K at birth. **Give 1 mg of parenteral vitamin K at birth to all children born to mothers taking enzyme-inducing AEDs.** (NICE CGN 137)

Risks of developing epilepsy

- The risk of unprovoked seizures is higher in offspring of parents with epilepsy onset before 20 years of age than in offspring of those with later onset epilepsy (9% vs 3%).
- Risk is also higher in offspring of parents with a history of absence seizures (9%) than in offspring of those with other generalized (3%) or partial (5%) seizures.

Choice of AED in pregnancy

- The choice of AED is determined primarily by the type of epilepsy.
- Choosing between AEDs is difficult as data for the relative risks of specific monotherapy regimens are limited. However, there is accumulating evidence of a greater risk with valproate exposure in utero for both MCMs and later development.
- In women with localization-related epilepsy there are many alternative drugs available, such as carbamazepine.
- For women with idiopathic generalized epilepsy carefully consider the balance vs risks for each individual.
- It is reasonable to switch WWE of childbearing potential to a less teratogenic regimen when possible. While VA is an effective AED, it is the AED with the greatest number of data showing an association with risk from in utero exposure.
- Although the evidence may not be adequate to justify switching every woman of childbearing age on VA to an alternative drug, lamotrigine may be a safer alternative for some. However, the long-term effects of this, or other newer AEDs, are not known.
- If possible, change from VA to another AED well before pregnancy to make sure the new treatment adequately prevents seizures.
- Changing to another AED during pregnancy poses risk of allergy, other serious adverse reactions, and polytherapy exposure. Once a patient is pregnant, changing from VA several weeks into gestation will not avoid the risk of MCMs. This may also apply to cognitive teratogenesis, since the timing of exposure related to this adverse outcome is unknown.
- Use of sodium valproate – higher doses of sodium valproate (more than 800 mg/day) and polytherapy, particularly with sodium valproate, are associated with greater risk. (NICE CGN 137)

Pre-conceptual counselling

- Offer it to all women of childbearing age.
- Give 5 mg/day of folic acid.
- Optimize treatment and where necessary review the need for continuation of AEDs.
- Withdrawal of AEDs in seizure-free women – plan it carefully months before conception, and discuss the implications for driving and risks of seizure recurrence.
- Discontinuing AEDs may not be a safe option, as it may expose the mother and fetus to physical injury from accidents arising from partial or generalized seizures.
- Provide information about the possibility of status epilepticus in those who plan to stop AED therapy.
- **Aim for seizure freedom before conception and during pregnancy (particularly for generalized tonic–clonic seizures) but consider the risk of adverse effects of AEDs and use the lowest effective dose of each AED, avoiding polytherapy if possible. (NICE CGN 137)**
- Consider genetic counselling if one partner has epilepsy, particularly if the partner has idiopathic epilepsy and a positive family history of epilepsy. Although there is an increased risk of seizures in children of parents with epilepsy, the probability that a child will be affected is generally low. However, this will depend on the family history. (NICE CGN 137)

Provide information and reassurance

- Generalized tonic–clonic seizures – inform that the fetus may be at relatively higher risk of harm during a seizure, although the absolute risk remains very low, and the level of risk may depend on seizure frequency.
- There is no evidence that focal absence and myoclonic seizures affect the pregnancy or developing fetus adversely unless the woman falls and sustains an injury.
- Increase in seizure frequency is generally unlikely in pregnancy or in the first few months after birth.
- The risk of a tonic–clonic seizure during labour and the 24 hours after birth is low (1–4%).
- Although women are likely to have healthy pregnancies, their risks of complications during pregnancy and labour are higher than for women without epilepsy.
- Majority of pregnancies proceed without difficulties; however discuss the risks of MCMs and potential longer term effects.

Antenatal care

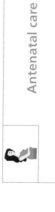

Maternal

- MDT – ensure close liaison between epilepsy team, obstetrician, and midwives to plan and provide care during the pregnancy (joint neurology and obstetric clinics).
- Do not abruptly withdraw or change medication even in women presenting with an unplanned pregnancy taking high-risk medication.
- Changes in medication after the first trimester, when organogenesis is complete, may be considered because of risks to neurodevelopmental delay; but consider the pros and cons carefully. Such changes can result in an increase in seizure frequency. In addition, the usual practice of overlapping the introduction of one antiepileptic with another during changes in monotherapy results in the fetus being exposed to polytherapy for a potentially significant period.

Fetal

- Women who are taking AEDs – offer a high resolution USS to screen for structural anomalies at 18–20 weeks of gestation but earlier scanning may allow major malformations to be detected sooner.
- Prenatal screening using serum alpha fetoprotein at 15–22 weeks combined with structural USS can identify 95% of fetuses with open NTDs.
- More detailed scanning with fetal echocardiography and imaging of the fetal face may be required.
- Increase surveillance for IUGR in later pregnancy if mother's fundal growth indicates FGR.

Labour and delivery

- Place of delivery – in a consultant-led obstetric unit with facilities for maternal and neonatal resuscitation.
- Provide adequate pain relief.
- Aim for vaginal delivery. Epilepsy in itself is not an indication for IOL or CS.
- Manage seizures during pregnancy and labour as in any person with epilepsy in collaboration with an epilepsy team.
- Recurrent or single prolonged tonic–clonic seizures can be terminated with sub-buccal midazolam, intravenous lorazepam or rectal diazepam.

Postnatal and breastfeeding

- An increase in seizures in the perinatal period can be treated with clobazam 10 mg twice daily if the mother is able to take oral medication. There is limited information on the use of clobazam in pregnancy but benzodiazepines can be associated with sedation in the newborn.
- The effect of AEDs on infants depends mainly on the AED level in breast milk and the metabolism and elimination half-life of the AED in the neonate. The excretion of AEDs in breast milk is variable, depending mainly on the degree of maternal serum protein binding.
- Phenytoin, carbamazepine, and valproate are only found in low concentrations in breast milk as they are all highly protein bound. In contrast, phenobarbital and primidone reach higher levels as they are less protein bound. Preliminary data suggest that lamotrigine and topiramate may be significantly excreted in breast milk, but no adverse effects have been reported.
- Relatively immature drug metabolism mechanisms and reduced serum protein binding in the infant may lead to drug accumulation particularly for phenobarbital and primidone.
- There is no evidence to determine if indirect exposure to maternally ingested AEDs has symptomatic effects on the newborns. Encourage breastfeeding as it has many positive effects for both mother and child.
- Advise mothers to look for appropriate weight gain and sleep patterns, excessive drowsiness or poor feeding. If there is any concern then measure the AED level in the infant.

Contraception

- Consider the possibility of interaction with oral contraceptives and assess the risks and benefits of treatment with individual drugs.
- If on enzyme-inducing AEDs –
  * If chooses to take the COCs, seek guidance about dosage from the SPC and current BNF.
  * The POP and POIM are not recommended.
  * Discuss use of additional barrier methods if seeking oral contraception or depot injections of progestogen.
  * If emergency contraception is required, the type and dose of emergency contraception should be in line with the SPC and current BNF.
- Discuss with women who are taking lamotrigine that the simultaneous use of any oestrogen-based contraceptive can result in a significant reduction of lamotrigine levels and lead to loss of seizure control. When a woman starts or stops taking these contraceptives, the dose of lamotrigine may need to be adjusted.

Newborn

- Give to all children born to mothers taking enzyme-inducing AEDs 1 mg of vitamin K parenterally at delivery.
- Introducing a few simple safety precautions may significantly reduce the risk of accidents and minimize anxiety. Inform about safety precautions to be taken when caring for the baby.
- The risk of injury to the infant caused by maternal seizure is low.

The Epilepsies: The Diagnosis and Management of the Epilepsies in Adults and Children in Primary and Secondary Care. NICE.

Adab N, Chadwick DW. Management of women with epilepsy during pregnancy. The Obstetrician & Gynaecologist 2006;8:20–25.

Harden CL, Hopp J, Ting TY, et al. Practice Parameter update: Management issues for women with epilepsy; Focus on pregnancy (an evidence-based review): Obstetrical complications and change in seizure frequency: Report of the Quality Standards Subcommittee and Therapeutics and Technology Assessment Subcommittee of the American Academy of Neurology and American Epilepsy Society. Neurology 2009;73:126.

Harden CL, Meador KJ, Pennell PB, et al. Practice Parameter update: Management issues for women with epilepsy; Focus on pregnancy (an evidence-based review): Teratogenesis and perinatal outcomes: Report of the Quality Standards Subcommittee and Therapeutics and Technology Assessment Subcommittee of the American Academy of Neurology and American Epilepsy Society. Neurology 2009;73:133.

Harden CL, Pennell PB, Koppel BS, et al. Practice Parameter update: Management issues for women with epilepsy; Focus on pregnancy (an evidence-based review): Vitamin K, folic acid, blood levels, and breastfeeding: Report of the Quality Standards Subcommittee and Therapeutics and Technology Assessment Subcommittee of the American Academy of Neurology and American Epilepsy Society. Neurology 2009;73:142.

Borthen I, Eide M, Veiby G, Daltveit A, Gilhus N. Complications during pregnancy in women with epilepsy: population-based cohort study. British Journal of Obstetrics & Gynaecology 2009; doi: 10.1111/j.1471-0528.2009.02354

CHAPTER 41   Haemoglobinopathies – sickle cell disease in pregnancy

- A heterogeneous group of single gene disorders, including structural haemoglobin variants and thalassaemias.
- More than 270 million people are carriers worldwide.

Haemoglobin (Hb) structure

- Hb – consists of 4 polypeptide chains, each of which is attached to a haem molecule. The polypeptide chains are – alpha, beta, gamma, delta, epsilon, and zeta.
- Adult Hb – HbA with $\alpha 2\beta 2$ chains; HbA2 with $\alpha 2\delta 2$ chains; HbF with $\alpha 2\gamma 2$.
- HbF ($\alpha 2\gamma 2$) – is the primary Hb of the fetus from 12 to 24 weeks of gestation.
- The genes that code for α-globin chains are located on the short arm of chromosome 16, and the β-globin gene is located on the short arm of chromosome 11.

The thalassaemias

- Disorders characterized by a reduced synthesis of globin chains, resulting in microcytic anaemia. These are classified according to the globin chain affected – α thalassemia and β thalassemia.

Sickle cell disease

- Autosomal recessive condition which affects haemoglobin structure.
- Abnormal Hb (HbS) – due to a single nucleotide substitution of thymine for adenine in the β-globin gene, resulting in substitution of valine for glutamic acid in the number 6 of β-globin polypeptide chain.
- HbS carriers – sickle cell trait; haemoglobin S combined with normal haemoglobin (A), asymptomatic, except for a possible increased risk of UTIs and microscopic haematuria.
- HbSS – affected: sickle cell anaemia.
- HbS and one other abnormality of β-globin structure or production also results in sickle cell disorder – HbSC, HbS/β thalassaemia and with haemoglobin D, E or O-Arab. These may result in vaso-occlusive phenomenon and haemolytic anaemia similar to HbSS.

- Clinical features are seen under conditions of decreased oxygen tension, as a consequence of polymerization of the abnormal haemoglobin in low-oxygen conditions in which the red blood cells become distorted into various shapes, some of which resemble sickles. These result in increased viscosity, haemolysis, and anaemia and further decrease in oxygenation.
- These cells are prone to increased breakdown, resulting in haemolytic anaemia. When sickling occurs in small blood vessels, it can interrupt blood supply to vital organs – vaso-occlusive crisis. Repeated vaso-occlusive crises result in widespread microvascular obstruction with interruption of perfusion and function of several organs, including the spleen, lungs, kidney, heart, and brain, resulting in acute painful crises.

- Adults are asplenic, having undergone autosplenectomy by adolescence.
- This results in increased incidence and severity of infections.
- Acute chest syndrome is characterized by a pulmonary infiltrate with fever leading to hypoxia and acidosis. The infiltrates are due to vaso-occlusion from sickling or embolization of marrow from long bones affected by sickling.
- Other complications of SCD include stroke, pulmonary hypertension, renal dysfunction, retinal disease, leg ulcers, cholelithiasis, and avascular necrosis (which commonly affects the femoral head and may necessitate hip replacement).
- SCD was previously associated with a high early mortality rate, but now the majority of children born with SCD in the UK live to reproductive age and average life expectancy is at least the mid-50s.

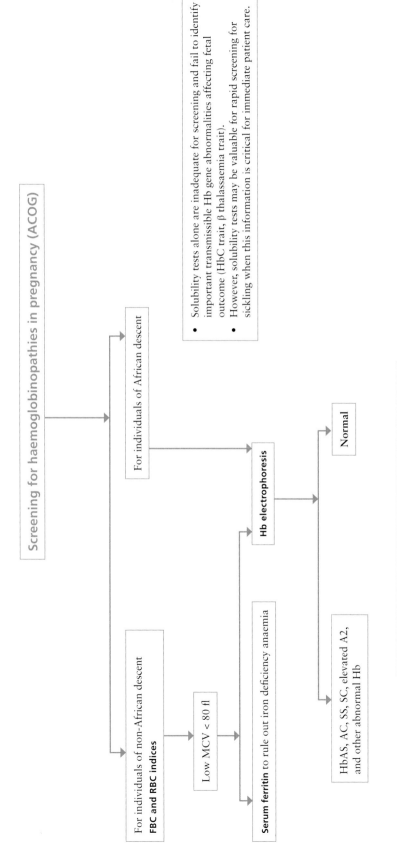

Screening for haemoglobinopathies in pregnancy (ACOG)

For individuals of non-African descent
FBC and RBC indices

Low MCV < 80 fl

Serum ferritin to rule out iron deficiency anaemia

For individuals of African descent

Hb electrophoresis

HbAS, AC, SS, SC, elevated A2, and other abnormal Hb

Normal

α thalassaemia cannot be diagnosed by electrophoresis. It can only be diagnosed by molecular genetic testing. If MCV is below normal, iron deficiency anaemia is ruled out, and the Hb electrophoresis is not consistent with β thalassaemia trait, then use DNA based testing to detect α globin gene deletions characteristic of α thalassaemia.

- Solubility tests alone are inadequate for screening and fail to identify important transmissible Hb gene abnormalities affecting fetal outcome (HbC trait, β thalassaemia trait).
- However, solubility tests may be valuable for rapid screening for sickling when this information is critical for immediate patient care.

Sickle cell disease (SCD) in pregnancy

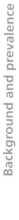

Background and prevalence

- SCD is the most common inherited condition worldwide.
- Most prevalent in individuals of African descent, in the Caribbean, Middle East, parts of India and the Mediterranean, and South and Central America.
- About 300 000 children with SCD are born each year; two-thirds of these are in Africa.
- In the UK there are 12 000–15 000 affected individuals and over 300 infants are born with SCD each year.
- There are approximately 100–200 pregnancies in women with SCD per year in the UK.

Risks or complications

- Increased risk of perinatal mortality, PTD, FGR, and acute painful crises during pregnancy.
- Possible increase in spontaneous miscarriage, antenatal hospitalization, maternal mortality, delivery by CS, infection, thromboembolic events, APH, PET, and PIH.
- Women with HbSC experience fewer adverse outcomes, but they are still at increased risk of painful crises during pregnancy, FGR, antepartum hospital admission, and postpartum infection. Therefore monitor women with HbSC in the same way as those with HbSS.
- There is a paucity of data on pregnancy outcomes in women with HbSβ thalassaemia, HbSD, HbSE or HbSO-Arab, but anecdotal evidence indicates that such women should also be monitored and treated with the same level of vigilance and care as those with HbSS.

Preconception care – specialist sickle cell clinic

- Reproductive planning and contraceptive choice should be part of the regular consultation.
- Provide information on how SCD affects pregnancy and how pregnancy affects SCD, and how to improve outcomes for mother and baby.
- Optimize management and screen for end-organ damage; advise about vaccinations, medications, and crisis avoidance.
- Advise women to have a low threshold for seeking medical help.
- Review women at least annually for the monitoring of chronic disease complications.

Inform women

- The role of dehydration, cold, hypoxia, overexertion, and stress in the frequency of sickle cell crises (SCC).
- Nausea and vomiting in pregnancy can result in dehydration and the precipitation of crises.
- The risk of worsening anaemia, increased risk of crises and acute chest syndrome (ACS) and increased risk of infection (especially UTI) during pregnancy.
- The increased risk of having a growth-restricted baby; fetal distress, IOL, and CS.

Genetic screening

To assess the chance of the baby being affected by SCD.
- Determine the haemoglobinopathy status of the partner.
- If a partner is a carrier, or affected by a major haemoglobinopathy ('at risk couple') – provide counselling and advice about the risk of having affected offspring. Discuss the reproductive options and risks including:
  * Prenatal diagnosis and TOP.
  * PGD.
- If the partner's status is unknown, treat the fetus as high risk for haemoglobinopathy.

Assess for chronic disease complications

- **Screen for pulmonary HT with echocardiography** – pulmonary HT is increased in patients with SCD and is associated with increased mortality. A tricuspid regurgitant jet velocity of >2.5 m/s is associated with a high risk of pulmonary HT.
- **BP and urinalysis** – to identify women with HT and/or proteinuria. Renal and liver function tests annually to identify sickle nephropathy and/or deranged hepatic function.
- **Retinal screening** – proliferative retinopathy is common in patients with SCD, especially patients with HbSC, and can lead to loss of vision. Screen these women preconceptually.
- **Screen for iron overload** – in women who have been multiply transfused in the past or who have a high ferritin level, cardiac MRI may be helpful to assess body iron loading. Aggressive iron chelation before conception is advisable in women who are significantly iron loaded.
- **Screen for red cell antibodies.**

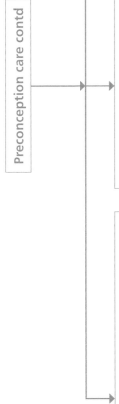

Preconception care contd

Antibiotic prophylaxis and immunization

Penicillin prophylaxis –

- Patients with SCD are hyposplenic and are at risk of infection, in particular from encapsulated bacteria such as *Neisseria meningitidis*, *Streptococcus pneumonia*, and *Haemophilus influenzae*.
- Penicillin prophylaxis is of benefit in young children with SCD, but there is no clear evidence in older patients or pregnant women.
- Provide daily penicillin prophylaxis to all patients with SCD. Give erythromycin if allergic to penicillin.

Vaccination – offer:

- *H. influenza* type b and the conjugated meningococcal C vaccine as a single dose if women have not received it as part of primary vaccination.
- Pneumococcal vaccine every 5 years.
- Hepatitis B vaccine and determine the woman's immune status preconceptually.
- Influenza and 'swine flu' vaccine annually.

Vitamin supplements

- Offer folic acid at a dosage of at least 1 mg daily for women with SCD outside pregnancy in view of their haemolytic anaemia, which puts them at increased risk of folate deficiency.
- Offer folic acid 5 mg once daily both preconceptually and throughout pregnancy to reduce the risk of neural tube defect and to compensate for the increased demand for folate during pregnancy.

Medications review

Hydroxycarbamide –

- Decreases the incidence of acute painful crises and ACS. It is teratogenic in animals. Advise women with SCD on hydroxycarbamide to use effective contraception. Stop hydroxycarbamide 3 months before conception.
- There are reports of women receiving hydroxycarbamide becoming pregnant, some of whom have continued the medication throughout pregnancy without adverse effects on the baby. If women become pregnant while taking hydroxycarbamide, stop it and arrange a level 3 USS to look for structural abnormality, but do not offer termination.

ACE inhibitors or angiotensin receptor blockers –

- Renal dysfunction, proteinuria, and microalbuminuria are common in SCD. ACE inhibitors or ARBs are used routinely in patients with SCD with significant proteinuria.
- These drugs are not safe in pregnancy, therefore stop in women who are trying to conceive.

Antenatal care

1. General aspects

- MDT – (obstetrician, midwife and a haematologist) or 'high-risk' teams. Medical review and screen for end-organ damage (if not undertaken preconceptually).
- Advise women to avoid precipitating factors of SCC such as exposure to extreme temperatures, dehydration, and over-exertion.
- All actions outlined in preconception care (vaccinations, review of iron overload, and red cell autoantibodies) – perform ASAP during antenatal care.

2. Haemoglobinopathy screening – offer partner testing (if not seen preconceptually). If the partner is a carrier, provide counselling ASAP – ideally by 10 weeks to allow the option of first-trimester diagnosis and TOP.

3. Medication during pregnancy

- Daily folic acid and prophylactic antibiotics.
- Stop the drugs that are unsafe in pregnancy.
- Assess iron status and give iron supplementation only if there is evidence of iron deficiency.
- Consider low-dose aspirin 75 mg once daily from 12 weeks to reduce the risk of PET.
- Incidence of VTE is increased therefore offer prophylactic LMWH during hospital admission.
- Prescribe NSAIDs for analgesia between 12 and 28 weeks only due to the concerns regarding adverse effects on fetal development.

Indications for blood transfusion in pregnancy complicated by SCD

- Women with previous serious medical, obstetric or fetal complications – exchange or top-up transfusion may be indicated depending on clinical indications. Decide in an MDT setting.
- Women who are on a transfusion regimen before pregnancy for primary or secondary stroke prevention or for the prevention of severe disease complications – continue transfusions during pregnancy.
- Twin pregnancies – consider prophylactic transfusion due to the high rate of complications in these women.
- Acute anaemia – top-up transfusion.
- Acute chest syndrome or acute stroke – exchange transfusion

4. Additional antenatal care for pregnancy

- Due to probable increased risk of PIH, assess BP and proteinuria at each visit. Women with pre-existing proteinuria or known renal impairment will require more frequent monitoring.
- Due to the increased risk of UTI and asymptomatic bacteriuria, perform urinalysis at each antenatal visit and send MSU for culture and sensitivity monthly.

5. Recommended schedule of USS

- A viability scan at 7–9 weeks.
- Routine first-trimester scan (11–14 weeks) and a detailed anomaly scan at 20 weeks.
- Serial growth scans every 4 weeks from 24 weeks due to the risk of FGR and PET.

6. Role of blood transfusion

- **Prophylactic transfusion – evidence:**
  - * Early studies recommended prophylactic transfusion during pregnancy as there was a decrease in maternal morbidity and perinatal mortality among transfused women.
  - * Recent studies – prophylactic transfusion decreases the incidence of maternal painful crises but does not influence fetal or maternal outcome.
  - * **Systematic review – there is insufficient evidence on the role of transfusion in pregnancy.**
  - * **Do not offer routine prophylactic transfusion.**
- Offer top-up transfusion for acute anaemia. Acute anaemia may be due to transient red cell aplasia, acute splenic sequestration or increased haemolysis and volume expansion encountered in SCD.
- There is no absolute level at which transfusion should be undertaken; decide in conjunction with clinical findings, but haemoglobin under 6 g/dl or a fall of over 2 g/dl from baseline is often used as a guide to transfusion requirement.
- Offer exchange transfusion for ACS and acute stroke. If acute exchange transfusion is required for the treatment of a sickle complication, it may be appropriate to continue the transfusion regimen for the remainder of the pregnancy.
- **Risks** associated with repeated transfusions – alloimmunization, delayed transfusion reactions, transmission of infection, and iron overload.
- Alloimmunization is common in SCD, occurring in 18–36% of patients. It can lead to delayed haemolytic transfusion reactions or haemolytic disease of the newborn and can render patients untransfusable. The most common antibodies are to the C, E, and Kell antigens. The risk of alloimmunization is significantly reduced by giving red cells matched for the C, E, and Kell antigens. **Blood should be matched for an extended phenotype including full rhesus typing (C, D, and E) and Kell typing. Blood used for transfusion should be cytomegalovirus negative.**

Antenatal care contd.

7. Management of acute painful crisis/sickle cell crisis

Assess

- Keep a low threshold for referring women to secondary care – all women with pain that does not settle with simple analgesia, who are febrile, have atypical pain or chest pain, or symptoms of SOB should be referred to secondary care.
- Take history to ascertain if this is typical sickle pain or not, and if there are precipitating factors.
- Examine with focus on the site of pain, any atypical features of the pain, and any precipitating factors, in particular for any signs of infection.
- Assess for medical complications such as ACS, sepsis or dehydration.
- Investigate – FBC, reticulocyte count and renal function, blood cultures, chest X-ray, urine culture, and LFTs.

- Acute painful crisis is the most frequent complication of SCD during pregnancy (27–50%) and it is the most frequent cause of hospital admission.
- Exclude sickle cell crisis urgently in women who become unwell.

Fluid and oxygen

- Fluid balance – ensure fluid intake of at least 60 ml/kg/24 hours.
- Monitor oxygen saturation and provide facial oxygen if oxygen saturation falls below the woman's baseline or <95%. Take early recourse to intensive care if satisfactory oxygen saturation cannot be maintained.
- Prescribe therapeutic antibiotics if the woman is febrile or there is a high clinical suspicion of infection. White blood cell counts are often raised in SCD and do not necessarily indicate infection.
- Thromboprophylaxis if admitted to hospital.
- Other adjuvants may be required to treat the adverse effects of opiates, such as antihistamines, laxatives, and antiemetics.

Analgesia

- Provide initial analgesia within 30 minutes and effective analgesia within 1 hour.
- Use the WHO analgesic ladder – start with paracetamol for mild pain; NSAIDs for mild to moderate pain between 12 and 28 weeks. Use weak opioids such as co-dydramol, co-codamol or dihydrocodeine for moderate pain, and stronger opiates such as morphine for severe pain.
- Mild pain – manage in the community with rest, oral fluids, and paracetamol or weak opioids.
- Opiates are not associated with teratogenicity or congenital malformation but may be associated with transient suppression of FMs and a reduced baseline variability of the FHR.
- Where a mother has received prolonged administration of opiates in late pregnancy, observe the neonate for signs of opioid withdrawal.
- Pethidine is contraindicated due to the risk of toxicity and seizures.

Monitoring

- Women whose pain settles following oral analgesia can be discharged home. Admit women who need strong opiate therapy.
- Monitor pain, sedation, vital signs, respiratory rate, and oxygen saturation every 20–30 minutes until pain is controlled and signs are stable, then monitor every 2 hours (hourly if receiving parenteral opiates).
- If respiratory rate is <10/minute, omit maintenance analgesia; consider naloxone.
- Consider reducing analgesia after 2–3 days and replacing injections with oral analgesia.
- Discharge the woman when pain is controlled and improving without analgesia or on acceptable doses of oral analgesia.
- Arrange any necessary home care and outpatient follow-up appointments.

Antenatal care contd
8. Other acute complications of SCD

Acute chest syndrome (ACS)

- ACS is the second most common complication (7–20% of pregnancies).
- It is characterized by tachypnoea, chest pain, cough, and SOB in the presence of a new infiltrate on the chest X-ray.
- Early recognition of ACS is the key. The signs and symptoms of ACS are the same as those of pneumonia, so treat both simultaneously.
- Acute severe infection with the H1N1 virus in pregnancy can cause a similar picture, therefore commence investigation and treatment for this.
- Treatment is with IV antibiotics, oxygen, and blood transfusion.
- Get urgent review by the haematology team for advice on transfusion. Top-up BT may be required if the haemoglobin is falling, or if the haemoglobin is < 65 g/l.
- If the woman is hypoxic, get critical care team review; ventilatory support may be required. In severe hypoxia, and if the haemoglobin level is maintained, exchange transfusion will be required.
- There is an increased risk of pulmonary embolism among women with SCD. In women presenting with acute hypoxia, consider pulmonary embolism. Commence therapeutic LMWH until definitive investigations are undertaken.

Acute stroke

- Acute stroke, both infarctive and haemorrhagic, is associated with SCD. Consider it in any woman with SCD who presents with acute neurological impairment.
- If a stroke is suspected, arrange an urgent brain imaging and seek haematologist advice for urgent exchange transfusion. It is a medical emergency and a rapid-exchange blood transfusion can decrease long-term neurological damage.
- Thrombolysis is not indicated in acute stroke secondary to SCD.

Acute anaemia

Erythrovirus infection –

- Acute anaemia in women with SCD may be due to erythrovirus infection. It causes a red cell maturation arrest and an aplastic crisis characterized by a reticulocytopenia. Therefore, request a reticulocyte count in any woman presenting with an acute anaemia and, if low, may indicate infection with erythrovirus.
- Treatment is with blood transfusion and isolation of the woman.
- There is risk of vertical transmission to the fetus, which can result in hydrops fetalis, therefore refer to the fetal medicine team.

Other causes of anaemia –

- Bleeding or any other causes of anaemia incidental to the SCD.
- Rare causes of anaemia in SCD include malaria and, occasionally, splenic sequestration in women with a mild phenotype.

Intrapartum care

Optimal timing and mode of delivery

- Studies have highlighted increased perinatal mortality, particularly during the later stages of pregnancy, in part owing to the complications of SCD. The risks of abruption, PET, peripartum cardiomyopathy, and acute SCC are increased and unpredictable. It is suggested that delivery at 38–40 weeks will prevent late pregnancy complications and associated adverse perinatal events.
- Women with normally grown fetus – offer elective IOL or elective CS if indicated after 38 weeks.
- SCD in itself is not a contraindication to vaginal delivery or VBAC.
- In women who have hip replacements (because of avascular necrosis) – discuss suitable positions for delivery.

Care and place of birth

- Deliver in hospitals that are able to manage the complications of SCD and high-risk pregnancies.
- Keep women warm and adequately hydrated.
- There is an increased frequency of SCC and ACS in the intrapartum period. The risk is increased with protracted labour (> 12 hours), which is often secondary to dehydration. If oral hydration is not tolerated or is inadequate, commence IV fluids and use a fluid balance chart to prevent fluid overload.
- Consider CS if labour is not progressing well and delivery is not imminent.
- Venous access can be difficult, especially if women have had multiple previous admissions – obtain anaesthetic review/IV access early.
- Demand for oxygen is increased and the use of pulse oximetry to detect hypoxia in the mother is appropriate. Perform arterial blood gas analysis and commence oxygen therapy if oxygen saturation is ≤ 94%.
- Routine antibiotic prophylaxis in labour is currently not supported by evidence.
- Hourly observations of vital signs.
- Investigate raised temperature (> 37.5°C). Keep a low threshold for commencing broad-spectrum antibiotics.
- Continuous EFM in labour should be used due to the increased rate of fetal distress, stillbirth, placental abruption, and compromised placental reserve.

Analgesia and anaesthesia

- Offer anaesthetic assessment in the third trimester of pregnancy.
- Pregnant women with SCD are at risk of end-organ damage as well as at risk of CS. GA carries additional risks therefore avoid where possible.
- Regional anaesthesia may reduce the necessity of general anaesthesia. It is also likely to reduce the need for high doses of opioids if the woman has sickle-related pain in the lower body. Regional analgesia is recommended for CS.
- Avoid pethidine because of the risk of seizures. Other opiates can be used.
- Indications for epidural analgesia in labour are the same as normal.

Postpartum care

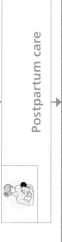

Optimum care post-delivery

- The risk of SCC remains increased in up to 25% of women and is more common following GA. Manage crises as for non-pregnant women.
- Maintain maternal oxygen saturation > 94% and adequate hydration.
- NSAIDs can be used in the postpartum period and during breastfeeding.
- Thromboprophylaxis – * Early mobilization. * Antithrombotic stockings. * LMWH while in hospital and 7 days postdischarge following vaginal delivery or for a period of 6 weeks following CS.
- Where the baby is at high risk of SCD, offer early testing for SCD.
- Encourage breastfeeding.

Contraceptive advice:

- Barrier methods are as safe and effective.
- The UK criteria (based on WHO criteria) for contraceptive use:
  * POP, Depo-Provera, the levonorgestrel IUS, and emergency contraception = category 1 (no restriction on their use).
  * Combined OCPs and copper IUD = category 2 (advantages outweigh disadvantages).
  * Combined OCPs – there is concern about an increased risk of VTE, but there is no evidence to confirm this risk.

Clinical Management Guidelines for Obstetricians and Gynaecologists: Haemoglobinopathies in pregnancy. ACOG No. 78; 2007.
Management of Sickle Cell Disease in Pregnancy. RCOG Green-top Guideline No. 61; July 2011.

Specific antenatal care for women with SCD

First appointment – Primary care/Hospital appointment

- Offer information, advice and support in relation to optimizing general health.
- Offer partner testing; review partner results if available and discuss Prenatal diagnosis if appropriate.
- Take a clinical history to establish extent of SCD and its complications.
- Review medications and its complications; stop hydroxycarbamide, ACE inhibitors or ARBs.
- 5 mg folic acid and antibiotic prophylaxis if no contraindication.
- Discuss vaccinations.
- Offer retinal and/or renal and/or cardiac assessments if not performed in the previous year.
- Document baseline oxygen saturations and BP; send MSU for culture.
- 7–9 weeks – Confirm viability in view of the increased risk of miscarriage.

Booking appointment – midwife with experience in high-risk obstetrics

- Discuss information, education, and advice about how SCD will affect pregnancy.
- Review partner results and discuss PND if appropriate.
- Baseline renal function test, urine protein/creatinine ratio, liver function test, and ferritin.
- Extended red cell phenotype if not previously performed.
- Confirm that all actions from first visit are complete.
- Consider low-dose aspirin from 12 weeks of gestation.

Midwife + MDT

Offer Routine ANC and repeat MSU at each visit –
- 16 weeks
- 20 weeks: USS anomaly scan; Repeat FBC

Midwife Appointments

Offer routine check including BP and urinalysis at –
- 26 weeks
- 30 weeks: Offer antenatal classes
- 34 weeks
- 39 weeks: recommend delivery by 40 weeks of gestation

MDT Appointments

Offer USS for fetal growth and AFV and Repeat MSU at –
- 24 weeks
- 28 weeks: Repeat FBC and group and antibody screen
- 32 weeks: Repeat FBC
- 36 weeks: Offer information and advice about: timing, mode and management of the birth, analgesia and anaesthesia; arrange anaesthetic assessment, care of baby after birth

Obstetrician Appointments

Offer routine check at –
- 38 weeks: Recommend IOL or CS between 38 and 40 weeks of gestation
- 40 weeks: Offer fetal monitoring if the woman declines delivery by 40 weeks.

CHAPTER 42 Haemoglobinopathies – beta thalassaemia in pregnancy

The thalassaemias – disorders characterized by a reduced synthesis of globin chains, resulting in microcytic anaemia. These are classified according to the globin chain affected. The basic defect is reduced globin chain synthesis with the resultant red cells having inadequate haemoglobin content and extravascular haemolysis due to the release into the peripheral circulation of damaged red blood cells and erythroid precursors because of a high degree of ineffective erythropoiesis.

α thalassaemia

- **α thalassaemia** – results from gene deletion of 2 or more copies of the 4 α globin chains.
  * Deletion of 1 α globin chain α -/ α α – clinically unrecognizable.
  * Deletion of 2 α globin chain - -/ α α or α -/ - α = α thalassaemia trait/minor – mild asymptomatic microcytic anaemia. These are carriers and are at increased risk of having a child with a more severe form of thalassaemia caused by deletion of 3 or 4 copies of α globin chain.
  * Deletion of 3 α globin chain - -/ - α = HbH disease is usually associated with mild to moderate haemolytic anaemia.
  * Deletion of 4 α globin chain - -/ - - = α thalassaemia major/ Hb Barts is associated with hydrops fetalis, IUD, and pre-eclampsia.
- **α thalassaemia trait** – the course of pregnancy is not significantly different from that of women with normal Hb.
- **HbH disease** – pregnancy in these women has been reported, and with the exception of mild to moderate chronic anaemia, outcomes are favourable.

β thalassaemia

- **β thalassaemia** – caused by a mutation in the β globin gene, that causes deficient or absent β chain production, which results in absence of HbA.
  * Heterozygous – β thalassaemia minor – depending on the amount of β chain production, it usually is associated with asymptomatic mild anaemia with favourable pregnancy outcome.
  * Homozygous – β thalassaemia major (Cooley's anaemia) – this results in a severe transfusion-dependent anaemia with extramedullary erythropoiesis. Elevated levels of HbF partially compensate for the absence of HbA; however death usually occurs by age 10 years unless treatment is begun early with periodic BT.
- The mainstay of modern treatment is blood transfusion and iron chelation therapy. Multiple transfusions cause iron overload resulting in hepatic, cardiac, and endocrine dysfunction. The anterior pituitary is very sensitive to iron overload and evidence of dysfunction is common. Puberty is often delayed and incomplete, resulting in low bone mass. Most of these women are subfertile due to hypogonadotrophic hypogonadism and therefore require ovulation induction therapy with gonadotrophins to achieve a pregnancy. Cardiac failure is the primary cause of death in over 50% of cases. Improved transfusion techniques and effective chelation protocols have improved the quality of life and survival of thalassaemia patients.
- Pregnancy is recommended only for those with normal cardiac function who have had prolonged hypertransfusion therapy to maintain Hb levels at 10g/dl and iron chelation therapy with desferoxamine.
- **β thalassaemia in pregnancy:**
  * Thalassaemia major women are those who require > 7 transfusions per year.
  * Thalassaemia intermedia women are those needing <7 transfusion episodes per year or those who are not transfused.
  * Thalassaemia trait women do not require transfusion.

Background and prevalence

- More than 70 000 babies are born with thalassaemia worldwide each year and there are 100 million individuals with asymptomatic thalassaemia trait.
- There are approximately 1000 individuals affected by thalassaemia trait in the UK.
- Previously, the community affected was principally from Cyprus and the Mediterranean. However, currently, the Asian communities of India, Pakistan, and Bangladesh account for 79% of thalassaemia births in the UK.
- The newborn sickle cell and thalassaemia screening programme in England during 2009/10 identified approximately 16 000 women as carriers of a haemoglobinopathy. 59% of screen-positive women had partner testing and 1006 couples were identified as being at high risk of having a child with a clinically significant haemoglobinopathy (SCD or thalassaemia). 396 couples took up the offer of prenatal diagnosis which revealed 23 pregnancies affected by thalassaemia, and 46 who were carriers of β thalassaemia; 91.7% of pregnancies affected by thalassaemia major were terminated.

Risks or complications

Maternal

- Subfertility – may occur in transfusion-dependent individuals where chelation has been sub-optimal with iron overload resulting in damage to the anterior pituitary. They require ovulation induction using injectable gonadotrophins to conceive.
- Cardiomyopathy due to iron overload.
- With around 9 months of little or no chelation women with thalassaemia major may develop diabetes mellitus, hypothyroidism, and hypoparathyroidism due to the increasing iron burden.
- Splenectomy is no longer the mainstay of treatment for these conditions but a considerable number of both thalassaemia major and intermedia patients have been splenectomized.

Fetal

- Increased risk of FGR.

CHAPTER 42   Beta thalassaemia in pregnancy

Preconception care – specialist MDT clinic

- **MDT** – obstetrician and midwife with expertise in managing high-risk pregnancies and a haematologist, cardiologist, and hepatologist.
- Inform about how thalassaemia affects pregnancy and vice versa. Discuss pregnancy and contraception well in advance because a prolonged period of iron chelation therapy may be required to control iron overload.
- Optimize management and screen for end-organ damage.
- Review transfusion requirements, compliance with chelation therapy, and assess body iron burden.
- Advise to use contraception despite the reduced fertility. There is no contraindication to the use of combined OCP, the POP, progesterone implant, and the IUS.

Genetic screening

- To assess the chance of the baby being affected by thalassaemia.
- Offer partner screening to determine his haemoglobinopathy status.
- Offer counselling if the partner is a carrier of a haemoglobinopathy that may adversely interact with the woman's genotype.
- Consider PGD in the presence of haemoglobinopathies in both partners (high-risk couples) to avoid a homozygous or compound heterozygous pregnancy.
- Discuss methods and risks of prenatal diagnosis and TOP.
- If partner is unavailable or unwilling to undergo preconceptual testing treat the fetus as high risk for a haemoglobinopathy and offer invasive tests.

Antibiotic prophylaxis and immunization

Women who are transfused regularly are at risk of transmitted infections; therefore ascertain infectivity and manage them. Women who had splenectomy are at risk of infection from encapsulated bacteria such as *N meningitidis*, *S. pneumoniae*, and *H. influenzae*.

Penicillin prophylaxis – provide daily penicillin prophylaxis if had splenectomy. Erythromycin if allergic to penicillin.

Vaccination – offer:

- *H. influenzae* type b (Hib) and the conjugated meningococcal C vaccine as a single dose if not received previously.
- Pneumococcal vaccine every 5 years.
- Hepatitis B vaccination in HBSAg negative women.
- Determine hepatitis C status for all women who are transfused. Refer to a hepatologist if positive.

Vitamin supplements – offer folic acid 5 mg daily both preconceptually and throughout pregnancy to reduce the risk of neural tube defects and to compensate for the increased demand for folate during pregnancy.

Thromboprophylaxis – these women have a prothrombotic tendency due to abnormal red cell membranes. The spleen normally helps to reduce the amounts of these in the circulation. Platelet counts are high in patients who have been splenectomized. Commence low-dose aspirin in women who have had a splenectomy or a platelet count > 600×10^9/l.

Assess for chronic disease complications

Liver –
- Assess for liver iron concentration using a Ferriscan® or liver T2*. Aim for liver iron < 7 mg/g (dry weight). If liver iron exceeds the target range, a period of intensive preconception chelation is required to optimize liver iron burden. If liver iron exceeds 15 mg/g (dw) prior to conception, the risk of myocardial iron loading increases so commence iron chelation with low-dose desferrioxamine between 20 and 28 weeks.
- Cholelithiasis is common due to the underlying haemolytic anaemia and women may develop cholecystitis in pregnancy. Liver cirrhosis and active hepatitis C (HCV) may run a more complex clinical course during pregnancy. Arrange liver and gall bladder (and spleen if present) USS – to detect cholelithiasis and liver cirrhosis. Refer to hepatologist where there is any evidence of cirrhosis either due to previous hepatitis or as a consequence of severe hepatic iron loading.

Heart (assessment by a cardiologist) –
- Organize an echocardiogram and an ECG, T2* cardiac MRI to determine the cardiac status of the woman and the severity of any cardiomyopathy. The aim is for no cardiac iron, but this can take years to achieve so individualize care. Aim for cardiac T2* > 20 ms.
- A reduced ejection fraction is a relative contraindication to pregnancy.

Pancreas –
- DM is common in these women, which is multifactorial; due to insulin resistance, iron-induced islet cell insufficiency, genetic factors, and autoimmunity.
- Good glycaemic control is essential prepregnancy.
- HbA1c < 6.1% is associated with a reduced risk of congenital abnormalities. Glycosylated haemoglobin is not a reliable marker of glycaemic control as this is diluted by transfused blood and results in underestimation, so serum fructosamine is preferred for monitoring. Aim for serum fructosamine concentrations < 300 nmol/l (equivalent to a HbA1c of 6.1%) for at least 3 months prior to conception in women with established DM.

Thyroid – Determine thyroid function. The woman should be euthyroid prepregnancy.

Bone density scan – Women are at high risk of osteoporosis secondary to underlying thalassaemic bone disease, chelation of calcium by chelation drugs, hypogonadism, and vitamin D deficiency. Offer a bone density scan to document preexisting osteoporosis. Optimize serum vitamin D concentrations with supplements if necessary.

Red cell antibodies – Measure ABO and full blood group genotype and antibody titres. Alloimmunity occurs in 8% to 21% of these patients. It may indicate a risk of haemolytic disease of the newborn and there may be issues around blood transfusion.

Medications review

- **Aggressive chelation** in the preconception stage can reduce and optimize body iron burden, reduce end-organ damage, and reverse cardiac iron load. Patients who are optimally chelated are less likely to suffer from endocrinopathies or cardiac problems.
- Due to lack of safety data, consider all chelation therapy as potentially teratogenic in the 1st trimester. Desferrioxamine is the only chelation agent with a body of evidence for use in the 2nd and 3rd trimester. The optimization of iron burden is therefore critical as the ongoing iron accumulation from transfusion in the absence of chelation may expose the pregnant woman to a high risk of new complications related to iron overload, particularly diabetes and cardiomyopathy.
- Review iron chelators and discontinue deferasirox and deferiprone ideally 3 months before conception. Avoid desferrioxamine in the 1st trimester; it has been used safely after 20 weeks of gestation at low doses.
- Desferrioxamine is safe during ovulation induction therapy.

Maternal – antenatal care

- MDT – an obstetrician, a midwife with experience of high-risk antenatal care, a haematologist with an interest in thalassaemia, and a diabetologist or cardiologist.
- **Haemoglobinopathy screening** – offer partner testing (if not seen preconceptually). If the partner is a carrier, provide counselling ASAP – ideally by 10 weeks to allow the option of first-trimester diagnosis and TOP.
- Assess for evidence of increasing anaemia or FGR.

Thalassaemia major –
- Review monthly until 28 weeks and fortnightly thereafter.
- Women with thalassaemia and diabetes – monthly assessment of serum fructosamine concentrations and review in the specialist diabetic pregnancy clinic.
- Specialist cardiac assessment at 28 weeks and thereafter as appropriate. Cardiac assessment is important to determine cardiac function, further iron chelation, and planning for labour.
- Monitor TFTs in hypothyroid patients and make appropriate dose changes.
- Individualize care depending on the degree of end-organ damage and women with diabetes or cardiac dysfunction may be reviewed more frequently.

Thalassaemia intermedia – review monthly by the MDT.

Recommended schedule of USS

- Viability scan at 7–9 weeks as there is a higher risk of early pregnancy loss.
- Routine 1st trimester scan (11–14 weeks) and a detailed anomaly scan at 18–20+6 weeks.
- Serial fetal biometry scans every 4 weeks from 24 weeks, because chronic anaemia affects placental transfer of nutrients and can therefore adversely affect fetal growth.

Antenatal thromboprophylaxis

There is a prothrombotic tendency due to the presence of abnormal red cell fragments especially if had splenectomy. These red cell fragments combined with a high platelet count significantly increase the risk of VTE.
- Give prophylactic LMWH during antenatal hospital admissions.
- All women who have undergone splenectomy – continue with low-dose aspirin if this was started preconceptually. Commence aspirin if the platelet count is > 600 × 10⁹/l.

Iron chelation therapy

Women with myocardial iron
- Regular cardiology review with monitoring of ejection fraction during the pregnancy, as signs of cardiac decompensation are the primary indications for intervention with chelation therapy.
- Iron replacement in women who have not had preconceptual assessment, or where there is concern about cardiac function.
  * Women with T2* MRI >20 ms do not require desferrioxamine chelation during pregnancy unless there is severe hepatic iron overload.
  * Women with thalassaemia major and T2* MRI of <10 ms are at high risk of cardiac decompensation. They may present with increasing breathlessness, paroxysmal nocturnal dyspnoea, orthopnoea, syncope, palpitations or peripheral oedema. Presentation in the 1st trimester is associated with adverse clinical outcomes.
- If a woman describes symptoms of palpitations then a cardiac assessment is appropriate. A falling ejection fraction or increasing ventricular volumes on echocardiography will suggest increasing risk of developing heart failure. If the woman complains of palpitations then a detailed history, ECG, and Holter monitor assessment is needed to confirm a pathological cause. In either circumstance desferrioxamine infusions may be indicated if there are concerns.
- Women at highest risk of cardiac decompensation – commence low-dose subcutaneous desferrioxamine (20 mg/kg/day) on a minimum of 4–5 days a week under joint haematology and cardiology guidance from 20 to 24 weeks.

Women with severe liver iron – high concentrations of liver iron (liver iron > 15 mg/g [dw] as measured by MRI) are associated with an increased risk of myocardial iron and in all women with thalassaemia major the therapeutic aim is to achieve a liver iron concentration below 15 mg/g (dw) to reduce the risk of myocardial iron overload. Review and consider low-dose desferrioxamine iron chelation from 20 weeks.

Transfusion regimen

Thalassaemia major –
- All women will be receiving blood transfusions on a regular basis aiming for a pretransfusion Hb of 100 g/l. These women will already be established on transfusion regimens which generally remain stable during pregnancy.

Thalassaemia intermedia – the decision to initiate a transfusion regimen is a clinical one based on the woman's symptoms and fetal growth.
- Women who are asymptomatic with normal fetal growth and low haemoglobin – individualize the plan with regard to blood transfusion in late pregnancy.
- If there is worsening maternal anaemia or evidence of FGR, commence regular transfusions aiming for maintenance pretransfusion haemoglobin concentration > 100 g/l.
- Initially administer a 2–3 unit transfusion with additional top-up transfusion if necessary the following week until the haemoglobin reaches 120 g/l. Monitor the haemoglobin after 2–3 weeks and transfuse 2 units if the haemoglobin has fallen < 100 g/l. Each woman's haemoglobin falls at different rates after transfusion so close surveillance of pretransfusion Hb concentrations is required.
- If the haemoglobin is > 80 g/l at 36 weeks in non-transfused women then transfusion can be avoided prior to delivery. Postnatal transfusion can be provided as necessary.
- If the haemoglobin is < 80 g/l then aim for a top-up transfusion of 2 units at 37–38 weeks.

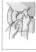

Intrapartum care

Optimal timing and mode of delivery

- There is no good evidence regarding the timing or mode of delivery for women with thalassaemia. The timing of delivery depends on the issues in pregnancy, e.g., diabetes or FGR, but if otherwise uncomplicated the delivery can be planned as per local guidelines.
- If there are medical complications such as cardiomyopathy – formulate a detailed management plan during the pregnancy.

Care and place of birth

- Birth in hospitals that are able to manage the complications and high-risk pregnancies.
- Cross-match for delivery if there are atypical antibodies present since this may delay the availability of blood. Otherwise a group and antibody will suffice.
- If the haemoglobin is <100 g/l, cross-match 2 units on admission to the labour ward.
- Women who are transfusion-dependent and not on a chelating agent will have high serum concentrations of toxic iron species non-transferrin bound iron. These may cause free radical damage and cardiac dysrhythmia when the body is subjected to stress such as labour. Therefore commence peripartum chelation therapy with IV desferrioxamine 2 g IV over 24 hours for the duration of labour.
- Continuous EFM.
- CS for obstetric indications.
- Active management of the third stage of labour to minimize blood loss.

Postpartum care

- At high risk of VTE due to the presence of abnormal red cells in the circulation. Provide appropriate prophylaxis whilst an inpatient and for 7 days post-discharge following vaginal delivery or for 6 weeks following CS.
- Encourage breastfeeding.
- Women who plan to breastfeed – restart desferrioxamine infusions on their previous iron chelation regimen as soon as the initial 24-hour infusion of IV desferrioxamine finishes after delivery as there is no evidence that desferrioxamine is excreted in breast milk.
- If the woman decides not to breastfeed, continue IV or subcutaneous desferrioxamine infusions until discharge from hospital or until resumption of her previous iron chelation regimen under haematology supervision, whichever is sooner.

Clinical Management Guidelines for Obstetricians and Gynaecologists: Haemoglobinopathies in pregnancy. ACOG No. 78; 2007.
Management of Beta Thalassaemia in Pregnancy. RCOG Green-top Guideline 66; 2014.

Specific antenatal care for women with thalassaemia

Midwife with experience in high-risk obstetrics

Booking appointment

- Offer information, advice and support to optimise general health; how thalassaemia will affect pregnancy
- Offer partner testing; review partner results if available and discuss Prenatal diagnosis if appropriate
- Take a clinical history to establish extent of thalassaemia complications.
- Women with diabetes referred to joint diabetes pregnancy clinic with haematology input.
- Review medications eg stop chelators Deferiprone, Deferasirox.
- 5 mg folic acid and antibiotic prophylaxis for Women who have had a splenectomy.
- Discuss vaccinations with those women who have had a splenectomy.
- Offer MRI heart and liver if not been performed in the previous year for thalassaemia major patients.
- Document BP; send MSU for culture; determine presence of any red cell antibodies

7–9 weeks: Confirm viability in view of the increased risk of miscarriage.
11–14 weeks: Confirm that all actions from first visit are complete.

Midwife + MDT

Offer Routine ANC and Diabetic care at each visit at –
- 16 weeks
- 20 weeks: USS anomaly scan.

Midwife Appointments

Offer routine check including BP and urinalysis at –
- 30 weeks: Offer antenatal classes
- 34 weeks
- 39 weeks

MDT Appointments

- 20 – 24 weeks:
  * Woman with risks of cardiac decompensation (T2*< 10ms) – start on low dose subcutaneous desferrioxamine (20mg/kg/day) on a minimum of 4 to 5 days a week from around 20–24 weeks.
  * Women with T2* > 10 but < 20ms – assess and consider starting desferrioxamine infusions if there are concerns.
  * Women with T2*>20ms – do not give any desferrioxamine unless severe hepatic iron overload.

Offer USS for fetal growth and AFV at –
- 24 weeks
- 28 weeks: Specialist cardiology review and formulation of delivery plan based on cardiac function.
- 32 weeks
- 36 weeks: Offer information and advice about: timing, mode and management of the birth, analgesia and anaesthesia; arrange anaesthetic assessment, care of baby after birth.

Obstetrician Appointments

Offer routine check at –
- 38 weeks: Recommend IOL or CS between 38 and 40 weeks of gestation.
- 40 weeks
- 41 weeks: For a non–diabetic woman with normal fetal growth and no complications, offer IOL at 42 weeks.

CHAPTER 43 Prevention and treatment of thrombosis and embolism during pregnancy and the puerperium

Prevalence and background – UK

- Pulmonary embolism (PE) – the leading direct cause of maternal death (1.56/100 000 maternities).
- Many PEs are preventable with appropriate thromboprophylaxis (TP).
- Incidence of antenatal PE – 1.3/10 000 maternities with a case fatality rate of 3.5%; 10 fatalities per year.
- Incidence of VTE in pregnancy and the puerperium is 1–2/1000. 700–1400 pregnancy-related VTE episodes/year in addition to those related to miscarriage and TOP.
- Overall case fatality for VTE in pregnancy is approximately 1%.
- VTE is up to 10 times more common in pregnant women than in non-pregnant women of the same age and can occur at any stage of pregnancy but the puerperium is the time of highest risk.
- 79% of the women who die from PE have identifiable risk factors.
- CS is a significant risk factor but women having vaginal deliveries are also at risk and 55% of the postpartum maternal deaths from VTE occur in women with vaginal delivery.
- LMWH reduces VTE risk in medical and surgical patients by 60% and 70%, respectively.

History and assessment of risk factors

Undertake an assessment of risk factors for VTE in early pregnancy or before pregnancy. Repeat:
- if a woman is admitted to hospital for any reason;
- if a woman develops other intercurrent problems;
- intrapartum and immediately postpartum.

Assess risk based on:
A. Risk factors for VTE in pregnancy.
B. Previous history of VTE.
C. Personal history of thrombophilias:
  a. asymptomatic heritable thrombophilia;
  b. acquired thrombophilia (antiphospholipid syndrome).
D. Family history of thrombophilia.

Risk factors for VTE in pregnancy

Pre-existing

- Previous venous thromboembolism.
- Thrombophilia:
  Heritable:
    Antithrombin deficiency; protein C deficiency
    protein S deficiency; Factor V Leiden
    prothrombin gene G20210A
  Acquired (antiphospholipid syndrome):
    Persistent lupus anticoagulant
    Persistent moderate/high-titre anticardiolipin antibodies
    or β2 glycoprotein 1 antibodies

- Medical comorbidities e.g., heart or lung disease, SLE, cancer, inflammatory conditions (inflammatory bowel disease or inflammatory polyarthropathy), nephrotic syndrome (proteinuria > 3 g/day), sickle cell disease.
- Intravenous drug use.
- Age > 35 years; • obesity (BMI > 30 kg/m²).
- Parity ≥ 3; • Smoking; • Paraplegia;
- Gross varicose veins (symptomatic or above knee or with associated phlebitis, oedema/skin changes).

Obstetric

- Multiple pregnancy.
- Assisted reproductive therapy.
- Pre-eclampsia.
- Caesarean section.
- PPH (> 1 l) requiring transfusion.
- Prolonged labour, mid-cavity rotational operative delivery.

New-onset/transient – potentially reversible

- Surgical procedure in pregnancy or puerperium (e.g., SMM, appendicectomy, postpartum sterilization).
- Hyperemesis • Dehydration • OHSS
- Admission or immobility (≥ 3 days bed rest), e.g., symphysis pubis dysfunction restricting mobility,
- Systemic infection (requiring antibiotics or admission to hospital), e.g., pneumonia, pyelonephritis.
- Postpartum infection • Long-distance travel (> 4 hours).

Timing of initiation of thromboprophylaxis

- Most VTE occurs antenatally, with an equal distribution throughout gestation. The CEMD UK (2003–2005) two-thirds of antenatal fatal pulmonary VTE occurred in the first trimester. Other studies reported almost 40–50% of antenatal VTE occur in first trimester.
- Undertake risk assessment before pregnancy and commence prophylaxis as early in pregnancy as practical.
- Additional risk factors may complicate the first trimester, such as hyperemesis, surgery for miscarriage, TOP, ectopic pregnancy or OHSS. OR for VTE with hyperemesis gravidarum is 2.5.

A. Previous VTE

- An increased risk of recurrence of VTE – 11% during and 4% outside pregnancy.
- The risk of recurrence appears to be constant over the whole period of pregnancy.
- Provide postpartum TP to all women with prior VTE, as this is the period of greatest risk.

Recurrent VTE

- At increased risk of recurrence and many will be on long-term warfarin.
- Refer to a clinician with expertise in haemostasis and pregnancy. For some women, higher doses of LMWH may be necessary.
- Counsel about the risks of warfarin to the fetus and advise to stop warfarin and change to LMWH as soon as pregnancy is confirmed, ideally within 2 weeks of the missed period and before the 6th week of pregnancy.
- Advise women who are not on warfarin to start LMWH as soon as they have a positive pregnancy test.

Single previous VTE

Temporary risk factor-associated

- The risk of antenatal recurrence is very low if the prior VTE was provoked by a transient major risk factor that is no longer present.

Unprovoked

- During pregnancy a recurrence rate of 4–6% is reported in women with a previous VTE episode that was either unprovoked or associated with thrombophilia compared with no recurrences in women with previous VTE associated with a temporary risk factor and who did not have thrombophilia.

Oestrogen-provoked

- Women with previous Oestrogen-related VTE are at higher risk of VTE in pregnancy and the puerperium.
- In one study, where the previous VTE was associated with use of oestrogen-containing OCPs, the recurrence rate of VTE in subsequent pregnancies was 9.5%. The risk was similar (9.8%) if the prior VTE occurred during previous pregnancy.

Thrombophilia-associated

Acquired

See next page

Heritable

- Heritable thrombophilia is found in 20–50% of women with pregnancy-related VTE.
- Data in pregnancy are extremely sparse. Heritable thrombophilia is a weak risk factor for recurrent VTE during pregnancy, with a RR of 1.9.
- Testing for thrombophilia will not usually influence TP in the current pregnancy unless detected in a woman with a prior VTE related to a temporary risk factor who would not otherwise receive TP. Consider investigating for thrombophilia where the temporary provoking stimulus was minor (long-distance travel) but not where it was major (surgery or major trauma with prolonged immobility).

- Women with antithrombin deficiency (particularly type 1) have a very high risk of recurrence and may require higher doses of LMWH in pregnancy. An intermediate or treatment dose of LMWH is required throughout pregnancy and postpartum for a minimum of 6 weeks or until converted back to long-term warfarin.

CHAPTER 43 Thrombosis and embolism

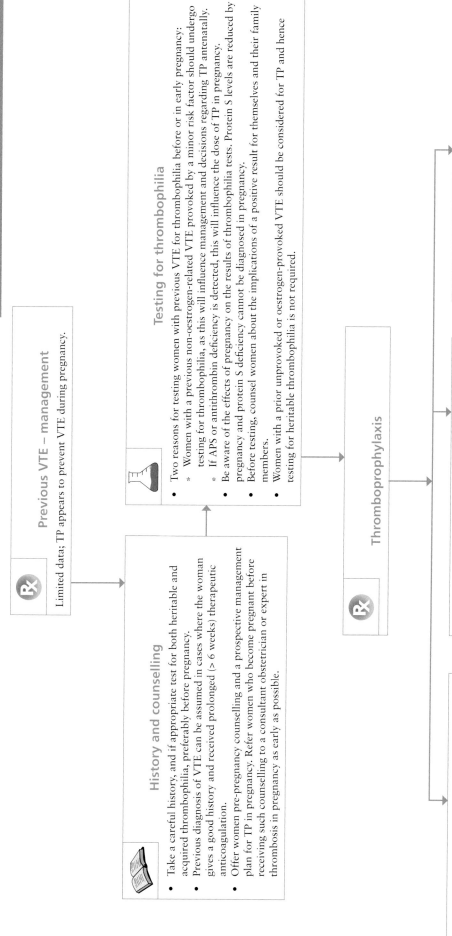

Previous VTE – management

Limited data; TP appears to prevent VTE during pregnancy.

History and counselling

- Take a careful history, and if appropriate test for both heritable and acquired thrombophilia, preferably before pregnancy.
- Previous diagnosis of VTE can be assumed in cases where the woman gives a good history and received prolonged (> 6 weeks) therapeutic anticoagulation.
- Offer women pre-pregnancy counselling and a prospective management plan for TP in pregnancy. Refer women who become pregnant before receiving such counselling to a consultant obstetrician or expert in thrombosis in pregnancy as early as possible.

Testing for thrombophilia

- Two reasons for testing women with previous VTE for thrombophilia before or in early pregnancy:
  * Women with a previous non-oestrogen-related VTE provoked by a minor risk factor should undergo testing for thrombophilia, as this will influence management and decisions regarding TP antenatally.
  * If APS or antithrombin deficiency is detected, this will influence the dose of TP in pregnancy.
- Be aware of the effects of pregnancy on the results of thrombophilia tests. Protein S levels are reduced by pregnancy and protein S deficiency cannot be diagnosed in pregnancy.
- Before testing, counsel women about the implications of a positive result for themselves and their family members.
- Women with a prior unprovoked or oestrogen-provoked VTE should be considered for TP and hence testing for heritable thrombophilia is not required.

Thromboprophylaxis

Very high risk

- Women with recurrent VTE associated with either antithrombin deficiency or APS (who will often be on long-term oral anticoagulation).
- Management by experts in haemostasis and pregnancy.
- TP – higher-dose LMWH antenatally and for 6 weeks postpartum or until converted back to warfarin after delivery.

High risk

- Women in whom the original VTE was:
  * Unprovoked.
  * Related to oestrogen (oestrogen-containing contraception or pregnancy).
  * Related to transient risk factor other than major surgery.
  * Who have other risk factors.
- TP with LMWH antenatally and for 6 weeks postpartum.

Intermediate risk

- Women in whom the original VTE was provoked by a transient major risk factor such as major surgery that is no longer present and who have no other risk factors.
- TP with LMWH for 6 weeks postpartum.
- TP with LMWH can be withheld antenatally until 28 weeks, provided that no additional risk factors are present (in which case they should be offered LMWH).
- Close surveillance for the development of other risk factors.

B. Asymptomatic heritable thrombophilia

- Detected because of screening following identification of heritable thrombophilia in a family member.
- Family history – the number of affected relatives, the age at which thrombosis developed, and the presence or absence of additional risk factors.
- Assess thrombophilia results in combination with the family history and other clinical risk factors, such as increasing age, obesity or immobility.

Factor V Leiden and prothrombin G20210A

- The most common heritable thrombophilias in the UK (3–5% and 1% of the population, respectively).
- Heterozygous are at 5-fold increased risk of VTE. With a background incidence of VTE in pregnancy of 1 in 1000 this would translate into an absolute risk of < 1%; and the benefit of TP at this level of risk would be limited.
- Absolute risk may be higher in women with family history of VTE and a thrombophilic genotype.
- The incidence of VTE in pregnancy in heterozygous V Leiden carriers with at least one symptomatic first-degree relative is 2%; risk during pregnancy is 0.4% and 1.7% in the postpartum period. Similar incidences for the prothrombin variant: 0.5% during pregnancy and 1.9% during the postpartum period.
- Compound heterozygotes for factor V Leiden and the prothrombin variant – risk is higher, with an absolute risk of about 4%.
- **Women who are homozygous for factor V Leiden or the prothrombin variant are at much higher risk of pregnancy-related VTE of 9–16%.**

Antithrombin, protein C, protein S deficiency, and MTHFR gene

- Women with protein C or protein S deficiencies who are asymptomatic have a moderately increased risk of VTE associated with pregnancy, with most events occurring postpartum.
- The risk associated with antithrombin deficiency varies according to the subtype but may be 15–50% higher than for other thrombophilias.
- The risk of VTE in pregnancy is 1/3 for type-1 antithrombin deficiency (with reduced activity and antigen level), 1/42 for type-2 antithrombin deficiency (with reduced activity and normal antigen level), 1/113 for protein C deficiency, and 1/437 for factor V Leiden.
- Women with hereditary antithrombin, protein C or protein S deficiency, pregnancy-related VTE episodes – 4 to 7% (two-thirds in the postpartum period).
- Homozygosity for methylene tetrahydrofolate reductase (MTHFR) gene – there is no evidence of an association with a clinically relevant increase in the risk of VTE in pregnancy.

Management

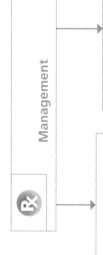

- Stratify according to level of risk associated with the thrombophilia and the presence or absence of a family history or other risk factors.
- Manage women without other risk factors with close surveillance antenatally but consider LMWH for at least 7 days postpartum.
- Exceptions are women with antithrombin deficiency or > 1 thrombophilic defect (homozygous factor V Leiden, homozygous prothrombin G20210A, and compound heterozygotes) or those with additional risk factors – seek advice of an expert and consider antenatal TP.
- If TP is given antenatally for a persisting risk factor, continue it postpartum for 6 weeks.

Antithrombin deficiency

- In women who are asymptomatic, an intermediate dose of heparin may be required. Heparins may not be as effective in antithrombin deficiency, as their mode of action is antithrombin-dependent and it is reasonable to monitor anti-Xa levels in this setting aiming for a level 4 hours following injection of 0.35–0.5 U/ml.
- Different subtypes of antithrombin deficiency are associated with different levels of VTE risk and therefore seek advice from an expert in this area.
- Commence treatment in early pregnancy and continue for 6 weeks postpartum.

C. Acquired thrombophilia (antiphospholipid syndrome – APS)

Definition

- APS – the presence of a lupus anticoagulant (LAC) and/or anticardiolipin (ACA) and/or β2-glycoprotein 1 antibodies of medium to high titre on 2 occasions 12 weeks apart in association with:
  * a history of thrombosis (arterial or venous) or
  * adverse pregnancy outcome:
    > ≥ 3 unexplained miscarriages before 10 weeks
    > a fetal death after 10 weeks of gestation or
    > a PTB (< 35 weeks) due to severe PET or IUGR.

Women with APS and prior VTE

- Manage with a haematologist and/or rheumatologist.
- Antiphospholipid antibody (APA) and LAC are associated with an increased risk of recurrent thrombosis. It is common for such women to be on long-term warfarin after a first thrombotic event.
- Give low-dose aspirin to all women.
- Give both antenatally and 6 weeks postpartum TP with LMW.
- Women on warfarin – convert to LMWH before 6th week of pregnancy.
- Women not on warfarin – commence LMWH in the first trimester ASAP after diagnosis of the pregnancy.
- For women with a single previous VTE event – a high prophylactic (12-hourly) dose of LMWH is often used.
- For women with a history of recurrent VTE – an intermediate (75% of treatment dose) or full treatment dose is used.
- After delivery – continue the appropriate dose of LMWH until re-established on long-term oral anticoagulation or for a minimum of 6 weeks if not on long-term therapy.

Women with APA or obstetric APS only

- The presence of APA alone, even if persistent, with no previous APS-classifiable pregnancy loss or thrombosis, does not equate to APS and such women do not require antenatal LMWH.
- APS (recurrent miscarriage or fetal loss) without VTE (obstetric APS) – the risk of postpartum VTE in these women is unclear but likely to be low. Provide postpartum TP for 6 weeks.
- Women with a persistent LAC or high-titre APA without prior VTE or recurrent miscarriage or fetal loss (i.e., without APS) – the risk of VTE is small; it is reasonable in the absence of additional risk factors to administer LMWH at a prophylactic dose for 7 days postpartum.
- Women with persistent APA with no previous VTE, and no other risk factors or fetal indications for LMWH – close surveillance antenatally but consider for LMWH for 7 days postpartum.

Other risk factors

Age and obesity

- Age over 35 years, obesity, and CS contribute most substantially to the rates of VTE because of their high (and increasing) prevalence.
- **Obesity** – 36% of women who died from PE in the UK between 2003 and 2005 were obese (BMI > 30). Obesity is associated with a higher risk of PE (OR 15) than of DVT (OR 4.4). The risk of VTE appears to increase further with increasing obesity. Thus, obesity is a moderate risk factor for VTE.
- Being overweight (BMI 25–30) is also a weak risk factor for pregnancy-related VTE.

Immobility, long distance travel, and others

- BMI > 25 and antepartum immobilization (strict bed rest 1 week or more before delivery) has a multiplicative effect on the risk for antepartum (OR 62) and postpartum VTE (OR 40).
- Assisted reproduction and multiple pregnancy have additive effects.
- All long distance (> 4 hours) travel (not exclusively by air) is a risk factor for VTE in pregnancy.

Admission to hospital

- NICE – consider giving VTE prophylaxis with LMWH to women who are pregnant or 6 or fewer weeks postpartum who are admitted to hospital and expected to be immobile for 3 or more days and assessed to be at increased risk of VTE.
- Undertake an assessment of thrombotic risk at each hospital admission as it is associated with increased risk of VTE.

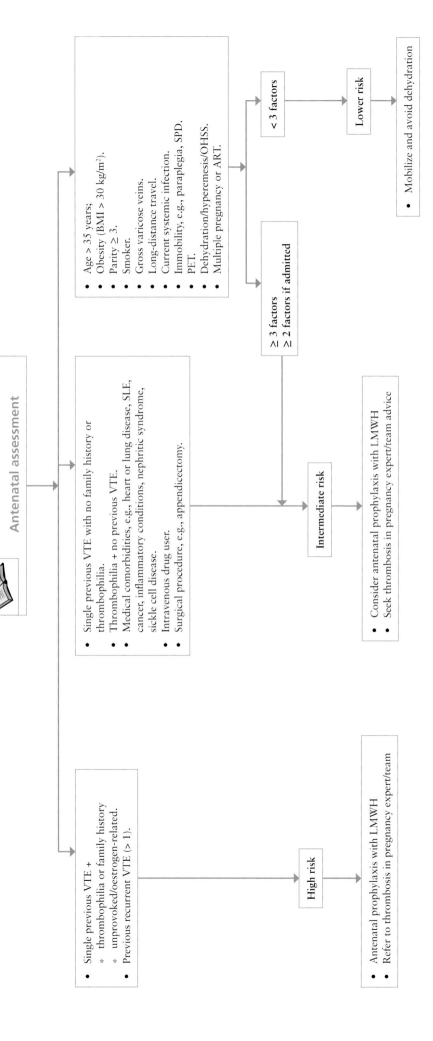

Antenatal assessment

- Single previous VTE +
  * thrombophilia or family history.
  * unprovoked/oestrogen-related.
- Previous recurrent VTE (> 1).

- Single previous VTE with no family history or thrombophilia.
- Thrombophilia + no previous VTE.
- Medical comorbidities, e.g., heart or lung disease, SLE, cancer, inflammatory conditions, nephritic syndrome, sickle cell disease.
- Intravenous drug user.
- Surgical procedure, e.g., appendicectomy.

- Age > 35 years;
- Obesity (BMI > 30 kg/m²).
- Parity ≥ 3.
- Smoker.
- Gross varicose veins.
- Long-distance travel.
- Current systemic infection.
- Immobility, e.g., paraplegia, SPD.
- PET.
- Dehydration/hyperemesis/OHSS.
- Multiple pregnancy or ART.

High risk

≥ 3 factors
≥ 2 factors if admitted

< 3 factors

Intermediate risk

Lower risk

- Antenatal prophylaxis with LMWH
- Refer to thrombosis in pregnancy expert/team

- Consider antenatal prophylaxis with LMWH
- Seek thrombosis in pregnancy expert/team advice

- Mobilize and avoid dehydration

Antenatal and postnatal prophylactic dose of LMWH
- Weight < 50 kg = 20 mg enoxaparin/2500 units dalteparin/3500 units tinzaparin daily.
- Weight 50–90 kg = 40 mg enoxaparin/5000 units dalteparin/4500 units tinzaparin daily.
- Weight 91–130 kg = 60 mg enoxaparin/7500 units dalteparin/7000 units tinzaparin daily.
- Weight 131–170 kg = 80 mg enoxaparin/10000 units dalteparin/9000 units tinzaparin daily.
- Weight > 170 kg = 0.6 mg/kg/day enoxaparin; 75 units/kg/day dalteparin; 75 units/kg/day tinzaparin.

TP during labour and delivery and use of regional anaesthesia and analgesia

- To allow for the use of regional analgesia or anaesthesia, advise women to discontinue LMWH at the onset of labour or prior to planned delivery.
- Advise women receiving antenatal LMWH if they have any vaginal bleeding or once labour begins. Reassess on admission to hospital.
- There is an increased risk of wound haematoma following CS with both unfractionated heparin and LMWH of around 2%.

- Regional anaesthesia or analgesia only after discussion with a senior anaesthetist.
- To minimize or avoid the risk of epidural haematoma:
  * Do not use regional techniques until at least 12 hours after the previous prophylactic dose of LMWH.
  * Do not use regional techniques until at least 24 hours after the previous therapeutic dose of LMWH.
  * Do not give LMWH for 4 hours after use of spinal anaesthesia or after the epidural catheter has been removed; do not remove the cannula within 10–12 hours of the most recent injection.
- If LMWH precludes regional techniques consider alternative analgesia such as opiate-based IV patient-controlled analgesia.
- Women at high risk of haemorrhage with risk factors including major APH, coagulopathy, progressive wound haematoma, suspected intra-abdominal bleeding, and PPH may be more conveniently managed with unfractionated heparin or graduated compression stockings.
- If a woman develops a haemorrhagic problem while on LMWH, stop the treatment and seek haematological advice.
- Excess blood loss and BT are risk factors for VTE, so consider TP or reinstitute as soon as the immediate risk of haemorrhage is reduced.

- Women receiving high prophylactic or therapeutic doses of LMWH – there may be an indication for IOL to help plan TP around delivery.
- Reduce the dose of heparin to its prophylactic dose on the day before IOL and if appropriate, continue with this dose during labour.
- For delivery by elective CS in women receiving antenatal LMWH – give the prophylactic dose of LMWH on the day before delivery. On the day of delivery, omit any morning dose and perform the operation that morning.
- Give the prophylactic dose of LMWH 4 hours postoperatively or 4 hours after removal of the epidural catheter.

Thromboprophylaxis after delivery

Perform risk assessment at least once following delivery.

Assessment of risk and management

- Women ≥ 2 persisting risk factors – give LMWH in prophylactic doses for 7 days.
- Occasionally one risk factor may be extreme without the presence of other risk factors. For example, all women with class 3 obesity (BMI > 40) – offer TP with LMWH even after a normal delivery and in the absence of other risk factors.
- Women undergoing surgery for any reason during the puerperium, those who develop severe infection, those who are readmitted or those who choose to travel long distance are at increased risk of VTE – extend TP for up to 6 weeks or until the additional risk factors are no longer present.

Thrombophilia or previous VTE

- History of previous VTE – offer TP with LMWH or warfarin for 6 weeks regardless of the mode of delivery.
- Women with thrombophilia without previous VTE – consider for LMWH for at least 7 days following delivery. This could be extended to 6 weeks if there is a family history or other risk factors are present.

Caesarean section

- Women delivered by elective CS have double the risk of VTE compared with vaginal birth. Women delivered by emergency CS have double the risk of VTE compared with elective CS.
- The numbers of VTE after elective and emergency CS are similar in weeks 1, 2, and 3 and thus it is important to extend the duration of prophylaxis in the presence of additional persistent (lasting > 7 days postpartum) risk factors for up to 6 weeks or until the additional risk factors are no longer present.
- Women who had an emergency CS – consider for TP with LMWH for 7 days.
- Women who had an elective CS, who have ≥ 1 additional risk factors (such as age > 35 years, BMI > 30) – consider for TP with LMWH for 7 days.

- The prothrombotic changes of pregnancy do not revert completely to normal until several weeks after delivery. The time of greatest risk for VTE associated with pregnancy is the early puerperium and the risk is greatest in the weeks immediately after delivery. The increased risk of VTE persists for 6 weeks postpartum, even though fewer cases are reported during weeks 5 and 6.
- In women at intermediate risk of VTE, there has been much debate as to the optimal duration of TP. Clinical data suggest that the highest risk lies in the first week postpartum. **Thus, a minimum of 7 days of TP is recommended.**
- Consider women with continuing additional risk factors as high risk and it may be necessary to extend prophylaxis **for up to 6 weeks.**
- Provide the first thromboprophylactic dose of LMWH ASAP after delivery provided that there is no PPH. If regional analgesia was used give LMWH 4 hours after removal of the epidural catheter.
- If the epidural catheter is left in place after delivery for the purpose of postpartum analgesia, remove it 12 hours after a dose and 4 hours before the next dose of LMWH.

Postnatal assessment

- Any previous VTE +.
- Anyone requiring antenatal LMWH.

- Caesarean section in labour.
- Asymptomatic thrombophilia (inherited or acquired).
- BMI > 40 kg/m².
- Prolonged hospital admission.
- Medical comorbidities, e.g., heart or lung disease, SLE, cancer, inflammatory conditions, nephritic syndrome, sickle cell disease.
- Intravenous drug user.

- Age > 35 years.
- Obesity (BMI > 30 kg/m²).
- Parity ≥ 3.
- Smoker.
- Gross varicose veins.
- Long-distance travel.
- Current systemic infection.
- Immobility, e.g., paraplegia, SPD.
- Pre-eclampsia.
- Elective caesarian section.
- Any surgical procedure in the puerperium.
- Mid-cavity rotational operative delivery.
- Prolonged labour (> 24 hours).
- PPH > 1 l or blood transfusion.

High risk

- At least 6 weeks postnatal prophylactic LMWH

Intermediate risk

- At least 7 days postnatal prophylactic LMWH
- If persisting or > 3 risk factors, consider extending thromboprophylaxis with LMWH

≥ 2 factors

< 2 factors

Lower risk

- Mobilization and avoidance of dehydration

Agents for thromboprophylaxis

Low-molecular-weight heparin (LMWH)

- Agent of choice for antenatal TP. They are as effective as and safer than unfractionated heparin.
- Risk of heparin-induced thrombocytopenia is low. Monitor platelet count only if the woman had prior exposure to unfractionated heparin. Prolonged unfractionated heparin use during pregnancy may result in osteoporosis and fractures but this risk is very low with LMWH; the incidence of osteoporotic fractures is 0.04% and of allergic skin reactions is 1.8%.
- Significant bleeding, usually related primarily to obstetric causes, can occur in 2% compared to 0.7% without the use of LMWH.
- Dose is based on weight, not BMI. Use booking weight to guide dose.
- Give higher doses to women of higher weight due to the risk of PE on standard dose. One can prescribe the usual prophylactic dose twice daily for women >90 kg.
- Monitoring of anti-Xa levels is not required, provided that the woman has normal renal function. Use lower doses of enoxaparin and dalteparin if the creatinine clearance is < 30 ml/minute. For tinzaparin, reduce the dose if the creatinine clearance is < 20 ml/minute.
- Women who are on long-term oral anticoagulants – higher prophylactic doses or therapeutic doses of LMWH may be appropriate.
- High prophylactic/intermediate dose LMWH – 40 mg enoxaparin BD or 5000 IU dalteparin BD, or tinzaparin 4500 IU BD.
- Therapeutic dose – 1 mg/kg enoxaparin BD or 100 IU/kg dalteparin BD or tinzaparin 175 IU/kg daily.
- In antithrombin deficiency, higher doses of LMWH (weight-adjusted: either 75% or 100% of treatment dose) may be necessary, as judged by anti-Xa levels.

Unfractionated heparin

- It has a shorter half-life than LMWH with more complete reversal of its activity by protamine sulphate.
- It may be used around the time of delivery in women at very high risk of VTE or in women at increased risk of haemorrhage.
- The required interval between a prophylactic dose of unfractionated heparin and regional analgesia or anaesthesia is less (4 hours) than with LMWH (12 hours) and there is less concern regarding neuraxial haematomas with unfractionated heparin.
- If no LMWH has been given for 24 hours but the woman has not yet delivered and there is concern about delaying further doses of LMWH, a prophylactic dose of 5000 IU unfractionated heparin could be used and repeated every 12 hours until LMWH can be resumed after delivery.
- Increased risk of heparin-induced thrombocytopenia (HIT).

Graduated elastic compression stockings (GECS)

- Cochrane review of GECS use for the prevention of DVT in non-pregnant hospitalized patients showed a significant reduction in incidence of DVT with the treatment group (OR 0.36).
- Following a symptomatic DVT – advise to wear a tighter-fitted GECS during the day, with an ankle pressure gradient of 30–40 mmHg for 2 years to prevent post-thrombotic syndrome (and continue for longer if post-thrombotic symptoms are present).
- GECS are used primarily for patients at high risk of bleeding (who are unable/contraindicated to receive pharmacological TP) and as an adjunct to anticoagulant TP where this has been shown to improve efficacy (surgical patients).
- Offer properly applied GECS of appropriate strength in pregnancy and the puerperium for:
  * Those who are hospitalized and have a contraindication to LMWH.
  * Those who are hospitalized post-CS (combined with LMWH) and considered to be at particularly high risk of VTE (such as previous VTE, > 3 risk factors).
  * Outpatients with prior VTE (usually combined with LMWH).
  * Women travelling long distance for more than 4 hours.
- More DVTs in pregnant women are iliofemoral compared with the non-pregnant population, where calf-vein DVTs are more common. Although NICE guidelines support the use of thigh-length GECS in inpatients undergoing surgery, other reviews outside pregnancy suggest equivalent efficacy of knee-length and thigh-length stockings and higher rates of compliance with the former.
- Therefore, on balance, properly applied thigh-length stockings are advocated for pregnant women but consider knee-length stockings if full-length stockings are ill fitting or compliance is poor.

Warfarin

- Its use in pregnancy is where heparin is considered unsuitable; for example, some women with mechanical heart valves.
- It crosses the placenta and is associated with the risk of congenital abnormalities – warfarin embryopathy in approximately 5% of fetuses exposed between 6 and 12 weeks of gestation. This incidence is dose-dependent, with a higher incidence in women taking > 5 mg/day.
- Other complications include an increase in the risk of spontaneous miscarriage, stillbirth, neurological problems in the baby, and fetal and maternal haemorrhage.

Low-dose aspirin

- No trials on the use of aspirin for TP in pregnancy. A meta-analysis of antiplatelet therapy in surgical and medical patients showed a significant reduction in DVT and PE with antiplatelet prophylaxis.

- **Fondaparinux** – A synthetic pentasaccharide that functions as an anticoagulant through specific inhibition of factor Xa via antithrombin. It is licensed in the UK for the prevention and treatment of VTE outside pregnancy and has a similar efficacy to LMWH. Limited experience of its use in pregnancy but it has been used in the setting of heparin intolerance. Its role in pregnancy should be reserved for women intolerant of heparin compounds.

- **Danaparoid** – A heparinoid that is used in patients intolerant of heparin either because of HIT or a skin allergy. It has both anti-IIa and anti-Xa effects, predominantly the latter with a long anti-Xa half-life of about 24 hours. Experience in the use of this agent is limited.

- **Lepirudin** – A direct thrombin inhibitor used in the management of patients with HIT. Few reports of its use in pregnancy but it can cross the placenta and has been reported to produce embryopathy when given in high doses to rabbits. Its use is best to avoid in pregnancy unless there is no acceptable alternative.

- **Dextran** – Avoid it because of the risk of anaphylactoid reaction, associated with uterine hypertonus, fetal distress, fetal neurological abnormalities, and death.

- **Oral thrombin and Xa inhibitors** – Dabigatran and rivaroxaban work through direct inhibition of thrombin and factor Xa, respectively. They are licensed for the prevention of VTE after major orthopaedic surgery. They are not licensed for use in pregnancy; therefore avoid in pregnant women.

Agents for thromboprophylaxis contd.

Agents for postpartum thromboprophylaxis

- LMWH is appropriate for postpartum TP although, if women are receiving long-term anticoagulation with warfarin, this can be started when the risk of haemorrhage is low, usually 5–7 days after delivery.
- Both warfarin and LMWH are safe when breastfeeding.
- LMWH is safe and easy to use and has the advantage of not requiring monitoring. For those women receiving LMWH antenatally (and 6 weeks postpartum) or for those requiring 7 days of postpartum TP it is the agent of choice.
- Warfarin requires close monitoring and visits to an anticoagulant clinic. It carries an increased risk of PPH and perineal haematoma compared with LMWH. It is not appropriate for those women requiring 7 days of postpartum prophylaxis. However, it is appropriate for those on maintenance warfarin outside pregnancy.
- Delay conversion from LMWH to warfarin for at least 5–7 days after delivery to minimize the risk of haemorrhage during the period of overlap of LMWH and warfarin.

Contraindications to LMWH

Women who are at risk of bleeding. Risk factors for bleeding are:

- women with active antenatal or postpartum bleeding;
- women considered at increased risk of major haemorrhage (such as placenta praevia);
- women with a bleeding diathesis, such as von Willebrand's disease, haemophilia or acquired coagulopathy;
- women with thrombocytopenia (platelet count < 75 × 10^9);
- acute stroke in the last 4 weeks (ischaemic or haemorrhagic);
- severe renal disease (glomerular filtration rate < 30 ml/minute/1.73 m^2);
- severe liver disease (prothrombin time above normal range or known varices);
- uncontrolled hypertension (BP > 200 mmHg systolic or > 120 mmHg diastolic).

Diagnosis of VTE – clinical suspicion

- Subjective clinical assessment of DVT and PE is unreliable in pregnancy and only a minority of women with clinically suspected VTE have the diagnosis confirmed with objective tests.
- Look for risk factors for VTE.
- Symptoms and signs – leg pain and swelling (usually unilateral), lower abdominal pain, low-grade pyrexia, dyspnoea, chest pain, haemoptysis, and collapse.
- When iliac vein thrombosis is suspected – back pain and swelling of the entire limb.

Investigations

- Perform objective tests expeditiously and treat with LMWH until the diagnosis is excluded, unless treatment is strongly contraindicated.
  - MDT - obstetrician, physician, haematologist, and radiologist.

D-dimer

- Do not perform to diagnose acute VTE in pregnancy.
- In pregnancy D-dimer can be elevated because of the physiological changes in the coagulation system.
- D-dimer levels are increased if there is a concomitant problem such as PET.
- A 'positive' D-dimer test in pregnancy is not necessarily consistent with VTE. However, a low level of D-dimer in pregnancy is likely to suggest that there is no VTE.

Acute DVT

- **Compression duplex USS – the primary diagnostic test:**
  * Confirms the diagnosis of DVT.
  * Negative USS and a high level of clinical suspicion – keep woman anticoagulated and repeat USS in 1 week or arrange an alternative diagnostic test. If repeat test is negative, discontinue anticoagulant treatment.
  * Negative USS with a low level of clinical suspicion – discontinue anticoagulant treatment.
- Iliac vein thrombosis – consider magnetic resonance venography or conventional contrast venography.

Acute PE

- **Chest X-ray** – features include atelectasis, effusion, focal opacities, regional oligaemia or pulmonary oedema. X-ray is normal in over 50% of pregnant women with objectively proven PE. The radiation dose to the fetus from a chest X-ray at any stage of pregnancy is negligible. It may identify other pulmonary disease such as pneumonia, pneumothorax or lobar collapse.
  * If the X-ray is abnormal with a high clinical suspicion of PE – perform CT pulmonary angiogram (CTPA).
  * If the X-ray is normal – perform bilateral Doppler USS leg studies. A diagnosis of DVT may indirectly confirm a diagnosis of PE and since anticoagulant therapy is the same for both conditions, further investigation may not be necessary. This would limit the radiation doses given to the mother and fetus.
  * If both tests are negative with persistent clinical suspicion – perform a ventilation–perfusion (V/Q) lung scan or a CTPA.

Ventilation–perfusion (V/Q) lung scan

- The ventilation component of the V/Q scan can be omitted during pregnancy, thereby minimizing the radiation dose for the fetus (which is in any event small and not associated with a substantial increased risk of complications) especially if the X-ray is normal.
- It has high NPV and is associated with a substantially lower radiation dose to pregnant breast tissue. Consider lung perfusion scans as the investigation of first choice, especially if there is a family history of breast cancer or the woman has had a previous chest CT scan.
- Pulmonary angiography carries the highest radiation dose (at least 0.5 mSv to the fetus and 5–30 mSv to the mother).

Computed tomography pulmonary angiogram (CTPA)

- CTPA is the first-line investigation for non-massive PE in non-pregnant women. Only around 5% of these investigations have a positive result.
- **Advantages over V/Q imaging** –
  1. Better sensitivity and specificity (non-pregnant women).
  2. Lower radiation dose to the fetus – the average fetal radiation dose with CTPA is < 10% of that with V/Q scan. The risk of fatal cancer to the age of 15 years is < 1/1 000 000 after in utero exposure to CTPA and 1/280 000 following a V/Q scan.
  3. It can identify other pathology such as aortic dissection.
- **Disadvantages – over V/Q imaging** –
  1. Relatively high radiation dose (20 mGy) to the mother's thorax and breast tissue, with an increased lifetime risk of breast cancer of 13.6% (background risk 1/200). It is suggested that this risk is an overestimate at least in the non-pregnant woman.
  2. May not identify small peripheral PE.
- Safety concerns of iodinated contrast medium with CTPA – can potentially alter fetal or neonatal thyroid function. Iodinated contrast media may be given to a pregnant woman when radiographic examination is essential but check thyroid function in the neonate.

- V/Q scanning carries a slightly increased risk of childhood cancer compared with CTPA but carries a lower risk of maternal breast cancer.
- Get informed consent before these tests.
- Carry out alternative or repeat tests where V/Q scan or CTPA and duplex Doppler are normal but the clinical suspicion of PE is high.
- Continue anticoagulant treatment until PE is definitively excluded.

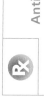

Confirmed VTE in pregnancy – therapeutic anticoagulation

Baseline blood investigations before initiating anticoagulant therapy

Initial blood tests

- **FBC, coagulation screen, urea and electrolytes, and LFTs.**
  As the use of anticoagulant therapy can be influenced by renal and hepatic function, confirm that these are normal before starting treatment.

Thrombophilia screen

- Do not routinely perform thrombophilia screen prior to therapy. The results of thrombophilia screen will not influence immediate management of acute VTE but can provide information that can influence the duration and intensity of anticoagulation.
- If a thrombophilia screen is performed be aware of the effects of pregnancy and thrombus:
  1. Protein S levels fall in normal pregnancy.
  2. Activated protein C (APC) resistance is found in around 40% of pregnancies.
  3. Antithrombin may be reduced when extensive thrombus is present.
  4. In nephrotic syndrome and PET antithrombin levels are reduced.
  5. In liver disease proteins C and S are reduced.

  Thrombophilia screens should be interpreted by haematologists with specific expertise in pregnancy.

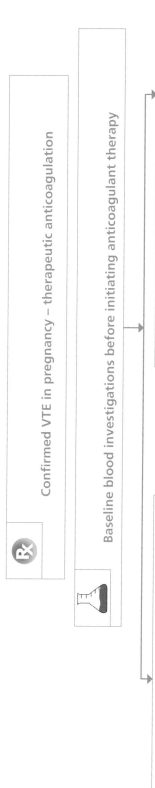

Anticoagulant treatment

LMWH

Safety and efficacy

- Compared with unfractionated heparin, LMWHs are more effective, associated with a lower risk of haemorrhagic complications and lower mortality in the initial treatment of DVT, and have equivalent efficacy in the initial treatment of PE.
- LMWHs do not cross the placenta. See risks – above.
- Four cases of osteoporotic fractures in association with LMWH use in pregnancy have been reported (tinzaparin and dalteparin), although in each case there were additional and significant risk factors for osteoporosis.
- Risk of recurrent VTE is 1.15% with treatment doses of LMWH.
- Women who develop HIT or have heparin allergy and require continuing anticoagulant therapy – manage with the heparinoid, danaparoid sodium or fondaparinux.

Therapeutic dose of LMWH

- Due to alterations in the pharmacokinetics of dalteparin and enoxaparin during pregnancy, give LMWH daily in two divided doses with dosage titrated against the woman's booking or most recent weight (enoxaparin 1 mg/kg BD; dalteparin 100 units/kg BD).
- Once-daily dose of tinzaparin (175 units/kg) may be appropriate but its safety and efficacy have not yet been substantiated in contrast to twice-daily dosing of enoxaparin and dalteparin.

Blood tests to monitor LMWH therapy

Anti-Xa levels – satisfactory anti-Xa levels are obtained using a weight-based regimen. There are concerns over the accuracy of anti-Xa monitoring. Do not routinely measure peak anti-Xa activity for patients on therapeutic LMWH. Perform it only in women at extremes of body weight (< 50 kg and ≥ 90 kg) or with other complicating factors (renal impairment or recurrent VTE) putting them at high risk. If LMWH therapy requires monitoring, the aim is to achieve a peak anti-Xa 3 hours postinjection, of 0.5–1.2 units/ml.

Platelet count – Do not routinely monitor platelet count as there have been no cases of HIT thrombosis in pregnancies managed with LMWH. Monitor **platelet count** if:
1. unfractionated heparin is used – monitor platelet count at least every other day until day 14 or until the unfractionated heparin is stopped, whichever occurs first;
2. patient is receiving LMWH after first receiving unfractionated heparin; or
3. patient has received unfractionated heparin in the past.

Maintenance therapy

- Continue with therapeutic doses of LMWH for the remainder of the pregnancy (LMWH BD):
  * LMWH is not associated with significant bleeding risk. There are significant risk factors for recurrence of VTE, including pregnancy-related changes in the coagulation system, reduced venous flow velocity, and in at least 50% a thrombophilia will be present.
  * The majority of DVTs in pregnancy are ileofemoral, with a greater risk of both embolization and recurrence.
- It is not yet established whether the dose of LMWH or unfractionated heparin can be reduced to an intermediate dose after an initial period of several weeks of therapeutic anticoagulation. This type of modified dosing regimen may be useful in pregnant women at increased risk of bleeding or osteoporosis.
- Outpatient follow-up with clinical assessment and monitoring of platelets and peak anti-Xa levels if appropriate.

Mobilization and compression therapy

- Pain and swelling in the affected leg are debilitating symptoms of DVT. With proximal DVT, pain and swelling improve faster in mobile patients wearing compression hosiery than in those resting in bed without any compression. This can also prevent the development of post-thrombotic syndrome.
- **In the initial management of DVT advise the patient to –**
  * **Elevate the leg.** * **Use GECS to reduce oedema.** * **Mobilize.**
- Early mobilization with compression therapy does not increase the likelihood of developing PE.
- Below-knee compression socks are acceptable for patients without thigh or knee swelling.
- For patients with persisting leg oedema after DVT, class II compression hosiery is more effective than class I stockings. Accurate fitting and correct application of the hosiery are essential to avoid discomfort and assist rather than prevent venous return. Class II compression socks and stockings should be taken off at night and do not need to be worn on the unaffected leg.

Embolectomy and inferior vena caval filter

- DVT threatens leg viability through venous gangrene – elevate the leg, give anticoagulation, and consider surgical embolectomy or thrombolytic therapy.
- Consider use of a temporary inferior vena caval filter in the perinatal period for women with iliac vein VTE, to reduce the risk of PE or in women with proven DVT and who have continuing PE despite adequate anticoagulation.
- There is evidence that the use of an inferior vena caval filter prior to labour or delivery reduces the risk of PE. However, when VTE occurs in the antepartum period, delay delivery if possible, to allow maximum time for anticoagulation, rather than putting in a filter.

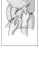

Therapeutic anticoagulant therapy during labour and delivery

Labour

- In order to avoid an unwanted anticoagulant effect during delivery, advise the woman that once she is established in labour or thinks that she is in labour, she should not inject any further heparin.
- Where delivery is planned, discontinue LMWH 24 hours before planned delivery (IOL or CS).
- If spontaneous labour occurs whilst on therapeutic dose of LMWH – monitor APTT. If it is markedly prolonged near delivery, protamine sulphate may be required to reduce the risk of bleeding.
- Discontinue SC unfractionated heparin 12 hours before and IV unfractionated heparin 6 hours before IOL or regional anaesthesia.

Regional anaesthesia

- Regional anaesthetic or analgesic techniques should not be undertaken until at least 24 hours after the last dose of therapeutic LMWH.
- Give a thromboprophylactic dose of LMWH by 3 hours after a CS (more than 4 hours after removal of the epidural catheter, if appropriate).
- Do not remove the epidural catheter within 12 hours of the most recent injection.

Specific surgical measures

- There is an increased risk of wound haematoma following CS with both unfractionated heparin and LMWH of around 2%. Consider wound drains (abdominal and rectus sheath) at CS and close the skin incision with staples or interrupted sutures to allow drainage of any haematoma.

- Any woman who is at high risk of haemorrhage and in whom continued heparin treatment is essential, manage with IV unfractionated heparin until the risk factors for haemorrhage have resolved.
- Risk factors include major APH, coagulopathy, progressive wound haematoma, suspected intra-abdominal bleeding, and PPH.
- If a woman develops a haemorrhagic problem while on LMWH, stop the treatment and seek expert haematological advice.

Postnatal anticoagulation

- Continue therapeutic LMWH for at least 6 weeks postnatally and until at least 3 months of treatment has been given in total.
- Both heparin and warfarin are satisfactory for use postpartum. Discuss the need for regular blood tests for monitoring of warfarin, particularly during the first 10 days of treatment.
- To continue with LMWH – can use antenatal dose or non-pregnant dose (enoxaparin 1.5mg/kg OD, dalteparin 10 000–18 000 units OD depending on body weight, tinzaparin 175 units/kg OD).
- Avoid postpartum warfarin until at least the third day and for longer in women at increased risk of PPH.
- Daily testing of the INR during the transfer from LMWH to warfarin to avoid over-anticoagulation. Check INR on day 2 of warfarin and titrate the dose to maintain the INR between 2 and 3. Continue heparin until the INR is > 2 on two successive days.

Postnatal clinic review

- Whenever possible in an obstetric medicine clinic or a joint obstetric haematology clinic.
- Before discontinuing treatment, assess the continuing risk of thrombosis including a personal and family history of VTE and any thrombophilia screen results.
- Assess post-thrombotic venous damage, thrombophilia tests (if necessary) after anticoagulants are stopped, review and repeat thrombophilia tests if necessary.
- Advise on the need for thromboprophylaxis in any future pregnancy and at other times of increased risk.
- Discuss contraception.

Prevention of post-thrombotic leg syndrome

- It is a common complication following DVT, found in over 60% of cases followed up over a median of 4.5 years.
- It is characterized by chronic persistent leg swelling, pain, a feeling of heaviness, dependent cyanosis, telangiectasis, chronic pigmentation, eczema, associated varicose veins, and in some cases lipodermatosclerosis and chronic ulceration. Symptoms are made worse by standing or walking and improve with rest and recumbancy.
- It is more common where there is a recurrent DVT, with obesity, and where there has been inadequate anticoagulation.
- GECS improve the microcirculation by assisting the calf muscle pump, reducing swelling and reflux, and reducing venous hypertension. Mild to moderate post-thrombotic syndrome decreases from 47% to 20% and severe post-thrombotic syndrome decreases from 23% to 11% with use of compression stockings over 2 years. GECS should be worn on the affected leg for 2 years after the acute event if swelling persists, to reduce the risk of post-thrombotic syndrome.

Massive life-threatening PE

Collapsed, shocked patients – ABC

- Get help – Multidisciplinary resuscitation team (senior physicians, obstetricians, and radiologists).
- Arrange an urgent portable echocardiogram or CTPA within 1 hour of presentation.
- Options – IV unfractionated heparin, thrombolytic therapy or thoracotomy and surgical embolectomy.
- If massive PE is confirmed or, in extreme circumstances prior to confirmation, consider immediate thrombolysis.

- **IV unfractionated heparin** – rapid effect and extensive experience of use in this situation.
- One regimen for the administration of IV unfractionated heparin is:
  * Loading dose of 80 units/kg, followed by a continuous IV infusion of 18 units/kg/hour.
  * If a woman has received thrombolysis, omit the loading dose of heparin and start an infusion at 18 units/kg/hour.
  * Measure APTT 4–6 hours after the loading dose, 6 hours after any dose change, and then at least daily when in the therapeutic range. The therapeutic target APTT ratio is 1.5–2.5 times the average laboratory control value. Adjust the infusion rate according to the APTT.
- APTT monitoring of unfractionated heparin is technically problematic, particularly in late pregnancy when an apparent heparin resistance occurs because of increased fibrinogen and factor VIII. This can lead to unnecessarily high doses of heparin being used, with subsequent haemorrhagic problems. Where such problems exist, seek a senior haematologist's advice. It may be useful to determine the anti-Xa level as a measure of heparin dose. With unfractionated heparin, a lower level of anti-Xa is considered therapeutic (target range 0.35–0.70 units/ml or 0.5–1.0 units/ml for women with life-threatening PE).

- **Thrombolytic therapy** (streptokinase, urokinase, recombinant tissue plasminogen activator) – it is more effective than heparin in reducing clot burden and rapidly improving haemodynamics. The studies, however, have not shown any better impact on long-term survival over the conventional therapy with heparin or LMWH.
- **Current recommendation – reserve thrombolytic therapy for women with severe PE with haemodynamic compromise.**
- After thrombolytic therapy has been given, an infusion of unfractionated heparin can be given but omit the loading dose.
- Data are limited in pregnancy and there have been concerns about maternal bleeding and adverse fetal effects. The maternal bleeding rate is 1–6%. Most bleeding events occur around catheter and puncture sites. In pregnant women, there have been no reports of intracranial bleeding.
- **Thoracotomy** – If the woman is not suitable for thrombolysis or is moribund, discuss with the cardiothoracic surgeons with a view to urgent thoracotomy.

The Acute Management of Thrombosis and Embolism During Pregnancy and the Puerperium. RCOG Green-top Guideline No. 37b; February 2007; Reviewed 2010. Reducing the Risk of Thrombosis and Embolism During Pregnancy and the Puerperium. RCOG Green-top Guideline No. 37a; November 2009. Please refer to the updated guidelines from April 2015.

CHAPTER 43   Thrombosis and embolism

CHAPTER 44 Pruritus in pregnancy

Prevalence and background

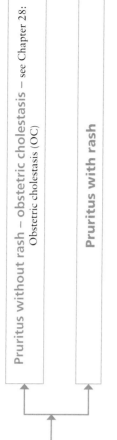

- Pruritus (itch) – a poorly localized, usually unpleasant sensation, which elicits a desire to scratch. The quality of itch is variable, and may be described as a burning, prickling, or crawling sensation.
- Causes – may be caused by a pre-existing or coincidental condition, or a condition specific to pregnancy. The most common of these are:
  * Without rash – intrahepatic cholestasis of pregnancy (see Chapter 28: Obstetric cholestasis [OC]).
  * With rash – polymorphic eruption of pregnancy, pruritic folliculitis of pregnancy, atopic eruption of pregnancy, and pemphigoid gestationis.
- Its incidence (any cause) is estimated to be as high as 18%.

Pruritus without rash – obstetric cholestasis – see Chapter 28: Obstetric cholestasis (OC)

Pruritus with rash

Risks

- Rarely associated with serious complications for the woman or the fetus.
- Itching can lead to sleep deprivation and loss of wellbeing during pregnancy.
- Bacterial infection (from superinfected excoriations caused by scratching).

History and examination

- Pruritus.
- Consequent sleep deprivation.
- Skin inspection – rash. Elicit timing of the onset of symptoms and the appearance of the rash.
- Skin trauma from intense scratching may be seen (excoriations).

Management

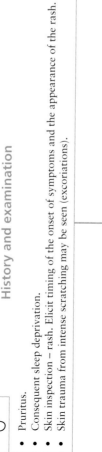

- **Symptomatic treatment –**
  * Emollients can be used liberally to soothe the skin.
  * Topical corticosteroids can be used to reduce inflammation.
  * A sedating antihistamine (e.g., chlorphenamine 4 mg 3–4 times a day) if difficulty sleeping.
- **Referral and admission to secondary care for women with suspected acute pustular psoriasis (impetigo herpetiformis)**.
- **Refer** to a dermatologist those women who are suspected of having severe atopic eruption of pregnancy; pruritic folliculitis of pregnancy; or if the diagnosis is uncertain.
- **Refer** to an obstetrician if pemphigoid gestation is suspected.

Differential diagnosis

DDx

- **Itch unrelated to pregnancy** – if the rash cannot be identified with certainty, consider a different cause that is not specific to pregnancy. Other causes of itch (that are not specific to pregnancy) are coincidental or pre-existing conditions.
- **Conditions that do not usually cause rash:**
  * Renal disease – around half of people with chronic renal disease experience itch.
  * Liver disease – itch is usually secondary to cholestasis, for example due to the formation of bile stones.
  * Haematological causes – iron deficiency (unusual cause), polycythaemia vera, or haemochromatosis (rarely causes itch).
  * Endocrine disorders – thyroid disorders (thyrotoxicosis causes itch more commonly than hypothyroidism).
  * Malignancy – Hodgkin's lymphoma, cutaneous T-cell lymphoma, leukaemia, and multiple myeloma.
  * Neurological disorders – multiple sclerosis.
  * Drugs – opioids.
  * Psychological causes – psychogenic pruritus.
- **Other skin conditions that can cause widespread itch and rash** – chickenpox, contact dermatitis, atopic eczema, insect bites and stings, scabies, urticaria, rubella may occasionally present with a mildly pruritic rash.
- **Pre-existing skin conditions** – atopic dermatitis, psoriasis, fungal infections, cutaneous tumours.
- **Other skin conditions in pregnancy not associated with rash** – impetigo herpetiformis

Pruritus with rash in pregnancy

	Polymorphic eruption of pregnancy (PEP)	Pemphigoid gestationis	Atopic eruption of pregnancy	Pruritic folliculitis of pregnancy
Incidence	Commonest pregnancy-specific dermatosis; 1 in 200–250 pregnancies.	Rare; 1 in 50 000 pregnancies. Serious condition.	1 in 300 pregnancies.	1 in 3000 pregnancies.
Also known as	Pruritic urticarial papules and plaques of pregnancy (PUPPP), toxic erythema of pregnancy, toxaemic rash of pregnancy, and late-onset prurigo of pregnancy.	Herpes gestationis.	Prurigo of pregnancy, prurigo gestationis, early onset prurigo of pregnancy, and eczema of pregnancy.	
Time of onset	Usually occurs in the third trimester after 35 weeks of gestation; it may occur in early pregnancy and in the postpartum period.	Rash can appear anytime but usually in third trimester.	Presents in first trimester or about 24–30 weeks of gestation.	Second or third trimester.
Association	More common in first pregnancy, in women with excessive weight gain, and in multiple pregnancy.	Associated with bullous pemphigoid. Associated with other autoimmune conditions, e.g., Grave's disease, insulin-dependent DM.	Mutiparous; more likely in women with a history of atopic eczema.	
Pathogenesis	The cause is not fully understood, but may be an abnormal dermatological response to abdominal distension. An increased incidence in women with multiple gestations suggests that skin stretching may play a role in inciting an immune-mediated reaction.	It is an autoimmune disorder – binding of IgG to the basement membrane triggers an immune response forming subepidermal vesicles.	Associated with atopy.	Possibly a hormone-induced acne.
Rash – type and distribution	Pruritic urticarial papules that coalesce into plaques. Typically starts on the abdomen (umbilical region is usually spared) along striae. It may remain localized or spread to the buttocks and proximal thighs, under the breasts and upper arms. It may develop into widespread non-urticated erythema, with eczematous lesions and vesicles (not bullae).	An intense itch often precedes the rash, which initially presents with erythematous urticarial papules and plaques on the abdomen (and nearly always the umbilicus) then spreads to cover the entire body and progresses to form tense blisters (bullae) including on the palms and soles. The woman is likely to have exacerbations and remissions throughout the pregnancy. In a few it may develop into bullous pemphigoid.	Consists of eczematous lesions and papular lesions. 1. Eczematous lesions affect atopic sites such as the face, neck, upper chest, and flexural surfaces of the limbs. 2. Papular lesions consist of small erythematous papules disseminated on the trunk and limbs, and larger 'prurigo nodules' mainly on the shins and extensor surfaces of the arms.	Multiple follicular papules affecting the upper back, arms, chest, and abdomen. These are not usually excessively itchy.
Effect on mother and baby	No serious risk to the woman or baby.	It can cause prolonged, distressing symptoms and often flares up postpartum. Fetus – risk of SGA but there is no increased risk of prematurity or stillbirth. 10% chance of mild transient skin lesions in the newborn.	No serious risk to the woman or her baby; the child may be at increased risk of developing atopic eczema.	
Treatment	Symptomatic treatment – emollients (1% menthol in aqueous cream); topical corticosteroids (1% hydrocortisone) to reduce inflammation. If the rash does not respond or is severe and generalized, consider a short course of oral corticosteroids (prednisolone 40–60 mg for 5 days); sedating antihistamine if difficulty sleeping.	Refer to dermatologist and obstetrician for confirmation of the diagnosis. Additional antenatal surveillance. Potent or very potent topical steroids or oral corticosteroids. Some may require topical or systemic immunosuppression with cyclosporine or tacrolimus. Further treatment may be required following childbirth.	Symptomatic treatment – • Emollients with an active ingredient (menthol 0.5% or 1% in aqueous cream). • Sedating antihistamine. • Moderately potent topical corticosteroids. If the rash is severe or unresponsive, seek specialist advice from a dermatologist. A short course of oral corticosteroids or phototherapy may be indicated.	Symptomatic treatment - topical benzoyl peroxide and mild potency topical corticosteroid (hydrocortisone 1%). If the rash is severe or resistant to treatment, or there is uncertainty in the diagnosis, consider referral to a dermatologist. Treatment options in secondary care include phototherapy.

Resolution	Symptoms last 4–6 weeks and usually resolve following birth.	Usually resolves within weeks to months following childbirth. Some women may experience further flares following menstruation or when using hormonal contraception, and a small number may experience persistence of skin lesions over several years.	It is benign and resolves spontaneously following childbirth.	It resolves 1–2 months following childbirth.
Recurrence		Recurrence is rare.	Usually recurs in future pregnancies. May recur with use of COC pills.	There is a risk of recurrence in future pregnancies.

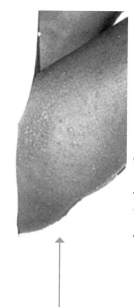

Impetigo herpetiformis.

Rash without pruritis – impetigo herpetiformis

- A form of pustular psoriasis, rare, appears in the second half of pregnancy.
- Systemic signs and symptoms include nausea, vomiting, diarrhea, fever, chills, and lymphadenopathy.
- **Pruritus is absent.**
- Medical complications (secondary infection, septicaemia, hyperparathyroidism with hypocalcaemia, hypoalbuminaemia) may occur.
- Treatment – systemic corticosteroids and antibiotics to treat secondarily infected lesions.
- Resolves after delivery; it may recur during subsequent pregnancies.
- Increased fetal morbidity has been reported, suggesting the need for increased antenatal surveillance.

Pre-existing skin conditions

- Pre-existing skin conditions (e.g., atopic dermatitis, psoriasis) may change during pregnancy. Atopic dermatitis and psoriasis may worsen or improve during pregnancy. Atopic changes may be related to prurigo of pregnancy and usually worsen, but may improve, during pregnancy. Psoriasis is more likely to improve than worsen.

Marc Tunzi and Gary. R. Gray. Common skin conditions during pregnancy. Family Medicine Residency Program, Natividad Medical Center, Salinas, California. American Family Physician. 2007 Jan 15;75(2):211–218.

Catherine Nelson-Piercy. Handbook of Obstetric Medicine. Chapter 13 – Skin diseases (4th edition); pages 263–271. Informa Healthcare.

www.crazygallery.info

www.consultantlive.com

Background

The nature and treatment of mental disorders in antenatal and postnatal period differ from the general population:

- The effects of disorders can be on the woman, fetus/infant, siblings, and other family members.
- In women with an existing disorder – there is an increased risk of women stopping medication abruptly which can precipitate or worsen an episode.
- The disorder may often require urgent intervention because of its effect on the fetus and on the woman's health.
- Postnatal psychotic disorders may have a more rapid onset with more severe symptoms than psychoses occurring at other times.
- The risk/benefit ratio of the use of psychotropic drugs in pregnancy and breastfeeding requires careful consideration.

Pre-pregnancy

- Ask women about:
  * Their past history of major mental disorders, particularly bipolar disorder, other serious affective disorder or schizophrenia.
  * Their current psychotropic medication and the details of current care providers.
- Women with serious mental disorders – refer for pre-pregnancy advice to specialized perinatal mental health services (PMHS) or to general psychiatric services.
- Be careful when prescribing to all women of childbearing age. Discuss the risks associated with becoming pregnant while taking psychotropic drugs and the risks from an untreated mental disorder and from stopping medication abruptly.

Antenatal booking visit

- Arrange antenatal booking visit before 12 weeks of pregnancy to identify women with or at high risk of major mental illness.
- Ask women about:
  * Previous or current major mental illness, particularly schizophrenia, bipolar disorder, other serious affective disorder, previous psychotic illness in the postnatal period or severe depression in the postnatal period.
  * Family history of bipolar disorder and of postpartum major mental illness (puerperal psychosis).
  * Previous treatment by mental health services, including periods of inpatient care.
  * Current treatment with psychotropic medication.
  * Any history of intimate partner violence, sexual abuse or assault, use of illegal drugs, self-harm, and lack of social support, as this group of women are at risk of depressive illness and suicide during pregnancy.
- Women identified as at high risk of postpartum major mental disorders – refer to specialized PMHS or otherwise to general psychiatric services.

Risks

- Serious consequences for the mother, infant, and other family members.
- Psychiatric disorders are the leading cause of maternal death in the UK.
- Depression is associated with the greatest number of suicides, although the rates for lifetime risk of suicide are lower than other less common disorders such as bipolar disorder.
- The majority of suicides in pregnant and postnatal women (about 60%) occur in the 6 weeks before delivery and the 12 weeks after delivery.
- Although suicide is the most common cause of death in the perinatal period and women with severe mental illnesses have high rates of suicide postnatally, the rates of suicide for women in the antenatal and postnatal periods are lower than that for the whole female population.
- Lack of recognition of high-risk factors, or failure to manage are major contributory factors in deaths from suicide.

Risk factors for the development of mental disorders in the postnatal period

- Past psychiatric history, including previous puerperal episodes, current disorder or symptomatology, and family history of psychosis in the postnatal period.
- Social factors such as women bringing children up alone, in poverty or in suboptimal accommodation may play an important role in maintenance of mental disorder in adults.
- Pre-existing bipolar disorder, other serious affective disorder, and personal history of puerperal psychosis predicts a 50% risk of early postpartum major mental illness.

Course and prognosis of mental disorders in the perinatal period

- The underlying course of most pre-existing mental disorders is not significantly altered, with the exception of bipolar disorder, which shows an increased rate of relapse and first presentation.
- The prognosis of disorders that develop during pregnancy or postnatally is not significantly different from those developing at other times.
- There is evidence of possible adverse outcomes for infants and siblings at this time.
- Maternal mental illness may negatively affect the woman's relationship with her partner and increase the partner's risk of mental illness.

Antenatal care throughout pregnancy

- At each antenatal clinic visit – ask women about their current mental health. Questions which may be used to detect depression include:
  * During the past month, have you often been bothered by feeling down, depressed or hopeless?
  * During the past month, have you often been bothered by having little interest or pleasure in doing things?
- If yes to either question, make further enquiry: is this something you feel you need or want help with?
- For subsequent assessment and for routine monitoring of outcomes, consider using self-report measures such as the Edinburgh Postnatal Depression Scale (EPDS), Hospital Anxiety and Depression Scale (HADS) or Patient Health Questionnaire 9 (PHQ9).
- Do not use other specific predictors, such as poor relationships with her partner, to predict development of a mental disorder.

Initial care

- **If the woman has a mental disorder or history of severe mental illness –**
  * Ask about her mental health at all subsequent contacts.
  * Develop a care plan, usually in the first trimester, covering pregnancy, delivery, and the postnatal period in conjunction with the woman, her family members/carers, and Secondary Mental Health Services (SMHS) and Perinatal Mental Health Services (PMHS). Record it in all versions of the woman's notes and communicate to the woman and all relevant HCPs.
- For women who develop mild/moderate depression or anxiety during pregnancy – consider self-help strategies (guided self-help, C-CBT or exercise).
- To minimize the risk of harm to the fetus or child, prescribe drugs cautiously. As a result, the thresholds for non-drug treatments, particularly psychological treatments, are likely to be lower.

Care during labour

- Clearly document whether women can continue to take their prescribed psychotropic medicines during labour.
- Inform the anaesthetist and neonatologist.

Early postpartum period

- Women identified as being at high risk of early postpartum mental illness (puerperal psychosis) – manage according to the detailed plan for late pregnancy and the early postpartum period, devised in collaboration with specialized PMHS.
- Observe the infants of mothers who have taken psychotropic medication in pregnancy for signs of neonatal adaptation syndrome. While usually mild and self-limiting, if they occur the infant will need neonatal assessment.
- Urgently discuss with specialized PMHS if any change in mental state.

Refer

- Women having current mild to moderate illness, and those with previous depressive/anxiety disorders – refer to their GP in the first instance.
- Refer to specialized PMHS or SMHS:
  * Women suffering from serious illness with symptoms of psychosis, suicidal ideation, self-neglect, evidence of harm to others or significant interference with daily functioning (psychotic disorders, severe anxiety or depression, obsessive–compulsive disorder, and eating disorders).
  * Woman with a history of bipolar disorder or schizophrenia.
  * Women with previous serious postpartum mental illness (puerperal psychosis).
  * Women on complex psychotropic medication regimens.
- Consider referral to PMHS or SMHS:
  * Women with illness of moderate severity developing in late pregnancy or early postpartum period.
  * Women with current illness of mild or moderate severity where there is a first-degree relative with bipolar disorder or puerperal psychosis. In the absence of current illness, such a family history indicates a raised, but low, absolute risk of early postpartum serious mental illness.
- Consider referring women who present with new symptoms in late pregnancy.
- Women with previous periods of inpatient mental health care should be screened by mental health services.
- In all cases inform the GP even if no further assessment or referral is made.

Women who need inpatient care for a mental disorder within 12 months of childbirth should be admitted to a specialist mother and baby unit.

Incidence and Prevelence of Perinatal Mental Health Disorders

Depression

- Prevalence for major depression among 16- to 65-year-olds in the UK is 21/1000, but if a broader category of 'mixed depression and anxiety' is included, these figures are 98/1000.
- Increased prevalence among separated and divorced females and couples with children.
- Point prevalence of major depression – 4% at the end of the first trimester, 5% at the end of the second, and 3% at the end of the third trimester; 1–6% in the first 12 months postnatally.
- Period prevalence – 13% during pregnancy, 6% from birth to 2 months postnatally, 7% at 6 months, and 22% at 12 months.

Psychosis

- Puerperal psychosis – psychosis in the early postnatal period (up to 3 months after delivery). However, it is unclear whether it is a distinct diagnosis.
- There appears to be an increase in rates of psychosis in the first 90 days after delivery. A study found 21-fold higher rates in this period compared with other times, with figures of around 1 per 1000. Childbirth is a risk factor for the onset of psychosis, albeit a very small one.
- Many women admitted with psychosis in the postnatal period have a pre-existing mental disorder, including bipolar disorder and schizophrenia.

Eating disorders

- Anorexia nervosa in pregnant women is less common than in the general population, due to the reduced fertility and fecundity associated with this disorder and its usual onset in adolescence.
- Pregnancy in women with bulimia nervosa is less rare since this disorder is less likely to cause infertility, although as many as 50% may suffer from amenorrhoea or oligoamenorrhoea at some point in the course of the illness. Oligoamenorrhoea or vomiting of oral contraceptives may increase the risk of unplanned pregnancy amongst women with bulimia nervosa.
- Factors associated with higher incidence in pregnancy include younger age (< 29 years), previous symptomatology, lower educational attainment, poorer housing, employment status, and previous miscarriage.
- Women with eating disorders during pregnancy are more likely to have obstetric problems, such as miscarriage, delivery by CS, and premature or small infants.

Anxiety disorders

- Anxiety disorders are often comorbid with depressive disorders.

Panic disorder

- There is no suggestion of a raised prevalence of panic disorder in pregnancy. The symptoms may improve in 40% of pregnancies and 38% may have postnatal onset.

Generalized anxiety disorder (GAD)

- Incidence – 15% at 18 weeks of gestation and 8% at 8 weeks postnatally with 2.4% de novo presentations. Despite the view that anxiety disorders only constitute mild mental health problems, they contribute significant disability to sufferers along with a possible negative effect on the fetus evident in infancy.

Obsessive-compulsive disorder (OCD)

- Some evidence of new onset of OCD associated with pregnancy and childbirth.
- OCD symptoms are much more common amongst women who are depressed postnatally than amongst those who are not (41% versus 6%).

Post-traumatic stress disorder (PTSD)

- Prevalence – 3–6% at around 6 weeks postnatally to 1.5% by 6 months postnatally.
- PTSD experienced by some women at this time may not be induced by traumatic delivery but will be pre-existing PTSD connected with traumatic events unrelated to the current context.
- Stillbirth may be a stressor for PTSD symptoms during subsequent pregnancy.

Consequences of mental disorder

Severe depression

- Increased rate of obstetric complications – SB, suicide attempts, postnatal specialist care for the infant, and LBW infants.
- Maternal depression postnatally may be associated with cognitive delay and a range of emotional and behavioural difficulties in young children.

Schizophrenia and bipolar disorder

- Increased rate of suicide, worsening of the disorder, poorer obstetric outcomes, increased PTD, LBW, and SGA infants.
- Maternal psychoses, including schizophrenia, increase the risk of infant mortality and SB.
- Maternal schizophrenia – parenting difficulties, high proportion of women lose care of their infant, and poor outcomes for the mental health of offspring.

Others

- Poor fetal outcomes with maternal eating disorders during pregnancy.
- Elevated risks of sudden infant death syndrome with postnatal depression and schizophrenia.
- Poorer long-term outcomes for children.
- Indirect effects such as social isolation and other disadvantages.

Pharmacological treatments

- Pharmacological treatments may be the only treatment, which in itself can carry a potential risk to the infant. The risks associated with most psychotropic drug exposure in pregnancy and breastfeeding are not well understood. Assessment of drug treatment risk is highly complex and there is a need to balance this against the harm of untreated disorder.
- In addition to possible teratogenic and other risks to the fetus, the altered physical state of the woman in pregnancy means that increased monitoring, for example, blood glucose during pregnancy, the impact of analgesic drugs during delivery, and the impact on breastfeeding, all need to be considered.

Consequences for the woman

- Impairment in social and personal functioning and the woman's ability to care effectively for herself and her children.
- Women are often concerned that their mental health problems may prevent them from actively caring for themselves, the unborn child or the infant. This can exacerbate an already troubling and disabling disorder.

Consequences for the infant and siblings

- Can affect the social and cognitive development of children and can also have long-term consequences on their mental health.
- Reduced IQ in children whose mothers had depression early in the postnatal period has been reported.
- Children may also be at risk of physical health problems. Considerable neglect of the child and active physical abuse can occasionally lead to tragic consequences.

Consequences for the wider family

- Mental health problems in pregnancy also present a burden to the wider family.

Prevention

Treat subthreshold symptoms in pregnant women – for symptoms of depression and/or anxiety that do not meet diagnostic criteria but significantly interfere with personal and social functioning, consider:

- **For women who have had a previous episode of depression or anxiety** – brief psychological treatment (4–6 sessions), such as interpersonal psychotherapy (IPT) or cognitive behavioural therapy (CBT).
- **For women who have not had a previous episode of depression or anxiety** – social support (regular informal individual sessions or group-based).

Routine antenatal and postnatal care – do not offer psychosocial interventions (for example, group psychoeducation) designed specifically to reduce the likelihood of the woman developing a mental disorder during pregnancy and the postnatal period as a part of routine antenatal and postnatal care.

Traumatic birth and stillbirth – do not routinely offer single-session formal debriefing focused on the birth to women who have experienced a traumatic birth. Provide support to women who wish to talk about their experience; encourage them to make use of support from family and friends. Do not routinely encourage mothers of infants who are stillborn or die soon after birth to see and hold the dead infant.

Management of Perinatal Mental Disorders

Balancing risks and benefits

All pregnancies carry a background risk, which may be increased by the presence of a mental disorder. Treatment can reduce the risk, but the use of some psychotropic drugs may increase it.

Discuss and balance risks – consider:

- the risk of relapse or deterioration in current symptoms and the woman's ability to cope with untreated or subthreshold symptoms;
- severity of previous episodes, response to treatment, and the woman's preference;
- the possibility that stopping a drug with teratogenic risk after pregnancy is confirmed may not remove the risk of malformations;
- the risks from stopping medication abruptly;
- the need for prompt treatment because of the potential impact of an untreated mental disorder on the fetus or infant;
- the increased risk associated with drug treatments during pregnancy and the postnatal period, including the risk in overdose;
- treatment options that would enable the woman to breastfeed if she wishes.

Discuss the absolute and relative risks associated with treating and not treating the mental disorder. Acknowledge the uncertainty surrounding the risks.

Existing risk to the fetus:

- Risk of congenital malformation in the general population is 2–4%. This risk increases where the woman has a mental disorder.

Risk of not treating mental disorder:

- Depends on the disorder and the woman's psychiatric history.
- Not treating the disorder poses a risk both to the woman's physical health as well as her ongoing mental health and wellbeing.
- There is also risk to the fetus and infant and there may be risks to family, fathers/partners, and carers.

Risk of treating mental disorder:

- The risks with psychotropic medication include side effects for the woman and possible malformation or developmental problems for the fetus, such as neurobehavioural teratogenicity. This varies between different drugs and, in some cases, is dose dependent.
- Risks for the infant immediately after delivery, including withdrawal effects and toxicity.

When prescribing a drug:

- choose drugs with lower risk profiles for the mother and fetus/infant;
- start at the lowest effective dose and slowly increase it; this is particularly important where the risks may be dose related;
- use monotherapy in preference to combination treatment;
- consider additional precautions for preterm, low birth weight or sick infants.

When stopping a drug, take into account:

- the risk to the fetus/infant during the withdrawal period;
- the risk from not treating the disorder.

Psychological treatments

- **Women requiring psychological treatment should be seen for treatment within 1 month of initial assessment, and no longer than 3 months afterwards.** This is because of the lower threshold for access to psychological therapies during pregnancy and the postnatal period arising from the changing risk–benefit ratio for psychotropic medication at this time.

Women taking psychotropic drugs

- In pregnant women who, at the time of conception and/or in the first trimester, were taking drugs with known teratogenic risk (lithium, valproate, carbamazepine, lamotrigine or paroxetine):
  * Confirm the pregnancy.
  * Offer screening and counselling about the continuation of the pregnancy, the need for additional monitoring, and the risks to the fetus if the woman continues to take medication.
  * Carry out a full paediatric assessment of the newborn infant.
  * Monitor the infant in the first few weeks after delivery for adverse drug effects, drug toxicity or withdrawal (for example, floppy baby syndrome, irritability, constant crying, shivering, tremor, restlessness, increased tone, feeding and sleeping difficulties, and, rarely, seizures); if the mother took antidepressants in the last trimester, these may result from serotonergic toxicity syndrome rather than withdrawal.
- Monitor infants of mothers who are breastfeeding while taking psychotropic medication for adverse drug reactions.
- **Specific risks of psychotropic medication**
  The risks of fetal malformations, problems for the neonate, and obstetric complications may be increased by the use of psychotropic drugs. For most drugs the risks are uncertain because there are limited data. If the level of risk is known, or it is known to be substantial, consider alternative treatment options.

Severe mental illness

Schizophrenia

Planning a pregnancy and during pregnancy –
- Consider switching from an atypical antipsychotic to a low-dose typical such as haloperidol, chlorpromazine or trifluoperazine.
- The perinatal period and breastfeeding – If taking depot medication the infant may show extrapyramidal symptoms several months after administration.

Bipolar disorder

Planning a pregnancy
- If antimanic medication is needed, choose a low-dose typical or atypical antipsychotic.
- If depression develops after stopping prophylactic medication, offer CBT.
- If an antidepressant is used, it should usually be an SSRI (but not paroxetine); monitor closely.

During pregnancy
- Maintain on antipsychotic if stable and likely to relapse without medication.
- If a woman has an unplanned pregnancy and is stopping lithium, offer an antipsychotic.

The perinatal period and breastfeeding
- After delivery, consider starting or restarting medication as soon as fluid balance is established if at high risk of an acute episode.
- Consider augmenting treatment with an antipsychotic if a woman maintained on lithium is at high risk of a manic relapse in the immediate postnatal period.
- If a prophylactic agent is needed offer an antipsychotic.

Acute mania
- Consider a typical or atypical antipsychotic.
- If taking prophylactic medication:
  * Check dose and adherence.
  * Increase dose if taking an antipsychotic or consider switching to an antipsychotic if not.
  * If no response and woman has severe mania, consider ECT, lithium, and rarely valproate.
- If there is no alternative to valproate consider augmenting it with antimanic medication (not carbamazepine).

Depressive symptoms
- For mild symptoms, consider in the following order:
  * Self-help approaches (guided self help and C-CBT).
  * Brief psychological treatments (counselling, CBT, and IPT).
- For moderate to severe symptoms, consider:
  * CBT for moderate depression.
  * Combined medication and CBT for severe depression.
  * When prescribing, consider quetiapine alone, or SSRIs (but not paroxetine) in combination with prophylactic medication. Monitor closely for signs of switching and stop the SSRI if manic or hypomanic symptoms develop.

The atypical antipsychotics (AAP) (also known as second generation antipsychotics) are a group of antipsychotic tranquillizing drugs used in the treatment of schizophrenia, acute mania, bipolar depression, and other indications. Both generations of medication tend to block receptors in the brain's dopamine pathways, but atypicals are less likely to cause extrapyramidal symptoms (EPS), which include unsteady Parkinson's disease-type movements, body rigidity, and involuntary tremors. Atypical antipsychotics are associated with: higher rate of responders, efficiency in patients with refractory disease, lower risk of suicides, better functional capacity, and an improved quality of life. Although atypical antipsychotics are thought to be safer than typical antipsychotics, they still have severe side effects, including tardive dyskinesia (a serious movement disorder), neuroleptic malignant syndrome, and increased risk of stroke, sudden cardiac death, blood clots, and diabetes. Significant weight gain may also occur. Examples: sulpiride, clozapine, olanzapine, risperidone.

Typical antipsychotics (first generation antipsychotics, conventional antipsychotics, classical neuroleptics, traditional antipsychotics, or major tranquillizers) are a class of antipsychotic drugs used to treat psychosis (in particular, schizophrenia), acute mania, agitation, and other conditions. The first typical antipsychotics to enter clinical use were the phenothiazines. Side effects include: dry mouth, muscle stiffness, muscle cramping, tremors, EPS, and weight gain. Traditional antipsychotics are classified as either high-potency or low-potency. High-potency: fluphenazine and haloperidol – more EPS and less histaminic (e.g., sedation), α-adrenergic (e.g., orthostatic hypotension), and anticholinergic effects (e.g., dry mouth). Low-potency: chlorpromazine – fewer EPS but more H1, α1, and muscarinic blocking effects.

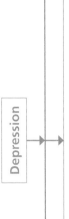

Depression

Mild depression

Planning a pregnancy
- Withdraw antidepressant and consider watchful waiting.
- If intervention is needed consider:
  * Self-help approaches (guided self-help, C-CBT, exercise).
  * Brief psychological treatments (counselling, CBT, and IPT).

During pregnancy and breastfeeding
- New episode of mild depression:
  * Self-help approaches.
  * Non-directive counselling at home.
  * Brief CBT/IPT.
- New episode of mild depression with a history of severe depression – consider antidepressant if psychological treatments declined or not responded to.

Moderate and severe depression

Planning a pregnancy
- Latest presentation was moderate depression – consider:
  * Switching to CBT/IPT if taking an antidepressant.
  * Switching to an antidepressant with lower risk.
- Latest presentation was severe depression – consider:
  * Combining CBT/IPT and antidepressant (switch to one with lower risk).
  * Switching to CBT/IPT.

During pregnancy and breastfeeding
- New episode of moderate depression – as for mild depression.
- Moderate depressive episode and a history of depression, or a severe depressive episode – consider:
  * CBT/IPT.
  * Antidepressant if preferred by the woman.
  * Combination treatment if there is no, or limited, response to psychological or drug treatment alone.

Treatment-resistant depression

During pregnancy and breastfeeding
- Consider a different single drug or ECT before combination drug treatment.
- Avoid lithium augmentation.

CBT – cognitive behavioural therapy.
C-CBT – computerized CBT.
IPT – interpersonal psychotherapy.
EMDR – eye movement desensitization and reprocessing.

Anxiety and eating disorders

Generalized anxiety disorder (GAD) and panic disorder
- Planning a pregnancy – consider:
  * Withdrawing medication and starting CBT if this has not already been tried.
  * Switching to a safer drug.
- During pregnancy –
  * **GAD** (new episode) – offer CBT.
  * **Panic disorder** (new episode) – consider:
    > CBT, self-help or C-CBT before starting drug treatment.
    > If medication is needed do not start paroxetine; consider a safer drug.

Obsessive–compulsive disorder (OCD)
- Planning a pregnancy and during pregnancy:
  * Consider:
    > Withdrawing medication and starting psychological therapy.
    > Starting psychological therapy before medication.
  * Withdraw paroxetine if the woman is taking it, and switch to a safer drug.
  * Breastfeeding
    * Avoid the combination of clomipramine and citalopram.

Post-traumatic stress disorder (PTSD)
- Planning a pregnancy and during pregnancy –
  * Withdraw antidepressant and offer trauma-focused CBT/EMDR.
  * Do not prescribe adjunctive olanzapine.
  * Breastfeeding
Refer to the NICE clinical guideline on post-traumatic stress disorder.

Eating disorders
- For anorexia – refer to the NICE clinical guideline on eating disorders.
- Planning a pregnancy and during pregnancy –
  Binge eating disorder – if taking an antidepressant, treat according to depression.
  Bulimia nervosa – consider: withdrawing medication gradually and referral for specialist treatment if problem persists.
  * Breastfeeding
    - **Bulimia nervosa** –
      * Offer psychological treatment rather than fluoxetine at 60 mg.
      * If the woman is taking fluoxetine at 60 mg, advise her not to breastfeed.

Psychotropic medication

Know your drug – antipsychotics

- Risks
  * Raised prolactin levels with some (amisulpride, risperidone, sulpiride).
  * Gestational diabetes and weight gain with olanzapine.
  * Agranulocytosis in the fetus (theoretical) and breastfed infant with clozapine.
  * EPS in the neonate especially with depot medication (self-limiting).
- Actions to take
  * Women taking antipsychotics planning a pregnancy – raised prolactin levels reduce the chances of conception. If levels are raised, consider an alternative drug.
  * If prescribing olanzapine to a pregnant woman, consider risk factors for gestational diabetes and weight gain, including family history, existing weight, and ethnicity.
  * Adjust dose and timing of the antipsychotic or switch to another drug to avoid side effects.
- Do not routinely prescribe:
  * Clozapine to women who are pregnant or breastfeeding; for those taking it, consider switching to another drug and monitor carefully.
  * Depot antipsychotics to pregnant women.
  * Anticholinergic drugs for extrapyramidal side effects of antipsychotics, except for short-term use.

Know your drug – lithium

- Risks
  * Fetal heart defects (risk rise from 8 in 1000 to around 60 in 1000).
  * Ebstein's anomaly (risk rise from 1 in 20000 to 10 in 20000).
  * High levels in breast milk.
- Actions to take
  * Do not routinely prescribe, particularly in the first trimester of pregnancy or during breastfeeding.
  * Advise a woman who is taking lithium and who is well and not at high risk of relapse, to stop the drug if planning a pregnancy.

If a woman taking lithium becomes pregnant

- If the pregnancy is confirmed in the first trimester, and the woman is well and not at high risk of relapse, stop the drug gradually over 4 weeks; this may not remove the risk of cardiac defects in the fetus.

- If she is not well or is at high risk of relapse, consider to:
  * switch over gradually to an antipsychotic; or
  * stop lithium and restart it in the second trimester if the woman is not planning to breastfeed and her symptoms have responded better to lithium than to other drugs in the past;
  * continue with lithium if she is at high risk of relapse.

If a woman continues taking lithium during pregnancy

- Check serum levels every 4 weeks, then weekly from the 36th week, and less than 24 hours after childbirth.
- Adjust the dose to keep serum levels towards the lower end of the therapeutic range.
- Make sure she maintains adequate fluid intake.
- Deliver in hospital and monitor during labour including fluid balance, because of the risk of dehydration and lithium toxicity (in prolonged labour, it may be appropriate to check serum lithium levels).

Psychotropic medication contd.

Know your drug – antidepressants

- Risks
  * Lowest known risks during pregnancy: tricyclic antidepressants (TCAs) such as amitriptyline, imipramine, nortriptyline; but are more likely to cause death if taken in overdose than selective serotonin reuptake inhibitors (SSRIs).
  * Lowest known risk with an SSRI during pregnancy: fluoxetine.
  * **Fetal heart defects with paroxetine if taken in the first trimester.**
  * Persistent pulmonary HT in the neonate with SSRIs taken after 20 weeks.
  * High BP with venlafaxine at high doses, together with higher toxicity in overdose than SSRIs and some TCAs and increased difficulty in withdrawal.
  * Withdrawal or toxicity in the neonate with all antidepressants (mild and self-limiting).
  * Lower than other antidepressants in breast milk: imipramine, nortriptyline, and sertraline.
  * Higher levels in breast milk: citalopram and fluoxetine.
- Actions to take
  * Advise a woman taking paroxetine who is planning pregnancy or has an unplanned pregnancy to stop the drug.

Know your drug – carbamazepine and lamotrigine

- Risks
  * Carbamazepine: neural tube defects (risk rise from 6 in 10 000 to 20–50 in 10 000) and other major fetal malformations including gastrointestinal tract problems and cardiac abnormalities.
  * Lamotrigine: oral cleft (9 in 1000), and dermatological problems (Stevens–Johnson syndrome) in the infant if taken while breastfeeding.
- Actions to take
  * Advise woman taking these drugs who is planning a pregnancy or has an unplanned pregnancy to stop them. Consider an alternative (such as an antipsychotic) if appropriate.
- Do not routinely prescribe:
  * Carbamazepine and lamotrigine for pregnant women
  * Lamotrigine for women who are breastfeeding.

Know your drug – valproate

- Risks
  * Neural tube defects (risk rise from 6 in 10 000 to 100–200 in 10 000).
  * Effects on the child's intellectual development.
  * Polycystic ovary syndrome in women younger than 18 years.
- Actions to take
  * Do not routinely prescribe to women of child-bearing age. If there is no effective alternative, explain risks during pregnancy and importance of using adequate contraception.
  * Do not prescribe to women younger than 18 years (increased risk of unplanned pregnancy).
  * If a woman taking valproate is planning a pregnancy or pregnant, advise her to stop the drug. In the treatment of bipolar disorder consider using an alternative drug (antipsychotic).
  * If there is no alternative to valproate, limit doses to a maximum of 1 g per day, in divided doses and in the slow-release form, with 5 mg per day folic acid.

Know your drug – benzodiazepines

- Risks
  * Cleft palate and other fetal malformations.
  * Floppy baby syndrome in the neonate.
- Actions to take
  * Do not routinely prescribe to pregnant women, except for the short-term treatment of extreme anxiety and agitation.
  * Consider gradually stopping in pregnant women.

Psychological and psychosocial interventions

Cognitive behavioural therapy

- Psychological distress is strongly influenced by patterns of thinking, beliefs, and behaviour. Depressed patients have patterns of thinking and reasoning that focus on a negative view of the world. Psychological distress may be alleviated by altering these thought patterns and behaviours.
- The key aspect of the therapy is an educative approach, where the patient learns to recognize their negative thinking patterns and how to re-evaluate them.

Debriefing

- In the antenatal and postnatal mental health setting, the term refers to treatment targeted at women who had traumatic births. The mother is encouraged to articulate her reactions to distressing traumatic aspects of the birth, and the treatment facilitates some normalization of the reactions to traumatic stimuli. It is offered to individuals and usually within 72 hours of birth.

Non-directive counselling (listening visits)

- Counsellors are trained to listen and reflect patient feelings and meaning. They are trained to help clients to gain better understanding of their circumstances and themselves. The therapist adopts an empathic and non-judgemental approach, listening rather than directing but offering non-verbal encouragement, reflecting back to assist the person in making decisions.

Interpersonal psychotherapy

- The patient and therapist work collaboratively to identify effects of key problem areas related to interpersonal conflicts, role transitions, grief and loss, and social skills, and their effects on current symptoms, feeling states, and/or problems.
- The treatment seeks to reduce symptoms by learning to cope with or resolve these interpersonal issues.

Psychodynamic psychotherapy

- The therapist and patient explore and gain insight into conflicts and how these are represented in current situations and relationships, including the therapy relationship.
- This leads to the patient being given the opportunity to explore feelings and conscious and unconscious conflicts originating in the past, with a focus on interpreting and working through them.

RCOG. Management of Women with Mental Health Issues during Pregnancy and the Postnatal Period. Good Practice No.14; June 2011.
NICE. Antenatal and Postnatal Mental Health; April 2007. Please refer to updated Guidelines 2014.
http://www.who.int/classifications/icd/en/bluebook.pdf

CHAPTER 46 Breech presentation

Background and prevalence

- The incidence of breech presentation decreases from about 20% at 28 weeks of gestation to 3–4% at term.
- It is more common where there has been a previous breech presentation.
- Persistent breech presentation may be associated with abnormalities of the baby, amniotic fluid volume, placental localization or of the uterus.

Risks or complications

- Higher perinatal mortality and morbidity with breech than cephalic presentation, due to prematurity, congenital malformations, and birth asphyxia or trauma.
- Irrespective of the mode of delivery, breech presentation is associated with increased risk of subsequent handicap. Failure to adopt the cephalic presentation may in some cases be a marker for fetal impairment.

Risk vs benefit – mode of delivery

Planned CS compared with planned vaginal birth.

Risk to baby

Systematic review –

- Planned CS has a reduced PNM and early neonatal morbidity for babies with a breech presentation at term compared with planned vaginal birth.
- After excluding the cases of: deliveries that occurred after a prolonged labour, labours that were induced or augmented with oxytocin or prostaglandins, cases where there was a footling or uncertain type of breech presentation at delivery, and those cases for whom there was no skilled or experienced clinician present at the birth –
  * Risk of PNM, neonatal mortality or serious neonatal morbidity with planned CS compared with planned vaginal birth was 1.6% vs 3.3% (P = 0.02).

Subanalysis –

- The benefits of delivery by CS were more significant in countries with a low PNMR.
- Adverse perinatal outcome was lowest with prelabour CS and increased with CS in early labour, in active labour, and vaginal birth.
- For women experiencing labour, adverse perinatal outcome was also associated with labour augmentation, birth weight <2.8 kg, longer time between pushing and delivery, and no experienced clinician at delivery.

Long term health of babies – no evidence that it is influenced by the mode of delivery. Two-year follow-up from Term Breech Trial – death or neurodevelopmental delay was similar between the two groups. The smaller number of peri-natal deaths with planned CS was balanced by a greater number of babies with neurodevelopmental delay. This was unexpected, as there had been fewer babies in the planned CS group with severe perinatal morbidity.

More recent study – in units where planned vaginal delivery is a common practice and when strict criteria are met before and during labour, planned vaginal delivery of singleton fetuses in breech presentation at term remains a safe option. In this study, 71% of women planned for vaginal delivery, delivered vaginally. The rate of neonatal morbidi-ty or death was considerably lower than the 5% in the Term Breech Trial (1.6%), and was not significantly different from the planned CS group.

Risk to mother

Immediate and short term

- Small increase in serious immediate complications.
- Significant increase in short-term serious maternal morbidity.
- Less urinary incontinence; more abdominal pain; and less perineal pain.

Long term – does not carry any additional risk to long-term health. Two-year follow-up of women (Term Breech Trial) – No differences were detected, except for more constipation in the planned CS group.

Long-term effects on future pregnancy outcomes are uncertain:

- For every infant potentially saved by a CS, 1 woman will experience a uterine rupture during a subsequent pregnancy (if VBAC is practised).
- In the 4 years following the Term Breech Trial, the increase of approximately 8500 planned CS probably prevented 19 perinatal deaths. However, it also resulted in 4 maternal deaths that may have been avoidable.
- In future pregnancies, 9 perinatal deaths are expected as a result of the uterine scar and 140 women will have potentially life-threatening complications from the uterine scar.
- The long-term risks of CS for the mother, such as scar dehiscence in a subsequent pregnancy, increased risk of repeat CS (up to 44%), and placenta accreta need to be taken into account when considering the risks and benefits of planned CS.

External cephalic version (ECV)

Background

- ECV – the manipulation of the fetus, through the maternal abdomen, to a cephalic presentation, to reduce the incidence of breech presentation at term and therefore the associated risks, particularly of avoidable CS.
- Spontaneous version rates for nulliparous women are approximately 8% after 36 weeks but < 5% after unsuccessful ECV.
- Spontaneous reversion to breech presentation after successful ECV occurs in < 5%.
- ECV – success rate of 30–80%. It reduces the incidence of non-cephalic presentation at delivery (RR 0.38, NNT 2).
- ECV reduces the CS rate by lowering the incidence of breech presentation (RR 0.55, NNT 6). The reduction in CS is seen in spite of a 2-fold increase in intrapartum CS for successfully turned babies, when compared with babies that were not breech at term.
- Labour with a cephalic presentation following ECV is associated with a higher rate of obstetric intervention than when ECV has not been performed. A small increase in instrumental delivery is also seen.
- ECV may not be performed because – breech is not diagnosed in about 25%, it is not offered/available, or refused.

Procedure and risks

- Place of ECV – ECV does not induce labour but may be associated with fetal bradycardia and a non-reactive CTG that are almost invariably transient. Perform ECV where facilities for monitoring and immediate delivery are available. The standard preoperative preparations for CS are not necessary.
- ECV is best performed at a weekly session with access to USS, CTG, and theatre facilities.
- Perform CTG after the procedure.
- Kleihauer testing is unnecessary but offer anti-D Ig to Rh-negative women.
- ECV can be painful, with few women experiencing no discomfort and around 5% reporting high pain scores. Data on analgesia for ECV are lacking.
- Very low complication rate – placental abruption, uterine rupture, and fetomaternal haemorrhage; 0.5% risk of emergency CS. No excess perinatal morbidity or perinatal mortality.

Alternatives to ECV

- Insufficient evidence to support the use of postural management as a method of promoting spontaneous version over ECV.
- Moxibustion, burning the tip of the fifth toe (acupuncture point BL67) has been used to promote spontaneous version of the breech, with some success, and appears to be safe. However, pooled data conclude that there is insufficient evidence to support its use. Do not offer as a method of promoting spontaneous version over ECV.

Contraindications

- **Absolute contraindications** (that are likely to be associated with increased mortality or morbidity): where CS is indicated; APH within the last 7 days; abnormal CTG; major uterine anomaly; ruptured membranes; multiple pregnancy.
- **Relative contraindications** (where ECV might be more complicated): SGA fetus with abnormal Doppler parameters; PET; oligohydramnios; major fetal anomalies; scarred uterus; unstable lie.
- ECV is contraindicated in only 4% of women with a breech presentation at term.
- Unstable lie – Perform ECV only in the context of a stabilizing induction. This may be associated with a significant intrapartum complication rate.
- After one CS – the available data on ECV are reassuring but are insufficient to confidently conclude that the risk is not increased.

Factors affecting outcome

- Race, parity, uterine tone, liquor volume, engagement of the breech, whether the head is palpable, and the use of tocolysis.
- Higher success – multiparous, non-white women, non-engaged breech, easily palpable head, good liquor volume. High liquor volume may be associated with spontaneous reversion.
- Maternal weight, placental position, gestation, and fetal size make less difference.
- Offer ECV from 36 weeks in nulliparous women and from 37 weeks in multiparous women. Due to a spontaneous version rate of 8% in nulliparous breeches after 36 weeks and the very low complication rate, ECV from 36 weeks in nulliparous women seems a reasonable compromise.
- ECV before 36 weeks of gestation is not associated with a significant reduction in non-cephalic births or CS. There is no upper time limit on the appropriate gestation for ECV. Success has been reported at 42 weeks of gestation and it can be performed in early labour provided that the membranes are intact.

Methods to increase the success rate of ECV

- A further second attempt later, particularly with a second operator or where the back has been in the midline, may lead to a small increase in overall success rates.
- Tocolysis with beta-sympathomimetics – is proven with glyceryl trinitrate patch/sublingually, or nifedipine. Consider tocolysis where an initial attempt at ECV without tocolysis has failed. A simple protocol is to offer salbutamol or terbutaline either routinely or if an initial ECV attempt has failed.
- Other methods include the application of noise to the abdomen (fetal acoustic stimulation) where the back is in the midline, and regional analgesia, including after a failed initial attempt. For the latter, an increase in success rate is evident with epidural but not spinal analgesia. As maternal pain might indicate a complication, concerns regarding safety remain.

Vaginal breech delivery

Assessment for selection for vaginal breech birth

- Clinical judgement is adequate for routine pelvic assessment.
- **X-ray pelvimetry** – studies are not able to confirm the value of this in selecting women who are more likely to succeed in a trial of labour or achieving any effect on perinatal outcome. Term Breech Trial – use of radiological pelvimetry was not linked to improved outcome.
- **MRI pelvimetry** – No difference was shown in the overall number of CS or in the perinatal outcome.
- **CT pelvimetry** – Retrospective study has suggested improved perinatal outcome for vaginal breech delivery in women with CT confirmed adequate pelvimetry.
- Routine radiological pelvimetry is not necessary.
- **Factors unfavourable for vaginal breech birth** –
  * Other contraindications to vaginal birth (placenta praevia, compromised fetal condition).
  * Clinically inadequate pelvis.
  * Previous CS.
  * Growth-restricted baby (< 2000 g).
  * Footling or kneeling breech presentation.
  * Large baby (> 3800 g).
  * Hyperextended fetal neck in labour (diagnosed with USS or X-ray).
  * Lack of presence of a clinician trained in vaginal breech delivery.
- Diagnosis of breech presentation for the first time during labour is not a contraindication for vaginal breech birth.

Selection criteria for trial of vaginal breech delivery –

- No medical or obstetric complications.
- No fetopelvic disproportion. A trial of vaginal breech delivery is more likely to be successful if both the mother's pelvis and the baby are of average proportions. A significantly higher risk of neurodevelopmental delay in children with birth weight > 3500 g is reported with planned vaginal birth.
- Frank or complete breech presentation. Non-frank breech presentations are at a high rate of cord prolapse (5.6%) but no increase in impaired perinatal outcome.
- No evidence of hyperextension of the fetal head.

Intrapartum management

- Do not routinely offer epidural analgesia – no evidence that epidural analgesia is essential.
- Maternal position – as most experience with vaginal breech birth is in the dorsal or lithotomy position, this position is advised. Some recommend use of upright postures to improve outcomes of vaginal breech birth. However, no studies have shown effectiveness of this position over traditional dorsal position.
- Continous electronic FHR monitoring.
- Term Breech Trial – most common reasons for emergency CS were 'failure to progress' (50%) and 'fetal distress' (29%).
- Do not perform FBS from the buttocks during labour.

IOL and augmentation

- Consider IOL if individual circumstances are favourable.
- Do not augment labour – augmentation of established labour is controversial as poor progress in established labour may be a sign of fetopelvic disproportion. In the Term Breech Trial cohort, labour augmentation was associated with adverse perinatal outcome.
- Delayed second stage of labour – consider CS if there is delay in the descent of the breech at any stage in the second stage of labour. This may be a sign of relative fetopelvic disproportion.
- Perform episiotomy when indicated to facilitate delivery.
- Do not undertake breech extraction routinely. Conventional teaching in the UK is that spontaneous delivery of the trunk and limbs is preferable, because breech extraction causes extension of the arms and head. There is insufficient evidence to support or refute the policy of routinely expediting vaginal breech delivery by extraction of the baby within a single uterine contraction.

Service provision

- An experienced practitioner with appropriate training.
- Place – in a hospital with facilities for emergency CS. Ready access to CS is important particularly in the event of poor progress in the second stage of labour.

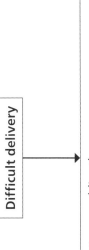

Difficult delivery

Delayed delivery of the arms – deliver the arms:
- by sweeping them across the baby's face and downwards; or
- by the Lovset manoeuvre (rotation of the baby to facilitate delivery of the arms).
- There is no evidence to indicate which method should be attempted first.

Delayed engagement in the pelvis of the aftercoming head –
- Suprapubic pressure to assist flexion of the head.
- The Mauriceau–Smellie–Veit manoeuvre – displacing the head upwards and rotating to the oblique diameter to facilitate engagement.
- There is no evidence to indicate which is the best method of assisting engagement of the head in the pelvis.

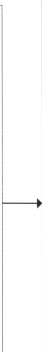

Aftercoming head – may be delivered:
- With forceps;
- By the Mariceau–Smellie–Veit manoeuvre; or
- By the Burns–Marshall method.
- There is no experimental evidence as to which method is preferable.
- Obstructed delivery of the aftercoming head – if conservative methods fail, symphysiotomy or CS.

What not to do

- Attempting vaginal breech birth in women with unfavourable clinical features.
- Routine radiological pelvimetry.
- Vaginal breech birth in previous CS.
- Routine epidural analgesia.
- Fetal blood sampling from the buttocks.
- Labour augmentation.
- Routine breech extraction.
- Routine CS for the delivery of preterm breech presentation.
- Routine CS for twin pregnancy with breech presentation of the second twin.

Management of the preterm breech and twin breech

Preterm babies in breech

- Do not offer routine CS for the delivery of preterm breech. Discuss the mode of delivery on an individual basis. In the absence of good evidence that a preterm baby needs to be delivered by CS, decide the mode of delivery after consultation with the woman and her partner.
- Evidence from the Term Breech Trial cannot be directly extrapolated to preterm breech delivery, which remains an area of clinical controversy.
- A retrospective cohort study – very-LBW breech or malpresenting neonates delivered by a primary CS had significantly lower adjusted RRs of death compared with those delivered vaginally. However, the poor outcome for very-LBW infants is mainly related to complications of prematurity and not the mode of delivery.
- Consider lateral incisions of the cervix where there is head entrapment during a preterm breech delivery to release the aftercoming head. Similar rates of head entrapment have been described for vaginal and abdominal delivery.

Twins in breech presentation

First twin in breech presentation at term

- In the absence of specific evidence on relative risks of planned vaginal birth and planned CS for the first twin in breech presentation, it is reasonable to use data from singleton breech presentation as a proxy to assist decision making.
- Although many choose CS when the first twin presents as a breech, because of concern about 'interlocking', this complication is extremely rare, with a reported rate of 1 in 817 twin pregnancies where the first twin was breech and the second cephalic.
- Be aware of this possible diagnosis if the delivery of the trunk is delayed and be prepared to displace the head of the second twin upwards or to perform rapid CS.

Second twin in breech presentation

- Do not offer routine CS for twin pregnancy with breech presentation of the second twin.
- The second twin is non-vertex in about 40% of cases. The presentation of the second twin at delivery is not always predictable. The chance of cephalic delivery may be improved by routinely guiding the head of the second twin towards the pelvis during and immediately after delivery of the first twin.
- Some prefer to routinely expedite delivery of the second twin by internal version and breech extraction irrespective of the presentation.

The Management of Breech Presentation. RCOG Guideline No. 20b; December 2006.
External Cephalic Version and Reducing the Incidence of Breech Presentation. RCOG Guideline No. 20a; December 2006; Reviewed 2010.
www.primary-surgery.org
hetv.org

CHAPTER 47 Caesarean section (CS)
About one in four women have a CS

Information to women

- Provide written information tailored to the woman's needs, taking into account the cultural needs of minority communities and women whose first language is not English or who cannot read, together with the needs of women with disabilities or learning difficulties.
- **Discuss antenatally:**
  - Indications for CS.
  - What the procedure involves.
  - Associated risks and benefits.
  - Implications for future pregnancies and birth after CS.
- **Plan mode of birth** – discuss the risks and benefits of CS and vaginal birth, taking into account their circumstances, concerns, priorities, and plans for future pregnancies.
- Planned CS (PCS) compared with planned vaginal birth (PVB) for women with an uncomplicated pregnancy –
  - **PCS may reduce the risk of:** perineal and abdominal pain during birth and 3 days postpartum, injury to vagina, early PPH, obstetric shock.
  - **PCS may increase the risk of:** NICU admission, longer hospital stay, hysterectomy caused by PPH, cardiac arrest.

Factors affecting likelihood of CS during intrapartum care

- Electronic FHR monitoring is associated with an increased likelihood of CS.

Factors which reduce the likelihood of CS

- **Place of birth** – planned home birth for healthy pregnant women with anticipated uncomplicated pregnancies.
- Continuous support during labour.
- In women with uncomplicated singleton pregnancy:
  - IOL >41 weeks.
  - A partogram with a 4-hour action line.
- Consultant obstetricians involved in the decision making.
- When CS is contemplated because of an abnormal FHR pattern, in cases of suspected fetal acidosis, FBS (if technically possible and there are no contraindications) reduces the risk of CS.

No influence on likelihood of CS

- **Place of birth** – planned childbirth in a 'midwifery-led' unit for healthy women with uncomplicated pregnancies.
- **Other factors** – walking in labour, non-supine position during the second stage of labour, immersion in water during labour, epidural analgesia during labour, use of raspberry leaves.
- **Complementary therapies** during labour (acupuncture, aromatherapy, hypnosis, herbal products, nutritional supplements, homeopathic medicines, and Chinese medicines) have not been properly evaluated.
- **Failure to progress in labour** – active management of labour and early amniotomy do not influence the likelihood of CS.

Planned CS (PCS)

Indicated

- Breech presentation – women with a singleton breech presentation at term, for whom ECV is contraindicated or has been unsuccessful.
- Multiple pregnancy – in twin pregnancies where the first twin is not cephalic the effect of CS in improving outcome is uncertain, but current practice is to offer a PCS.
- Placenta praevia – women with a placenta that partly or completely covers the internal cervical os (minor or major placenta praevia).
- Morbidly adherent placenta. See Chapter 30 Antepartum haemorrhage (APH).
- Mother-to-child transmission of maternal infections –
  - Hepatitis C virus – for women co-infected with hepatitis C virus and HIV, PCS reduces mother-to-child transmission of both hepatitis C virus and HIV.
  - HIV – consider either a vaginal birth or a CS for women on antiretroviral treatment (ART) with a viral load of 50–400 copies per ml because there is insufficient evidence that a CS prevents mother-to-child transmission of HIV. Offer CS to women with HIV who are not receiving any ART or are receiving ART with a viral load of ≥400 copies per ml.
  - Herpes simplex virus (HSV) – for women with primary genital HSV infection in the third trimester, offer PCS because it decreases the risk of neonatal HSV infection.

Not indicated

- Multiple pregnancy – in otherwise uncomplicated twin pregnancies at term where the presentation of the first twin is cephalic, PNM and morbidity are increased for the second twin. However, the effect of PCS in improving outcome for the second twin remains uncertain.
- Preterm birth – do not offer CS routinely.
- SGA – the risk of neonatal morbidity and mortality is higher with 'SGA' babies. However, the effect of PCS in improving these outcomes remains uncertain.
- Predicting CS for cephalopelvic disproportion in labour – pelvimetry, shoe size, maternal height, and estimations of fetal size (USS or clinical examination) do not accurately predict cephalopelvic disproportion and are not useful in predicting 'failure to progress' in labour.
- Mother-to-child transmission of maternal infections –
  - Hepatitis B and C viruses – insufficient evidence that this reduces mother-to-child transmission.
  - Recurrent herpes simplex virus at birth.
  - HIV – do not offer a CS to women on HAART with a viral load of < 400 copies per ml or women on any ART with a viral load of < 50 copies per ml. The risk of HIV transmission is the same for a CS and a vaginal birth.
  - BMI – do not use a BMI of > 50 alone as an indication for PCS.

231

CHAPTER 47 Caesarean section (CS)

Maternal request for CS – needs discussion

- Explore, discuss, and record the specific reasons for the request; discuss the overall risks and benefits of CS compared with vaginal birth; include a discussion with other members of the obstetric team if necessary to explore the reasons for the request; and ensure the woman has accurate information.
- When a woman requests a CS because she has anxiety about childbirth, refer to a HCP with expertise in providing perinatal mental health support to help her address her anxiety in a supportive manner.
- If after discussion and offer of support a vaginal birth is still not an acceptable, offer a PCS.

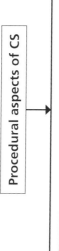

Procedural aspects of CS

Timing of PCS – the risk of respiratory morbidity is increased in babies born by CS before labour, but this risk decreases significantly after 39 weeks. Therefore do not offer PCS routinely before 39 weeks.

Preoperative testing and preparation for CS

- Haemoglobin assessment to identify those who have anaemia.
- Pregnant women having CS for APH, abruption, uterine rupture, and placenta praevia are at increased risk of blood loss of > 1000 ml, therefore carry out CS at a maternity unit with on-site blood transfusion services.
- Pregnant women who are healthy with uncomplicated pregnancies – do not routinely offer:
  * Grouping and saving of serum.
  * Cross-matching of blood.
  * A clotting screen.
  * Preoperative USS for localization of the placenta, because this does not improve CS morbidity outcomes.

Classification of urgency

- **Category 1** – when there is immediate threat to the life of the woman or fetus.
- **Category 2** – when there is maternal or fetal compromise which is not immediately life-threatening.
- **Category 3** – No maternal or fetal compromise but needs early delivery. Delivery timed to suit woman or staff.
- **Decision-to-delivery interval for unplanned CS:**
  * Perform category 1 and 2 CS – ASAP after making the decision.
  * Perform category 1 CS within 30 minutes.
  * Perform category 2 CS in most situations within 75 minutes of making the decision.

Anaesthesia and other issues

- **Offer –**
  * Antacids and drugs to reduce gastric volumes and acidity before CS, to reduce the risk of aspiration pneumonitis.
  * Antiemetics to reduce nausea and vomiting during CS.
  * IV ephedrine or phenylephrine, and volume pre-loading with crystalloid or colloid to reduce the risk of hypotension during CS.
  * Prophylactic antibiotics before skin incision – this reduces the risk of maternal infection more than prophylactic antibiotics given after skin incision, and no effect on the baby has been demonstrated. Choose antibiotics effective against endometritis, and urinary tract and wound infections. Do not use co-amoxiclav for prophylaxis.
  * Thromboprophylaxis to reduce the risk of DVT.
- Test umbilical artery pH after all CS for suspected fetal compromise, to allow review of fetal wellbeing and guide ongoing care of the baby.
- Methods to prevent HIV transmission in theatre – wear double gloves and follow general recommendations for safe surgical practice.

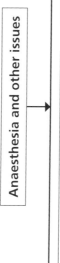

- **Regional anaesthesia** – offer regional anaesthesia because it is safer and results in less maternal and neonatal morbidity than GA (including women with placenta praevia).
  * Leave an indwelling urinary catheter to prevent over-distension of the bladder because the anaesthetic block interferes with normal bladder function.
- **General anaesthesia (GA):**
  * For unplanned CS – preoxygenation, cricoid pressure, and rapid sequence induction to reduce the risk of aspiration.
  * Practice training drill for failed intubation during obstetric anaesthesia.
- IV ephedrine/phenylephrine to manage hypotension during CS.
- Operating table to have a lateral tilt of 15°, since this reduces maternal hypotension.
- Provide post-CS analgesia.

Surgical techniques

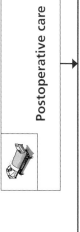

- Transverse abdominal incision – less postoperative pain and an improved cosmetic effect compared with a midline incision.
- The transverse incision of choice – the Joel Cohen incision (a straight skin incision, 3 cm above the symphysis pubis; subsequent tissue layers are opened bluntly and, if necessary, extended with scissors and not a knife) – shorter operating times and reduced postoperative febrile morbidity.
- The use of separate surgical knives to incise the skin and the deeper tissues at CS is not necessary because it does not decrease wound infection.
- When there is a well-formed lower uterine segment, blunt rather than sharp extension of the uterine incision reduces blood loss, incidence of PPH, and the need for transfusion at CS.
- Use forceps only if there is difficulty delivering the baby's head. The effect on neonatal morbidity of the routine use of forceps at CS remains uncertain.
- Oxytocin 5 IU by slow IV injection to encourage contraction of the uterus and to decrease PPH.
- Remove placenta using controlled cord traction and not manual removal as this reduces the risk of endometritis.

- Perform intraperitoneal repair of the uterus. Exteriorization of the uterus is associated with more pain and does not improve operative outcomes such as haemorrhage and infection.
- The effectiveness and safety of single layer closure of the uterine incision is uncertain. Suture the uterine incision in two layers.
- Do not suture the visceral or the parietal peritoneum because this reduces operating time and the need for postoperative analgesia, and improves maternal satisfaction.
- If a midline abdominal incision is used – use mass closure with slowly absorbable continuous sutures because this results in fewer incisional hernias and less dehiscence than layered closure.
- Do not routinely close the subcutaneous tissue space, unless the woman has > 2 cm subcutaneous fat, because it does not reduce the incidence of wound infection.
- Do not use superficial wound drains because they do not decrease the incidence of wound infection or wound haematoma.
- The effects of different suture materials or methods of skin closure at CS are not certain.

Postoperative care

Care of the woman

- Observe on a one-to-one basis until women have regained airway control, cardiorespiratory stability, and are able to communicate. After recovery continue observations every half hour for 2 hours, and hourly thereafter provided that the observations are stable or satisfactory.
- Women who have had intrathecal opioids – minimum hourly observation of respiratory rate, sedation, and pain scores for at least 12 hours for diamorphine and 24 hours for morphine.
- Women who have had epidural opioids or patient-controlled analgesia with opioids – routine hourly monitoring of respiratory rate, sedation, and pain scores throughout treatment and for at least 2 hours after discontinuation of treatment.
- Offer diamorphine (intrathecally) for intra- and postoperative analgesia because it reduces the need for supplemental analgesia after a CS. Epidural diamorphine (2.5–5 mg) is an alternative.
- Offer patient-controlled analgesia using opioid analgesics because it improves pain relief.
- Provided there is no contraindication, offer NSAIDs as an adjunct to other analgesics, because they reduce the need for opioids.
- Women can eat and drink when they feel hungry or thirsty.
- Remove urinary catheter once woman is mobile after a regional anaesthetic and not sooner than 12 hours after the last epidural 'top up' dose.
- Do not offer routine respiratory physiotherapy after a CS under general anaesthesia, because it does not improve respiratory outcomes such as coughing, phlegm, body temperature, chest palpation, and auscultatory changes.
- Length of hospital stay – offer early discharge to women who are recovering well, are apyrexial, and do not have complications (after 24 hours), and follow-up at home, because this is not associated with more infant or maternal readmissions.

Care of the baby

- An appropriately trained practitioner skilled in the resuscitation of the newborn should be present at CS performed under GA or where there is evidence of fetal compromise.
- Babies born by CS are more likely to have a lower temperature; ensure thermal care of the newborn baby.
- Encourage early skin-to-skin contact between the woman and her baby because it improves maternal perceptions of the infant, mothering skills, maternal behaviour, and breastfeeding outcomes, and reduces infant crying.
- Offer additional support to help them to start breastfeeding ASAP after the birth of their baby. This is because women who have had a CS are less likely to start breastfeeding in the first few hours after the birth, but, when breastfeeding is established, they are as likely to continue as women who have a vaginal birth.

Follow-up

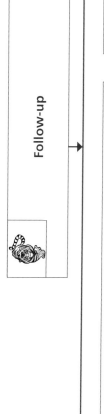

Recovery following CS

- Regular analgesia for postoperative pain:
  * Severe pain – co-codamol with added ibuprofen.
  * Moderate pain – co-codamol.
  * Mild pain – paracetamol.
- CS wound care: remove the dressing 24 hours after the CS; monitor for fever; assess the wound for signs of infection (increasing pain, redness or discharge), separation or dehiscence; clean and dry the wound daily; remove sutures or clips.
- Women who have urinary symptoms – consider the possible diagnosis of:
  * UTI.
  * Stress incontinence (about 4% of women).
  * Urinary tract injury (1 per 1000 CS).
- Women who have heavy and/or irregular vaginal bleeding – this is more likely to be due to endometritis than retained products of conception.
- Women are at increased risk of VTE – pay attention to women who have chest symptoms (such as cough or shortness of breath) or leg symptoms (such as painful swollen calf).
- Women can resume activities such as driving a vehicle, formal exercise, and sexual intercourse once they have fully recovered from the CS.
- After a CS the women are not at increased risk of difficulties with breastfeeding, depression, post-traumatic stress symptoms, dyspareunia, or faecal incontinence.

Pregnancy and childbirth after CS

- When advising about the mode of birth after a previous CS consider:
  * Maternal preferences and priorities.
  * The risks and benefits of repeat CS.
  * The risks and benefits of VBAC, including the risk of unplanned CS.
- Women who have had up to and including 4 CS – the risk of fever, bladder injuries, and surgical injuries does not vary with planned mode of birth. The risk of uterine rupture, although higher for planned vaginal birth, is rare.
- Offer women planning a VBAC:
  * Electronic fetal monitoring during labour.
  * Immediate access to CS and on-site blood transfusion services.
  * IOL – monitor closely because they are at increased risk of uterine rupture.
- Pregnant women with both previous CS and a previous vaginal birth are more likely to achieve a vaginal birth than women who have had a previous CS but no previous vaginal birth.

What not to do

- PCS routinely before 39 weeks.
- Pregnant women who are healthy with uncomplicated pregnancies – * Serum group and screen. * Blood cross-match. * Clotting screen. * Preoperative USS for localization of the placenta.
- Co-amoxiclav for antibiotic prophylaxis.
- Single layer closure of the uterine incision.
- Suturing of the visceral or the parietal peritoneum.
- Routine closure of the subcutaneous tissue space.
- Superficial wound drains.
- Routine respiratory physiotherapy.

Consent – caesarean section

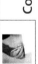

Discuss

- Explain the procedure.
- **Intended benefits** – to secure the safest and/or quickest route of delivery in the circumstances present at the time the decision is made, where the anticipated risks to mother and/or baby of an alternative mode of delivery outweigh those of CS.
- **Procedure, the benefits and risks of any available alternative treatments, including no treatment** –
  - If either a midline abdominal incision or a classical uterine incision is being considered, inform the woman along with the reasons and the added risks.
  - Forceps may be used to deliver the head, especially with breech presentations.
  - Discuss the reason for the CS and the risks to mother and/or baby of not performing the CS.
  - An informed, competent pregnant woman may choose the no-treatment option; that is, she may refuse CS, even when this would be detrimental to her own health or the wellbeing of her fetus.
- Other procedures, which may be appropriate but not essential at the time, such as ovarian cystectomy/oophorectomy – discuss and record woman's wishes.
- Plan form of anaesthesia.

Extra procedures

- Any extra procedures which may become necessary:
  - * Hysterectomy.
  - * Blood transfusion.
  - * Repair of damage to bowel, bladder or blood vessels.
- If any other procedures are anticipated, these must be discussed and a separate consent obtained. A decision for sterilization should not be made while the woman is in labour or immediately prior to the procedure. An additional specific consent form should be used for sterilization at CS.

Complications from Emergency CS are greater than elective CS (24/100 compared with 16/100 women). Complication rates are higher at 9–10 cm dilatation when compared with 0–1 cm (33/100 compared with 17/100 women).

Serious risks:

Maternal –

- Emergency hysterectomy – 7–8/1000 women.
- Need for further surgery at a later date, including curettage – 5/1000.
- Admission to ICU (highly dependent on reason for CS) – 9/1000.
- VTE – 4–16/10000.
- Bladder injury – 1/1000.
- Ureteric injury – 3/10000.
- Death – approximately 1/12000.

Future pregnancies –

- Uterine rupture during subsequent pregnancies/deliveries – 2–7/1000.
- Antepartum stillbirth – 1–4/1000.
- Placenta praevia and placenta accreta – 4–8/1000.

Frequent risks:

Maternal –

- Persistent wound and abdominal discomfort in the first few months after surgery – 9/100.
- Repeat CS with attempted VBAC – 1 in 4.
- Readmission to hospital – 5/100.
- Haemorrhage (>1000 ml) – 4–8/100.
- Infection (endometritis, UTI, wound) – 6–8/100.
- Stress incontinence – 4/100.

Fetal –

- Lacerations – 1–2/100 babies.
- Length of hospital stay is likely to be longer after a CS (average 3–4 days) than after a vaginal birth (average 1–2 days).
- Surgical and anaesthetic risks are increased with obesity and in those who have significant pathology, who have had previous surgery or who have pre-existing medical conditions.

Risks	
Very common	1/1 to 1/10
Common	1/10 to 1/100
Uncommon	1/100 to 1/1000
Rare	1/1000 to 1/10000
Very rare	Less than 1/10000

Caesarean section. NICE Clinical Guideline 132; November 2011.
Caesarean section. RCOG Consent Advice No. 7; October 2009.

CHAPTER 48 Induction of labour (IOL)

Prevalence and background

- IOL is required when the outcome of the pregnancy will be better if it is artificially interrupted rather than being left to follow its natural course.
- 1 in 5 deliveries in the UK are induced.
- IOL using pharmacological methods – about two-thirds of women give birth without further intervention, 15% with instrumental births, and 22% with emergency CS.
- Induced labour may be less efficient and more painful than spontaneous labour, and epidural analgesia and assisted delivery are more likely to be required.

Information and decision making

- Most women go into labour spontaneously by 42 weeks.
- Membrane sweeping makes spontaneous labour more likely, and reduces the need for IOL to prevent prolonged pregnancy; discomfort and vaginal bleeding are possible from the procedure.
- Options – * IOL between 41+0 and 42+0 weeks; and * expectant management.
- Explain the following to women being offered IOL:
  * The reasons for induction.
  * When, where, and how induction could be carried out.
  * Pain relief.
  * The alternative options if the woman chooses not to have IOL.
  * The risks and benefits of IOL in specific circumstances and the proposed induction methods.
  * That induction may not be successful and what the woman's options would be.

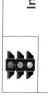

Indications

Prolonged pregnancy

- Offer women with uncomplicated pregnancies IOL between 41+0 and 42+0 weeks to avoid the risks of prolonged pregnancy.
- From 42 weeks, women who decline IOL – offer increased antenatal monitoring consisting of at least twice-weekly CTG and USS estimation of maximum amniotic pool depth.

Preterm PROM

- Do not offer IOL before 34 weeks unless there are additional obstetric indications (infection or fetal compromise).
- PROM after 34 weeks:
  * Risks to the woman (sepsis, possible need for CS).
  * Risks to the baby (sepsis, problems relating to preterm birth).

Prelabour rupture of membranes at term

- Offer a choice of IOL or expectant management. IOL is appropriate approximately 24 hours after prelabour rupture of membranes at term.

Previous caesarean section

- Offer IOL with vaginal PGE2, CS or expectant management on an individual basis.
- Inform of the following risks with IOL:
  * Increased risk of need for emergency CS.
  * Increased risk of uterine rupture.

Intrauterine fetal death

- Offer a choice of immediate IOL or expectant management if the woman is physically well, her membranes are intact, and there is no evidence of infection or bleeding.
- Offer immediate IOL if ruptured membranes, infection or bleeding.

Others

- **Maternal request** – do not offer IOL routinely on maternal request alone. However, consider IOL under exceptional circumstances at or after 40 weeks.
- **Breech presentation** – IOL is not generally recommended. If ECV is unsuccessful, declined or contraindicated, and the woman chooses not to have an elective CS, offer IOL if delivery is indicated, after discussing the associated risks with the woman.
- **FGR** – do not offer IOL if there is severe FGR with confirmed fetal compromise.
- **History of precipitate labour** – do not routinely offer IOL to avoid an unattended birth to women with a history of precipitate labour.
- **Suspected fetal macrosomia** – in the absence of any other indications, do not offer IOL for suspected large for gestational age (macrosomic) baby.

Methods for induction of labour

Membrane sweeping

- Membrane sweeping involves the examining finger passing through the cervix to rotate against the wall of the uterus, to separate the chorionic membrane from the decidua. If the cervix will not admit a finger, massaging around the cervix in the vaginal fornices may achieve a similar effect.
- Membrane sweeping is regarded as an adjunct to IOL rather than an actual method of IOL.
- Prior to formal IOL, offer vaginal examination for membrane sweeping:
  * At 40- and 41-week antenatal visits for nulliparous women.
  * At the 41-week antenatal visit for parous women.
- Offer additional membrane sweeping if labour does not start spontaneously.

Pharmacological methods

- Vaginal PGE2 is the preferred method of IOL, unless there are specific clinical reasons for not using it (risk of uterine hyperstimulation). It can be administered as a gel, tablet or controlled-release pessary.
- The recommended regimens are:
  * One cycle of vaginal PGE2 tablets or gel: one dose, followed by a second dose after 6 hours if labour is not established (up to a maximum of two doses).
  * One cycle of vaginal PGE2 controlled-release pessary: one dose over 24 hours.
  * Risk of uterine hyperstimulation.
  * Offer misoprostol as a method of IOL to women who have IUFD or only in the context of a clinical trial.

Amniotomy

- Do not use amniotomy, alone or with oxytocin, as a primary method of induction unless there are specific reasons for not using PGE2. Avoid if baby's head is high.
- To avoid cord prolapse:
  * Assess engagement of presenting part before induction.
  * Palpate for umbilical cord presentation during preliminary vaginal examination (avoid dislodging baby's head).

Methods not recommended for IOL

- **Pharmacological methods** – oral PGE2, IV PGE2, extra-amniotic PGE2, intracervical PGE2, IV oxytocin alone, hyaluronidase, corticosteroids, oestrogen, vaginal nitric oxide donors.
- **Non-pharmacological methods** – herbal supplements, acupuncture, homeopathy, castor oil, hot baths, enemas, sexual intercourse.
- **Mechanical methods** – mechanical procedures (balloon catheters and laminaria tents).

Bishop score

It is based on the station, dilation, effacement (or length), position, and consistency of the cervix. A score of eight or more indicates that the cervix is ripe, or 'favourable' with a high chance of spontaneous labour, or response to IOL.

Monitoring and pain relief

Monitoring

- Assess Bishop score and confirm a normal FHR pattern with EFM before IOL.
- After administration of vaginal PGE2, when contractions begin, assess fetal wellbeing with continuous EFM. Once the CTG is confirmed as normal, use intermittent auscultation unless there are clear indications for continuous EFM.
- Reassess Bishop score 6 hours after vaginal PGE2 tablet/gel administration or 24 hours after vaginal PGE2 controlled-release pessary insertion, to monitor progress.

Setting and timing

- Outpatient setting – carry out IOL only if safety and support procedures are in place. Audit the practice of IOL in an outpatient setting continuously.
- Inpatient setting – carry out IOL using vaginal PGE2 in the morning because of higher maternal satisfaction.

Pain relief

- IOL is likely to be more painful than spontaneous labour.
- Provide appropriate pain relief – range from simple analgesics to epidural analgesia.
- Encourage women to use their own coping strategies for pain relief.
- Labour in water is recommended for pain relief.

Prevention and management of complications

Failed induction

- Labour not starting after one cycle of treatment for IOL. Reassess the woman's condition and the pregnancy in general and fetal wellbeing using EFM.
- The subsequent management options include:
    * A further attempt to induce labour (the timing depends on the clinical situation and the woman's wishes).
        * CS.

Cord prolapse

- To reduce the likelihood of cord prolapse, which may occur at the time of amniotomy, undertake the following precautions:
    * Before induction, assess engagement of the presenting part. Avoid amniotomy if the baby's head is high.
    * Palpate for umbilical cord presentation during the preliminary vaginal examination and avoid dislodging the baby's head.
    * Check for any signs of a low-lying placental site before membrane sweeping and IOL.

Others

- **Uterine hyperstimulation** – consider tocolysis.
- **Uterine rupture** – deliver the baby by emergency CS.

What not to do

- IOL before 34 weeks in absence of any additional obstetric indications.
- IOL for maternal request.
- IOL for breech presentation.
- IOL for fetal growth restriction with confirmed fetal compromise.
- IOL for history of precipitate labour.
- IOL for suspected fetal macrosomia.
- Amniotomy, alone or with oxytocin, as a primary method of IOL.

Induction of Labour. Clinical Guideline; NICE CGN 70; July 2008.

Prevalence and background

- About 600 000 women give birth in England and Wales each year.
- About 40% are nulliparous and almost 90% of women have singleton delivery after 37 weeks of pregnancy with cephalic presentation.
- About two-thirds go into labour spontaneously.
- Care during labour has physical and emotional impact in the short and longer term.

General care throughout labour

- Mobilization – encourage and help women to mobilize and adopt whatever positions they find most comfortable throughout labour.
- Provide one-to-one care; encourage support by birth partner(s) of their choice.
- Do not give routine H2-receptor antagonists or antacids to low-risk women. Consider these for women who receive opioids or who have or develop risk factors that make a GA more likely.
- Women may drink during established labour; isotonic drinks may be more beneficial than water.
- Women may eat a light diet in established labour unless they have received opioids or they develop risk factors that make a GA more likely.

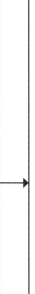

Planning place of birth – birth at home, in a midwife-led unit (MLU) or in an obstetric unit.

Determined by risk factors in the index pregnancy or medical history.

Medical conditions indicating increased risk suggesting birth at an obstetric unit

Cardiovascular	* Confirmed cardiac disease
	* Hypertensive disorders
Respiratory	* Asthma requiring an increase in treatment or hospital treatment
	* Cystic fibrosis
Haematological	* Haemoglobinopathies – sickle-cell disease, β-thalassaemia major
	* History of thromboembolic disorders
	* Immune thrombocytopenia purpura or other platelet disorder or platelet count below 100×10^9/l
	* von Willebrand's disease
	* Bleeding disorder in the woman or unborn baby
	* Atypical antibodies which carry a risk of HDN
Infective	* Risk factors associated with GBS
	* Hepatitis B/C with abnormal liver function tests, HIV
	* Toxoplasmosis – women receiving treatment
	* Current active infection of chickenpox/rubella/genital herpes in the woman or baby
	* Tuberculosis under treatment
Immune	* Systemic lupus erythematosus; scleroderma
Endocrine	* Hyperthyroidism, diabetes
Renal	* Abnormal renal function, renal disease requiring supervision by a renal specialist
Neurological	* Epilepsy; myasthenia gravis, previous cerebrovascular accident
Gastrointestinal	* Liver disease associated with current abnormal liver function tests
Psychiatric	* Psychiatric disorder requiring current inpatient care

Other factors indicating increased risk suggesting birth at an obstetric unit

Previous complications	* Unexplained stillbirth/neonatal death or previous death related to intrapartum difficulty
	* Previous baby with neonatal encephalopathy
	* Pre-eclampsia requiring preterm birth; eclampsia
	* Placental abruption with adverse outcome
	* Uterine rupture
	* Primary PPH requiring additional treatment or blood transfusion
	* Retained placenta requiring manual removal in theatre
	* Caesarean section; shoulder dystocia
Current pregnancy	* Multiple birth * Placenta praevia; placental abruption
	* PET or PIH * PTL or PPROM
	* Anaemia – haemoglobin < 85 g/l at onset of labour
	* IUD * IOL * Malpresentation – breech or transverse lie
	* Substance misuse * Alcohol dependency requiring treatment
	* GDM * BMI at booking of > 35 kg/m²
	* Recurrent APH
Fetal indications	* SGA (< 5th centile or reduced growth velocity on USS)
	* Abnormal fetal heart rate (FHR)/Doppler studies
	* Ultrasound diagnosis of oligo-/polyhydramnios
Previous gynaecological history	* Myomectomy. * Hysterotomy.

Indications for individual assessment

Medical conditions indicating individual assessment when planning place of birth

Cardiovascular	*	Cardiac disease without intrapartum implications
Haematological	*	Atypical antibodies not putting the baby at risk of HDN
	*	Sickle-cell trait
	*	Thalassaemia trait
	*	Anaemia – haemoglobin 8.5–10.5 g/dl at onset of labour
Infective	*	Hepatitis B/C with normal liver function tests
Immune	*	Non-specific connective tissue disorders
Endocrine	*	Unstable hypothyroidism such that a change in treatment is required
Skeletal/neurological	*	Spinal abnormalities
	*	Previous fractured pelvis
	*	Neurological deficits
Gastrointestinal	*	Liver disease without current abnormal liver function
	*	Crohn's disease
	*	Ulcerative colitis

Other factors indicating individual assessment when planning place of birth

Previous complications	*	Stillbirth/neonatal death with a known non-recurrent cause
	*	Pre-eclampsia developing at term
	*	Placental abruption with good outcome
	*	History of previous baby > 4.5 kg
	*	Extensive vaginal, cervical, or third- or fourth-degree perineal trauma
	*	Previous term baby with jaundice requiring exchange transfusion
	*	Antepartum bleeding of unknown origin (single episode >24 weeks)
Current pregnancy	*	BMI at booking of 30–34 kg/m^2
	*	BP of 140 mmHg systolic or 90 mmHg diastolic on two occasions
	*	Clinical or ultrasound suspicion of macrosomia
	*	Para 6 or more, age over 40 at booking
	*	Recreational drug use, under current outpatient psychiatric care
Fetal indications	*	Fetal abnormality
Previous gynaecological history	*	Major gynaecological surgery, fibroids
	*	Cone biopsy or large loop excision of the transformation zone

- In women who plan to give birth at home or in a MLU there is a higher likelihood of a normal birth, with less intervention. If something does go unexpectedly seriously wrong during labour at home or in a MLU, the outcome for the woman and baby could be worse than if they were in the obstetric unit with access to specialized care.
- If a woman has a pre-existing medical condition or has had a previous complicated birth that makes her at higher risk of developing complications during her next birth, advise to give birth in an obstetric unit.

Indications for intrapartum transfer

- Indications for EFM including abnormalities of the FHR on intermittent auscultation.
- Significant meconium-stained liquor.
- Malpresentation or breech presentation diagnosed for the first time at the onset of labour.
- Uncertainty about the presence of a fetal heartbeat.
- Maternal request for epidural pain relief.
- Delay in the first or second stages of labour.
- Obstetric emergency – APH, cord presentation/prolapse, PPH, maternal collapse or a need for advanced neonatal resuscitation.
- Retained placenta.
- Maternal pyrexia in labour (38.0°C once or 37.5°C on two occasions 2 hours apart).
- Either raised DBP (> 90 mmHg) or raised SBP (> 140 mmHg) on two consecutive readings taken 30 minutes apart.
- Third- or fourth-degree tear or other complicated perineal trauma requiring suturing.

Coping with pain in labour

| Non-epidural | Regional analgesia |

Pain-relieving strategies

- Breathing and relaxation techniques, massage techniques.
- Offer labour in water for pain relief. Monitor the temperature of the woman and the water hourly to ensure that the woman is comfortable and not becoming pyrexial.
- The use of injected water papules is not recommended.
- Do not offer acupuncture, acupressure, and hypnosis but women may wish to use these techniques.
- Support playing of music of the woman's choice.
- Do not offer transcutaneous electrical nerve stimulation (TENS) to women in established labour.

Pharmacological

Inhalational analgesia
- Entonox (a 50:50 mixture of oxygen and nitrous oxide) may reduce pain in labour, but it may make women feel nauseous and light-headed.

Intravenous and intramuscular opioids
- Pethidine, diamorphine or other opioids provide limited pain relief and may have significant side effects for both the woman (drowsiness, nausea, and vomiting) and baby (short-term respiratory depression and drowsiness) which may last several days.
- Pethidine, diamorphine or other opioids may interfere with breastfeeding.
- If an IV or IM opioid is used, administer with an antiemetic.

The risks and benefits

- Regional analgesia provides more effective pain relief than opioids.
- It is associated with a longer second stage of labour and an increased chance of vaginal instrumental birth.
- It is not associated with long-term backache.
- It is not associated with a longer first stage of labour or an increased chance of CS.
- It will be accompanied by a more intensive level of monitoring and IV access.
- Modern epidural solutions contain opioids and, whatever the route of administration, all opioids cross the placenta and in larger doses (> 100 μg in total) may cause short-term respiratory depression in the baby and make the baby drowsy.

Care and observations

- Do not deny women who request regional analgesia in labour. This includes women in the latent first stage of labour.
- Preloading and maintenance fluid infusion need not be administered routinely before establishing low-dose epidural analgesia and combined spinal–epidural analgesia.
- During establishment of regional analgesia or after further boluses (10 ml or more of low-dose solutions) measure BP every 5 minutes for 15 minutes.
- If the woman is not pain-free 30 minutes after each administration of local anaesthetic/opioid solution, recall the anaesthetist.
- Hourly assessment of the level of the sensory block.
- Continue regional analgesia until after completion of the third stage of labour and any necessary perineal repair.
- Upon confirmation of full cervical dilatation, unless the woman has an urge to push or the baby's head is visible, delay pushing for at least 1 hour and longer if the woman wishes.
- Following the diagnosis of full dilatation, ensure that birth will have occurred within 4 hours regardless of parity.
- Oxytocin should not be used as a matter of routine in the second stage of labour.
- Continuous EFM for at least 30 minutes during establishment and after administration of each further bolus.

Establishing and maintaining

- Either epidural or combined spinal–epidural analgesia.
- If rapid analgesia is required – combined spinal–epidural analgesia with bupivacaine and fentanyl.
- Epidural analgesia – a low-concentration local anaesthetic and opioid solution (10–15 ml of 0.0625–0.1% bupivacaine with 1–2 μg per ml fentanyl).
- Maintainance of epidural analgesia – low-concentration local anaesthetic and opioid solutions (0.0625–0.1% bupivacaine or equivalent combined with 2.0 μg per ml fentanyl).
- Either patient-controlled epidural analgesia or intermittent boluses are the preferred modes of administration for maintenance of epidural analgesia.

Normal labour: first stage

Definition of the first stage

- **Latent first stage of labour** – a period of time, not necessarily continuous, when there are painful contractions, and there is some cervical change, including cervical effacement and dilatation up to 4 cm.
- **Established first stage of labour** – when there are regular painful contractions, and there is progressive cervical dilatation from 4 cm.
- **Duration of the first stage** – while the length of established first stage of labour varies between women, first labours last on average 8 hours and are unlikely to last over 18 hours. Second and subsequent labours last on average 5 hours and are unlikely to last over 12 hours.
- **Delay in the established first stage** – consider all aspects of labour:
  * Cervical dilatation of < 2 cm in 4 hours for first labours.
  * Cervical dilatation of < 2 cm in 4 hours or a slowing in the progress of labour for second or subsequent labours.
  * Descent and rotation of the fetal head.
  * Changes in the strength, duration, and frequency of uterine contractions.

The initial assessment of a woman:

- Take a history; review her clinical records.
- Temperature, pulse, BP, urinalysis.
- Length, strength, and frequency of contractions.
- Abdominal palpation – fundal height, lie, presentation, position, and station.
- Assess woman's pain.
- Vaginal loss – show, liquor, blood.
- FHR – for a minimum of 1 minute immediately after a contraction.
- Offer a vaginal examination.
- Women who seek advice or attend hospital with painful contractions but who are not in established labour – offer individualized support, occasionally analgesia, and encourage to remain at or return home.
- Do not offer admission CTG in low-risk pregnancy.

Observations during the established first stage

- Use partogram once labour is established with a 4-hour action line.
- **Observations include:**
  * 4-hourly temperature and BP; hourly pulse.
  * Half-hourly – frequency of contractions.
  * Frequency of emptying the bladder.
  * Vaginal examination 4-hourly, or where there is concern about progress.
  * Intermittent auscultation of the FHR after a contraction for at least 1 minute, at least every 15 minutes, and record the rate as an average.

FHR assessment and reasons for transfer to continuous EFM

- Intermittent auscultation of FHR for low-risk women in established labour.
- Once in established labour – intermittent auscultation of the fetal heart after a contraction.
- **Change from intermittent auscultation to continuous EFM in low-risk women if:**
  * Significant meconium-stained liquor; consider for light meconium-stained liquor.
  * Abnormal FHR on intermittent auscultation (< 110 bpm; > 160 bpm; any decelerations after a contraction).
  * Maternal pyrexia (38.0°C once or 37.5°C on 2 occasions 2 hours apart).
  * Fresh bleeding in labour, oxytocin use for augmentation, the woman's request.

Possible routine interventions in the first stage

- Do not routinely offer active management of labour (one-to-one continuous support, strict definition of established labour, early routine amniotomy, routine 2-hourly vaginal examination, oxytocin if labour becomes slow).
- In normally progressing labour, do not perform amniotomy routinely.
- Do not use combined early amniotomy with use of oxytocin routinely.

Complicated labour: first stage

Perceived delay in the established first stage

- Consider: parity; cervical dilatation and rate of change; uterine contractions; station and position of presenting part.
- Consider amniotomy if intact membranes, as it will shorten labour by about an hour and may increase the strength of contractions.
- Perform a vaginal examination 2 hours later and if progress is < 1 cm make a diagnosis of delay.
- Amniotomy alone for suspected delay is not an indication to commence continuous EFM.

Confirmed delay in established first stage of labour

- Nulliparous women – consider oxytocin. Use of oxytocin following spontaneous or artificial rupture of the membranes will bring forward time of birth but will not influence the mode of birth or other outcomes.
- Multiparous women – full assessment before making a decision about the use of oxytocin.
- **Oxytocin and further assessment** – oxytocin will increase the frequency and strength of the contractions.
  * Offer epidural before oxytocin is started.
  * Where oxytocin is used, the time between increments of the dose should be no more frequent than every 30 min. Increase oxytocin until there are 4–5 contractions in 10 min.
  * Perform vaginal examination 4 hours after commencing oxytocin in established labour. If there is < 2 cm progress after 4 hours of oxytocin, consider CS.

Normal labour: second stage

Definition of the second stage

- **Passive second stage of labour:** finding of full dilatation of the cervix prior to or in the absence of involuntary expulsive contractions.
- **Onset of the active second stage of labour:** the baby is visible; expulsive contractions with full dilatation of the cervix or other signs of full dilatation of the cervix; active maternal effort following confirmation of full dilatation of the cervix in the absence of expulsive contractions.
- **Duration and definition of delay in the second stage**
  - *Nulliparous women:*
    > Birth is expected to take place within 3 hours of the start of the active second stage in most women.
    > Delay in the active second stage – when it has lasted 2 hours. Undertake an operative vaginal birth if birth is not imminent.
  - *Parous women:*
    > Birth is expected to take place within 2 hours of the start of the active second stage in most women.
    > Delay in the active second stage – when it has lasted 1 hour. Undertake an operative vaginal birth if birth is not imminent.
- If full dilatation of the cervix has been diagnosed in a woman without epidural analgesia, but she does not get an urge to push, assess further after 1 hour.
- **Oxytocin in the second stage** – consider oxytocin for nulliparous women if contractions are inadequate at the onset of the second stage.

- **Observations:**
  - ☆ Hourly BP and pulse.
  - ☆ 4-hourly temperature.
  - ☆ Vaginal examination – hourly in the active second stage.
  - ☆ Half-hourly frequency of contractions.
  - ☆ Frequency of emptying the bladder.
  - ☆ Assessment of progress – maternal behaviour, effectiveness of pushing, and fetal wellbeing in relation to fetal position and station at the onset of the second stage.
- **Intermittent auscultation of FHR** – after a contraction for at least 1 minute, at least every 5 minutes.
- **Women's position and pushing in the second stage** Discourage women from lying supine or semi-supine and encourage to adopt any other position that they find most comfortable. Guide women by their own urge to push. If pushing is ineffective or if requested by the woman, assist birth by changing position, emptying the bladder, and encouragement.
- **Water birth** – there is insufficient evidence to either support or discourage giving birth in water.

Intrapartum interventions to reduce perineal trauma

- **Do not offer perineal massage.**
- Either the 'hands on' (guarding the perineum and flexing the baby's head) or the 'hands poised' (with hands off the perineum and baby's head but in readiness) technique can be used to facilitate spontaneous birth.
- Do not use lignocaine spray to reduce pain.
- **Do not perform a routine episiotomy** during spontaneous vaginal birth. Where an episiotomy is performed, the recommended technique is a mediolateral episiotomy originating at the vaginal fourchette and directed to the right side. The angle to the vertical axis should be between 45 and 60 degrees.
- **Perform an episiotomy** if there is a clinical need such as instrumental birth or suspected fetal compromise. Provide effective analgesia prior to episiotomy, except in an emergency due to acute fetal compromise.
- **Women with a history of severe perineal trauma** – inform that the risk of repeat severe perineal trauma is not increased in a subsequent birth, compared with women having their first baby. Do not offer episiotomy routinely following previous 3rd/4th degree trauma.
- **Women with infibulated genital mutilation** – inform of the risks of difficulty with vaginal examination, catheterization, and application of fetal scalp electrodes; the risks of delay in the second stage and spontaneous laceration together with the need for an anterior episiotomy and the possible need for defibulation in labour.

Complicated labour: second stage

Maternal care

- Support and provide analgesia/anaesthesia.
- Nulliparous women – if after 1 hour of active second stage progress is inadequate, suspect delay. Offer amniotomy if the membranes are intact.
- Women with confirmed delay in the second stage – assess but do not commence oxytocin; with ongoing obstetric review every 15–30 minutes.
- Consider instrumental birth if there is concern about fetal wellbeing, or for prolonged second stage.
- If a woman declines anaesthesia, use a pudendal block combined with local anaesthetic to the perineum.
- CS if vaginal birth is not possible.

Immediate care of newborn

- Initiate basic resuscitation of newborn babies with air.
- Oxygen for babies who do not respond once adequate ventilation has been established.

243

CHAPTER 49 Intrapartum care

Normal labour: third stage

Definition of the third stage

- The time from the birth of the baby to the expulsion of the placenta and membranes.
- **Active management** of the third stage involves:
  - Routine use of uterotonic drugs.
  - Early clamping and cutting of the cord.
  - Controlled cord traction.
- **Physiological management** of the third stage involves:
  - No routine use of uterotonic drugs.
  - No clamping of the cord until pulsation has ceased.
  - Delivery of the placenta by maternal effort.
- **Prolonged third stage** – if not completed within 30 minutes of the birth of the baby with active management and 60 minutes with physiological management.

Observations

- General physical condition.
- Vaginal blood loss.
- In the presence of haemorrhage, retained placenta or maternal collapse, frequent observations to assess the need for resuscitation.

Physiological and active management of the third stage

- Offer active management of the third stage as it reduces the risk of maternal haemorrhage and shortens the third stage.
- Support women at low risk of PPH who request physiological management of the third stage.
- Change from physiological management to active management of the third stage in the case of:
  * Haemorrhage.
  * Failure to deliver the placenta within 1 hour.
  * The woman's desire to artificially shorten the third stage.
- Pull the cord or palpate the uterus only after administration of oxytocin as part of active management.
- Do not use umbilical oxytocin infusion or prostaglandin routinely.

Complicated labour: third stage

Retained placenta

- IV access – do not use IV infusion of oxytocin to assist the delivery of the placenta.
- Use oxytocin injection into the umbilical vein with 20 IU of oxytocin in 20 ml of saline followed by proximal clamping of the cord.
- If the placenta is still retained 30 minutes after oxytocin injection, or sooner if there is concern about the woman's condition, assess for removal of the placenta.
- Provide adequate analgesia or anaesthesia.
- Manual removal of the placenta – carry out under effective regional anaesthesia (or GA when necessary).

Risk factors for PPH. See Chapter 54 Prevention and management of postpartum haemorrhage (PPH).

Management of PPH. See Chapter 54 Prevention and management of postpartum haemorrhage (PPH).

- Immediate – call for help; uterine massage; IV fluids; uterotonics.
- Treatment combinations for PPH – repeat bolus of oxytocin (IV), ergometrine (IM, or cautiously IV), IM oxytocin with ergometrine (Syntometrine), misoprostol, oxytocin infusion (Syntocinon) or carboprost (IM).
- Additional therapeutic options – tranexamic acid (IV) and rarely, in the presence of otherwise normal clotting factors, rFactor VIIa.
- No particular surgical procedure can be recommended above another for the treatment of PPH.

Repair of the perineum

- Undertake ASAP to minimize the risk of infection and blood loss.
- Effective analgesia with infiltration with up to 20 ml of 1% lignocaine or equivalent, or topping up the epidural.
- First-degree trauma – undertake suturing in order to improve healing, unless the skin edges are well opposed.
- Second-degree trauma – undertake suturing of the muscle in order to improve healing. If the skin is opposed following suturing of the muscle, there is no need to suture it.
- Where the skin does require suturing – undertake a continuous subcuticular technique.
- Use a continuous non-locked suturing technique for the vaginal wall and muscle layer.
- Use an absorbable synthetic suture material to suture the perineum.

- Offer rectal NSAIDs routinely following perineal repair of first- and second-degree trauma provided they are not contraindicated.
- Observe the following basic principles when performing perineal repairs:
  * Aseptic technique.
  * Check and count equipment, swabs, and needles before and after the procedure.
  * Ensure good lighting to see and identify the structures involved.
  * Repair difficult trauma in theatre under regional or general anaesthesia. Insert an indwelling catheter for 24 hours to prevent urinary retention.
  * Aim for a good anatomical alignment of the wound.
  * Carry out a rectal examination after completing the repair to ensure that suture material has not been accidentally inserted through the rectal mucosa.
- Inform woman of the extent of the trauma, pain relief, diet, hygiene, and the importance of pelvic-floor exercises.

Care of the baby and woman immediately after birth

Initial assessment of the newborn baby and mother–infant bonding

- Record the Apgar score at 1 and 5 minutes.
- If the baby is born in poor condition (the Apgar score at 1 minute is 5 or less) – record the time to the onset of regular respirations and double clamp the cord to allow paired cord blood gases to be taken. Continue to record Apgar scores until the baby's condition is stable.
- Encourage women to have skin-to-skin contact with their babies ASAP after the birth. Encourage initiation of breastfeeding ASAP after the birth, ideally within 1 hour.
- Keep the baby warm and dry.
- Avoid separation of a woman and her baby within the first hour of the birth for routine postnatal procedures, for example weighing, measuring, and bathing unless these are necessary for the immediate care of the baby or requested by mother.
- Record head circumference, body temperature, and birth weight.
- Perform an initial examination to detect any major physical abnormality and to identify any problems that require referral.

Observations

- Maternal observation – temperature, pulse, BP, uterine contraction, lochia.
- Examination of placenta and membranes – assessment of their condition, structure, cord vessels, and completeness
- Successful voiding of the woman's bladder.

Perineal care

If genital trauma is identified following birth:

- Offer inhalational analgesia and provide effective local or regional analgesia.
- Ensure good lighting and lithotomy to allow adequate visual assessment.
- Assess the extent of perineal trauma to include the structures involved, the apex of the injury, and bleeding.
- Perform a rectal examination to assess whether there has been any damage to the external or internal anal sphincter, if there is any suspicion that the perineal muscles are damaged.
- Document fully, possibly pictorially.

Prelabour rupture of the membranes at term (PROM)

Maternal

- Women with an uncertain history of PROM – speculum examination to confirm.
- Avoid vaginal examination in the absence of contractions.
- No need to carry out a speculum examination with a certain history of rupture of the membranes at term.
- Risk of serious neonatal infection is 1% compared with 0.5% for women with intact membranes.
- 60% of women with PROM will go into labour within 24 hours. IOL is appropriate 24 hours after PROM.
- Until the induction is commenced or if expectant management beyond 24 hours is chosen by the woman: offer lower vaginal swabs and maternal CRP to detect any infection that may be developing. Advise women to record their temperature every 4 hours and to report immediately any change in the colour or smell of their vaginal loss.
- Bathing or showering are not associated with an increase in infection, but having sexual intercourse may be.
- Assess fetal movement and heart rate at initial contact and then every 24 hours following ROM while the woman is not in labour, and advise the woman to report immediately any decrease in FMs.
- If labour has not started 24 hours after PROM – advise to give birth where there is access to neonatal services and to stay in hospital for at least 12 hours following the birth.
- If there is evidence of infection in the woman, prescribe a full course of broad-spectrum IV antibiotics.

Neonatal

- Advise women to inform if any concerns about their baby's wellbeing in the first 5 days following birth, particularly in the first 12 hours when the risk of infection is greatest.
- Do not perform blood, CSF, and/or surface cultures in an asymptomatic baby.
- Asymptomatic term babies born to women with PROM (> 24 hours before labour) – closely observe at 1 and 2 hours and then 2-hourly until 12 hours of age. These observations include: general wellbeing; chest movements and nasal flare; skin colour including perfusion, by testing capillary refill; feeding; muscle tone; temperature; heart rate and respiration.
- A baby with any symptom of possible sepsis, or born to a woman who has evidence of chorioamnionitis – immediately refer to a neonatal care specialist.

Meconium-stained liquor (MSL)

Monitoring and treatment of women

- Defined as either dark green or black amniotic fluid that is thick or tenacious, or any meconium-stained amniotic fluid containing lumps of meconium.
- Continuous EFM.
- Consider continuous EFM for women with light MSL depending on a risk assessment of stage of labour, volume of liquor, parity, and the FHR.
- Do not use amnioinfusion.

Resuscitation of babies

- If significant MSL – HCPs trained in advanced neonatal life support should be available for the birth.
- Do not carry out suctioning of the nasopharynx and oropharynx prior to birth of the shoulders and trunk.
- Suction of the upper airways only if the baby has thick or tenacious meconium present in the oropharynx.
- If the baby has depressed vital signs, undertake laryngoscopy and suction under direct vision.
- If there has been significant meconium staining and the baby is in good condition – observe closely for signs of respiratory distress at 1 and 2 hours and then 2-hourly until 12 hours of age.
- If there has been light meconium staining – observe at 1 and 2 hours and review by a neonatologist if the baby's condition causes concern at any time.

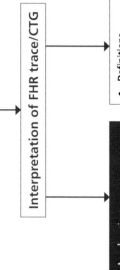

Complicated labour: electronic fetal monitoring of babies in labour – EFM

Interpretation of FHR trace/CTG

Feature	Baseline (bpm)	Variability (bpm)	Decelerations	Accelerations
Reassuring	110–160	≥ 5	None	Present
Non-reassuring	100–109 161–180	< 5 for 40–90 minutes	Typical variable decelerations with over 50% of contractions, occurring for > 90 minutes Single prolonged deceleration for up to 3 minutes	The absence of accelerations with otherwise normal trace is of uncertain significance
Abnormal	< 100 > 180 Sinusoidal pattern ≥ 10 minutes	< 5 for 90 minutes	Either atypical variable decelerations with over 50% of contractions or late decelerations, both for > 30 minutes Single prolonged deceleration for > 3 minutes	

- **Definitions**
  - ∗ Normal – FHR trace in which all four features are classified as reassuring.
  - ∗ Suspicious – FHR trace with one feature classified as non-reassuring and the remaining features classified as reassuring.
  - ∗ Pathological – FHR trace with two or more features classified as non-reassuring or one or more classified as abnormal.
- **Further information about classifying FHR traces**
  - ∗ If repeated accelerations are present with reduced variability, the FHR trace is reassuring.
  - ∗ True early uniform decelerations are rare and benign, and therefore they are not significant.
  - ∗ Most decelerations in labour are variable.
  - ∗ If a bradycardia occurs in the baby for > 3 minutes, urgent assessment and preparations to urgently expedite the birth of the baby, classified as a category 1 birth. This includes moving the woman to theatre if the fetal heart has not recovered by 9 minutes. If the fetal heart recovers within 9 minutes reconsider the decision to deliver in conjunction with the woman if reasonable.
  - ∗ A tachycardia in the baby of 160–180 bpm, where accelerations are present and no other adverse features appear, is not suspicious. However, an increase in the baseline heart rate, even within the normal range, with other non-reassuring or abnormal features should increase concern.

- Ensure accurate record-keeping
  - ∗ The date and time clocks on the EFM machine should be correctly set.
  - ∗ Traces should be labelled with the mother's name, date, and hospital number.
  - ∗ Any intrapartum events that may affect the FHR should be noted at the time on the FHR trace, which should be signed and the date and time noted (for example, vaginal examination, FBS or siting of an epidural).
  - ∗ Any member of staff who is asked to provide an opinion on a trace should note their findings on both the trace and the woman's medical records along with the date, time, and signature.
  - ∗ Following birth, the HCP should sign and note the date, time, and mode of birth on the FHR trace.
  - ∗ The FHR trace should be stored securely with the woman's medical records at the end of the monitoring process.

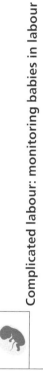

Complicated labour: monitoring babies in labour

Continuous EFM

- Systematic assessment based on the above definitions and classifications every hour.
- If woman is lying supine change to left-lateral position.
- Prolonged use of maternal facial oxygen therapy may be harmful to the baby.
- In the presence of abnormal FHR patterns and uterine hypercontractility not secondary to oxytocin infusion, consider tocolysis (SC terbutaline 0.25 mg).
- In cases of suspected or confirmed acute fetal compromise, deliver within a time appropriate for the clinical condition.
- **Continuous EFM in the presence of oxytocin:**
  * If the FHR trace is normal, continue oxytocin until 4–5 contractions every 10 minutes. Reduce oxytocin if contractions > 5 in 10 minutes.
  * If the FHR trace is suspicious, continue to increase oxytocin to achieve 4–5 contractions every 10 minutes.
  * If the FHR trace is pathological, stop oxytocin and undertake a full assessment of the fetal condition before oxytocin is recommenced.

Adjuncts to the use of continuous EFM including FBS

- Digital stimulation of the fetal scalp during a vaginal examination is an adjunct to continuous EFM.
- If fetal death is suspected despite the presence of an apparently recorded FHR, then confirm fetal viability with real-time USS.
- FBS – if a pathological FHR trace, unless there is clear evidence of acute compromise.
- Where assisted birth is contemplated because of an abnormal FHR pattern, in cases of suspected fetal acidosis undertake a FBS in the absence of technical difficulties or any contraindications.
- Where there is clear evidence of acute fetal compromise (prolonged deceleration > 3 minutes), FBS is not necessary – make urgent preparations to expedite birth.
- Take FBSs with the woman in the left-lateral position.
- **The classification of FBS results:**
  * ≥ 7.25 – normal FBS result
  * 7.21–7.24 – borderline FBS result
  * ≤ 7.20 – abnormal FBS result.
- Interpret these results taking into account the previous pH measurement, the rate of progress in labour, and the clinical features of the woman and baby.
- **Contraindications to FBS:**
  * maternal infection (for example, HIV, hepatitis viruses, and herpes simplex virus);
  * fetal bleeding disorders (for example, haemophilia);
  * prematurity (less than 34 weeks).

- Abnormal FBS result – deliver.
- Normal FBS result – repeat FBS no longer than 1 hour later if the FHR trace remains pathological, or sooner if there are further abnormalities.
- Borderline FBS result – repeat FBS no longer than 30 minutes later if the FHR trace remains pathological or sooner if there are further abnormalities.
- Consider the time taken to take a FBS when planning repeat samples.
- If the FHR trace remains unchanged and the FBS result is stable after the second test, a third/ further sample may be deferred unless additional abnormalities develop on the trace.
- Where a third FBS is considered necessary, seek consultant obstetric opinion.

What not to do

- Acupuncture, acupressure, and hypnosis for pain relief.
- Transcutaneous electrical nerve stimulation in established labour.
- Women should not enter water (a birthing pool or bath) within 2 hours of opioid administration or if they feel drowsy.
- Oxytocin routinely in the second stage of labour.
- Use of admission CTG in low-risk pregnancy.
- Routine active management of labour, amniotomy, combined early amniotomy with use of oxytocin or episiotomy.
- Routine episiotomy following previous 3rd/4th degree trauma.
- Routine umbilical oxytocin infusion or prostaglandin.

Intrapartum Care: Care of Healthy Women and Their Babies During Childbirth. NICE CGN Clinical Guideline 55; September 2007.

Background and prevalence

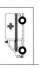

- The goal of OVD is to mimic spontaneous vaginal birth, thereby expediting delivery with a minimum of maternal or neonatal morbidity.
- OVD rates – 10–13%.

Risks or complications

- Short-term and long-term morbidity of pelvic floor injury.
- Neonatal intracranial and subgaleal haemorrhage.
- Neurodevelopmental problems for children.
- CS in the second stage of labour is an alternative approach but also carries significant morbidity and implications for future births.
- Two maternal deaths have been described in association with tearing of the cervix at vacuum delivery and a maternal death has been described following uterine rupture in association with forceps delivery.

Classification for OVD

- **Outlet** Fetal scalp visible without separating the labia
  Fetal skull has reached the pelvic floor
  Sagittal suture is in the anterio-posterior diameter or right or left occiput anterior or posterior position (rotation does not exceed 45°)
  Fetal head is at or on the perineum
- **Low** Leading point of the skull (not caput) is at station plus 2 cm or more and not on the pelvic floor
  Two subdivisions:
  * rotation of 45° or less from the occipito-anterior position
  * rotation of more than 45° including the occipito-posterior position
- **Mid** Fetal head is no more than 1/5th palpable per abdomen
  Leading point of the skull is above station plus 2 cm but not above the ischial spines
  Two subdivisions:
  * rotation of 45° or less from the occipito-anterior position
  * rotation of more than 45° including the occipito-posterior position
- **High** Not included in the classification as OVD is not recommended in this situation where the head is 2/5th or more palpable abdominally and the presenting part is above the level of the ischial spines

Strategies that can reduce OVD

- Continuous support during labour.
- Use of upright or lateral positions in the second stage of labour compared with supine or lithotomy positions.
- Avoiding epidural analgesia – epidural analgesia compared with non-epidural methods is associated with an increased incidence of OVD but provides better pain relief than non-epidural analgesia.
- Delayed pushing for 1 to 2 hours or until woman has a strong urge to push, in primiparous women with an epidural can reduce the need for rotational and midcavity deliveries.
- Using a partogram does not lead to a reduction in the incidence of OVDs.
- In primiparous women with an epidural, starting oxytocin in the second stage of labour may reduce the need for non-rotational forceps delivery. NICE recommends not to use oxytocin as a matter of routine in the second stage of labour. Use oxytocin with extreme caution in the second stage of labour in multiparous women. Assess each woman individually for the management of the second stage of labour.
- There is insufficient evidence to suggest that discontinuing epidural analgesia reduces the incidence of OVD but there is evidence that it increases a woman's pain.
- There is no difference between the rates of OVD for combined spinal–epidural and standard epidural techniques or patient-controlled epidural analgesia and standard epidural technique.

Indications for OVD

- **Fetal** – presumed fetal compromise.
- **Maternal** – to shorten and reduce the effects of the second stage of labour on medical conditions (e.g., cardiac disease class III or IV, hypertensive crises, myasthenia gravis, spinal cord injury patients at risk of autonomic dysreflexia, proliferative retinopathy).
- **Inadequate progress:**
  * Nulliparous – lack of continuing progress for 3 hours (total of active and passive second-stage labour) with regional anaesthesia, or 2 hours without regional anaesthesia.
  * Multiparous – lack of continuing progress for 2 hours (total of active and passive second-stage labour) with regional anaesthesia, or 1 hour without regional anaesthesia.
- **Maternal fatigue/exhaustion.**

- OVD is used to shorten the second stage of labour. Balance the risks and benefits of continuing pushing versus OVD.
- Maternal morbidity increases significantly after 3 hours of the second stage and further increased after 4 hours.
- Discuss the benefits of a shortened second stage for certain medical conditions in the antenatal period.
- There is no evidence that elective OVD for inadvertent dural puncture is of benefit, unless the woman has a headache that worsens with pushing.
- There is a minimal risk of fetal haemorrhage if the extractor is applied following FBS or application of a spiral scalp electrode.
- Forceps can be used for the after-coming head of the breech and in situations where maternal effort is impossible or contraindicated.

Contraindications

- Do not use vacuum extractor at < 34 weeks + 0 days of gestation because of the susceptibility of the preterm infant to cephalohaematoma, intracranial haemorrhage, subgaleal haemorrhage, and neonatal jaundice.
- Do not use vacuum extractors with a face presentation.
- Do not perform OVD before full dilatation of the cervix if the criteria for safe delivery have not been met.

- Use vacuum extraction at between 34 weeks + 0 days and 36 weeks + 0 days of gestation with caution as the safety is uncertain.
- Fetal bleeding disorders (e.g., alloimmune thrombocytopenia) or a predisposition to fracture (e.g., osteogenesis imperfecta) are relative contraindications. However, there may be considerable fetal risk if the head has to be delivered abdominally from deep in the pelvis.
- Blood-borne viral infections of the mother are not a contraindication to OVD. However, avoid difficult OVD where there is an increased chance of fetal abrasion or scalp trauma and avoid fetal scalp clips or FBS during labour.

Careful assessment to fulfil prerequisites for OVD

Prerequisites –
- **Abdominal and vaginal examination**
  * Head is ≤ 1/5th palpable per abdomen.
  * Vertex presentation.
  * Cervix is fully dilated and the membranes ruptured.
  * Exact position of the head can be determined.
  * Assessment of caput and moulding. Irreducible moulding may indicate cephalo–pelvic disproportion.
  * Pelvis is adequate.
- **Preparation of mother**
  * Clear explanation and informed consent.
  * Appropriate analgesia is in place for mid-cavity rotational deliveries. This will usually be a regional block. A pudendal block may be appropriate, particularly in urgent delivery.
  * Empty maternal bladder. Remove in-dwelling catheter.

- **Preparation of staff**
  * Operator must have the knowledge, experience, and skill necessary.
  * Adequate facilities (appropriate equipment, bed, lighting).
  * Back-up plan in place in case of failure to deliver. When conducting mid-cavity deliveries, theatre staff should be available to allow a CS to be performed without delay (< 30 minutes).
  * Anticipation of complications that may arise (e.g., shoulder dystocia, PPH).
  * Personnel present that are trained in neonatal resuscitation.
  * At present there is insufficient evidence to recommend routine use of USS to determine fetal head position as part of assessment for OVD.

OVD – procedure

Consent

- Inform women in the antenatal period about OVD, especially during their first pregnancy, when the risk of requiring a forceps or ventouse delivery is higher.
- For deliveries in the delivery room, obtain verbal consent. If circumstances allow, written consent may also be obtained.
- Obtain written consent for trial of OVD in theatre.
- Document the decision, reasons for proceeding to OVD and an accurate record of the OVD.

Operator

- Neonatal trauma is associated with initial unsuccessful attempts at OVD by inexperienced operators. Operator must have the knowledge, experience, and skills necessary to assess and to use the instruments and manage complications that may arise.

Place

- For OVD that has a higher risk of failure, consider a trial and conduct in a place where immediate recourse to CS is available.
- OVD in operating theatre compared with deliveries in the labour room has a doubling in the decision-to-delivery interval. There are no significant differences in the neonatal outcomes. Therefore, balance the risks of failed OVD in the labour room with the risks associated with the transfer time when the delivery is conducted in an operating theatre.
- Fetal injuries have been attributed to delay between a failed OVD and CS.
- There is little evidence of increased maternal or neonatal morbidity following failed OVD compared with immediate CS where immediate recourse to CS is available.
- The alternative view is that when an OVD is conducted in an operating theatre, there may be a delay associated with transfer that may have a negative impact on the neonatal outcome.

Episiotomy

- In the absence of robust evidence to support routine use of episiotomy in OVD, restrictive use of episiotomy, using the operator's judgement, is supported.

Prophylactic antibiotics

- Insufficient data to justify the use of prophylactic antibiotics.

Instruments

- Choose the instrument most appropriate to the clinical circumstances and to the level of skill.
- Failed delivery is more likely with vacuum extraction. Soft vacuum extractor cups compared with rigid cups are associated with a significant increase in the rate of failure but a significant reduction in puerperal scalp trauma.
- The Kiwi OmniCup is safe and effective. However, it is less successful in achieving a vaginal delivery with a reported failure rate of 13%.
- The options available for rotational delivery include Kielland forceps, manual rotation followed by direct traction forceps or rotational vacuum extraction.
- Rotational delivery with the Kielland forceps carries additional risks and requires specific expertise and training.
- There is insufficient evidence to favour either a rapid (over 2 minutes) or a stepwise increment in negative pressure with vacuum extraction.
- Vacuum extraction compared with forceps is associated with:
  * More failure, cephalhaematoma, retinal haemorrhage, maternal worries about baby.
  * Less maternal perineal and vaginal trauma.
  * No more likelihood of delivery by CS, low 5-minute Apgar scores, the need for phototherapy.
- In view of the reduction of maternal pelvic floor injuries, the vacuum is advocated as the instrument of first choice. The downside is the increased risk of failed OVD and of sequential use of instruments (vacuum followed by forceps) with inherent additional risks to the mother and infant. Therefore, select the instrument best suited to the individual circumstances.
- A RCT has reported that symptoms of altered faecal continence are significantly more common following forceps delivery compared with vacuum extraction. However, a 5-year follow-up did not show any significant differences in long-term outcome between the two instruments for either the mother or the child.

Higher rates of failure

- **Higher rates of failure are associated with:**
  * Maternal BMI > 30.
  * Estimated fetal weight > 4000 g or clinically big baby.
  * Occipito-posterior position.
  * Mid-cavity delivery or when 1/5th of the head is palpable per abdomen (at mid-cavity the biparietal diameter is still above the level of the ischial spines).

CHAPTER 50   Operative vaginal delivery (OVD)

251

Place for sequential use of instruments

- Sequential use compared with forceps alone is associated with an increased risk of need for mechanical ventilation, intracranial haemorrhage, retinal haemorrhage, and feeding difficulty. CS in the second stage of labour is associated with an increased risk of major obstetric haemorrhage, prolonged hospital stay, and admission of the baby to the SCBU compared with completed instrumental delivery.
- Balance the risks of CS following failed vacuum extraction with the risks of forceps delivery following failed vacuum extraction. The use of outlet/low-cavity forceps following failed vacuum extraction may be judicious in avoiding a potentially complex CS.
- Attempt only if experienced and avoid if possible.
- Inform the neonatologist.

When to abandon OVD

- Abandon if there is no evidence of progressive descent with moderate traction during each contraction or where delivery is not imminent following 3 contractions of a correctly applied instrument.
- There is increased risk of neonatal trauma and admission to the SCBU following excessive pulls (> 3) and sequential use of instruments. The risk is further increased where delivery is completed by CS following a protracted attempt at OVD.
- The rate of subdural or cerebral haemorrhage in vacuum deliveries (1 in 860) is similar to forceps use (1 in 664) or CS during labour (1 in 954). However, risk is significantly increased following use of both vacuum and forceps (1 in 256).
- Take paired cord blood samples.

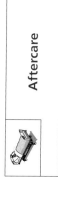

Aftercare

Advise women for future deliveries

- Encourage women to aim for a spontaneous vaginal delivery in a subsequent pregnancy as there is a high probability of success. The likelihood of achieving a spontaneous vaginal delivery is approximately 80% even for women who have required more complex OVD in theatre.
- Discuss at the earliest opportunity as there is evidence to suggest that women decide on the future mode of delivery soon after delivery.

What not to do

- Routine use of USS to determine fetal head position as part of assessment for OVD.
- Elective OVD for inadvertent dural puncture.
- A vacuum extractor at < 34 weeks + 0 days of gestation and for face presentation.
- Forceps and vacuum extractor deliveries before full dilatation of the cervix.
- Midwife-led debriefing to reduce maternal depression following OVD.
- Sequential instrumental delivery by an inexperienced operator.

- Thromboprophylaxis – reassess for risk factors for VTE and prescribe appropriate thromboprophylaxis. Mid-cavity delivery, prolonged labour, and immobility are risk factors for VTE.
- Analgesia – provide regular paracetamol and diclofenac.
- Care of the bladder – monitor the timing and volume of the first void urine. Measure post-void residual if retention is suspected. Women who have had a spinal anaesthetic or an epidural that has been topped up for a trial may be at increased risk of retention, which can be associated with long-term bladder dysfunction. Leave an indwelling catheter in place for at least 12 hours post-delivery to prevent asymptomatic bladder overfilling.
- Offer physiotherapy to prevent urinary incontinence.
- Reduce psychological morbidity for the mother – OVD can be associated with fear of subsequent childbirth and in a severe form may manifest as a post-traumatic stress-type syndrome termed tocophobia.
- There is no evidence to support that midwifery-led debriefing to discuss the indication for OVD following OVD.
- Review prior to hospital discharge to discuss the indication for OVD, management of any complications, and the prognosis for future deliveries.

Consent – operative vaginal delivery (OVD) (vacuum-assisted delivery and/or forceps delivery)

Discuss

- **Describe** the nature of vacuum-assisted/forceps delivery.
- Inform –
  - Episiotomy may be required, particularly with forceps delivery.
  - For trial of OVD – vaginal delivery is not certain and get consent for proceeding to CS if necessary.
- **Explain** the procedure.
- Intended benefits –
  To secure the safest and/or quickest route of delivery in the circumstances present at the time the decision is made, where the anticipated risks to mother and/or baby of OVD outweigh those of an alternative mode of delivery. The benefits may include:
  - Expedited delivery where fetal compromise is suspected.
  - Relief where the second stage of labour is delayed owing to maternal exhaustion or other reasons.
  - Safer delivery in cases where maternal pushing is not advisable – such as cerebral aneurysm, proliferative retinopathy or cardiac problems.
- **What the procedure is likely to involve, the benefits and risks of any available alternative treatments, including no treatment** – delivery of the baby vaginally by means of forceps or a vacuum device. A clinical assessment is performed before the instrument is applied. The operator will choose the instrument most appropriate to the clinical circumstances and their competence. A CS performed when the baby's head is low in the birth canal could be more traumatic for mother and baby than an operative vaginal delivery.
- Woman may decline OVD even when this would be detrimental to her own health or the wellbeing of her baby.
- Accept and document if the woman objects to the use of a particular instrument.
- Plan form of anaesthesia.

Risks

- Higher rates of failure and serious or frequent complications are associated with:
  - Higher maternal BMI.
  - Ultrasound-EFW > 4000 g or clinically large baby.
  - Occipito-posterior position.
  - Mid-cavity delivery or when 1/5 fetal head palpable abdominally.

- **Serious risks**

  Maternal:
  - Third- and fourth-degree perineal tear:
    - 1–4/100 with vacuum-assisted delivery.
    - 8–12/100 with forceps delivery.
  - Extensive or significant vaginal/vulval tear:
    - 1 in 10 with vacuum.
    - 1 in 5 with forceps.

  Fetal:
  - Subgaleal haematoma 3–6/1000.
  - Intracranial haemorrhage 5–15/10000.
  - Facial nerve palsy (rare).

- **Frequent risks**

  Maternal:
  - PPH 1–4 in 10;
  - Vaginal tear/abrasion (very common).
  - Anal sphincter dysfunction/voiding dysfunction.

  Fetal:
  - Forceps marks on face (very common).
  - Chignon/cup marking on the scalp (practically all cases of vacuum-assisted delivery) (very common).
  - Cephalhaematoma 1–12/100.
  - Facial or scalp lacerations 1 in 10.
  - Neonatal jaundice /hyperbilirubinaemia 5–15/100.
  - Retinal haemorrhage 17–38/100.
- Surgical and anaesthetic risks are increased with obese patients, those who have significant pathology, those who have had previous surgery or those who have pre-existing medical conditions.

Extra procedures

- Any extra procedures which may become necessary:
  - Episiotomy (5–6 in 10 for vacuum-assisted delivery, 9 in 10 for forceps).
  - Manoeuvres for shoulder dystocia.
  - Caesarean section.
  - Blood transfusion.
  - Repair of perineal tear.
  - Manual rotation prior to forceps or vacuum-assisted delivery.

Risks

Very common	1/1 to 1/10
Common	1/10 to 1/100
Uncommon	1/100 to 1/1000
Rare	1/1000 to 1/10000
Very rare	Less than 1/10000

Operative Vaginal Delivery. RCOG Green-top Guideline No. 26; January 2011.
Operative Vaginal Delivery (Vacuum-Assisted Delivery and/or Forceps Delivery) RCOG Consent Advice No. 11; July 2010.

CHAPTER 51 Vaginal birth after previous caesarean section (VBAC)

Background and definitions

Planned VBAC – any woman who has experienced a prior CS and who plans to deliver vaginally.

Successful and unsuccessful VBAC – a vaginal birth (spontaneous or assisted) in a woman undergoing planned VBAC is a successful VBAC. Birth by emergency CS during the labour is an unsuccessful VBAC.

Maternal outcomes

- *Uterine rupture* – a disruption of the uterine muscle extending to and involving the uterine serosa or disruption of the uterine muscle with extension to the bladder or broad ligament.
- *Uterine dehiscence* – a disruption of the uterine muscle with intact uterine serosa.
- *Other outcomes* – hysterectomy, VTE, haemorrhage, blood transfusion, viscus injury (bowel, bladder, ureter), endometritis, maternal death.

Fetal outcomes

- *Term perinatal mortality (PNM)* – stillbirths (SB) (antepartum and intrapartum) + neonatal deaths (NND) (death of a live born infant from birth to age 28 days) per 10 000 live births (LB) and SBs at or beyond 37 completed weeks of gestation.
- *Term delivery-related perinatal death* – intrapartum SB + NNDs /10 000 LB and SB, at or beyond 37 completed weeks of gestation. Birth related PNMR exclude antepartum SBs.
- *Neonatal respiratory morbidity* – the combined rate of transient tachypnoea of the newborn (TTN) and respiratory distress syndrome (RDS).
- *Hypoxic-ischaemic encephalopathy (HIE)* – hypoxia resulting from a decrease in the blood supply to a bodily organ, tissue, or part caused by constriction or obstruction of the blood vessels, which results in compromised neurological function manifesting during the first few days after birth. HIE refers to a subset of the much broader category of neonatal encephalopathy, in which the aetiology is felt to be intrapartum hypoxic–ischaemic injury.

Factors associated with successful VBAC:

- Previous vaginal birth, particularly previous VBAC, is the single best predictor for successful VBAC and is associated with an approximately 87–90% success rate.
  - No previous vaginal birth.

Risk factors for unsuccessful VBAC are:

- Induced labour.
  - Previous CS for dystocia.
- BMI >30.
- When all these factors are present, successful VBAC is achieved in only 40% of cases.

Factors associated with a decreased likelihood of planned VBAC success:

- VBAC at or after 41 weeks of gestation.
  - Birth weight >4000 g.
- No epidural anaesthesia.
  - Previous preterm CS.
- Cervical dilatation at admission <4 cm.
  - <2 years from previous CS.
- Advanced maternal age.
  - Non-white ethnicity.
- Short stature.
  - A male infant.
- Several preadmission and admission-based multivariate models have been developed to predict the likelihood of VBAC success; however their usefulness remains to be determined.

Absolute contraindications

- Women with:
  - A prior history of one classical CS.
  - Previous uterine rupture – risk of recurrent rupture is unknown.
  - Previous high vertical classical CS – 200–900/10000 risk of uterine rupture where the uterine incision has involved the whole length of the uterine corpus.
  - ≥ 3 previous CS deliveries – risk of rupture unknown.
- In certain extreme circumstances (miscarriage, IUFD) for some women in this group, the vaginal route (although risky) may not necessarily be contraindicated.
- Others associated with an increased risk of uterine rupture:
  - Women with a prior inverted T or J incision – 190/10000 rupture risk.
  - Women with prior low vertical incision – 200/10000 rupture risk.
- Women with a previous uterine incision other than an uncomplicated low transverse CS incision who wish to consider vaginal birth – assess with full access to the details of the previous surgery.

Antenatal assessment and counselling

- Women with a prior history of one uncomplicated lower-segment transverse CS, in an otherwise uncomplicated pregnancy at term, with no contraindication to vaginal birth – discuss the options of planned VBAC or elective repeat caesarean section (ERCS).
- Counsel about the maternal and perinatal risks and benefits of VBAC and ERCS.
- Review the operative notes of the previous CS to identify the indication, type of uterine incision, and any perioperative complications.
- Finalize a plan for mode of birth before the EDD (ideally by 36 weeks).
- Also plan for the event of labour starting prior to the scheduled date as up to 10% of women scheduled for ERCS go into labour before the 39th week.
- The chances of successful planned VBAC are 72–76%.

Relative contraindications

- Women with 2 previous uncomplicated low transverse CS, in uncomplicated pregnancy at term, with no contraindication for vaginal birth may be considered for planned VBAC.
- There is no significant difference reported in the rates of uterine rupture in VBAC with ≥ 2 previous CS compared with a single previous CS. However, the rates of hysterectomy and transfusion are increased in the former group.
- Reported rate of VBAC success with 2 previous CS is 62–75%, similar to single prior CS.
- Therefore, provided that the woman has been fully informed of these increased risks and a comprehensive individualized risk analysis has been undertaken of the indication for and the nature of the previous CSs, then planned VBAC may be supported in women with two previous low transverse CSs.
- There is insufficient and conflicting information on whether the risk of uterine rupture is increased in women with previous myomectomy or prior complex uterine surgery.

Risks and benefits of VBAC – maternal

- **Planned VBAC carries a risk of uterine rupture of 22–74/10000. There is virtually no risk of uterine rupture in women undergoing ERCS.**
- Uterine rupture in an unscarred uterus – 0.5–2.0/10000 deliveries; mainly confined to multiparous women in labour.
- Uterine rupture is associated with significant maternal and perinatal morbidity and PNM.
- Women who experienced both intrapartum and postpartum fever in their prior CS are at increased risk of uterine rupture in their subsequent planned VBAC.
- There is conflicting evidence on whether single-layer compared with double-layer uterine closure may increase the risk of uterine rupture in subsequent planned VBAC.

- **Planned VBAC compared with ERCS carries around 1% additional risk of either blood transfusion or endometritis.**
- There is no statistically significant difference in hysterectomy, VTE or maternal death.
- The vast majority of cases of maternal death in women with prior CS arise due to medical disorders.
- Maternal death from uterine rupture in planned VBAC occurs in <1/100000 cases.
- The increased risk of morbidity among women attempting VBAC is due to higher rates among women with unsuccessful VBAC.
- Unsuccessful planned VBAC compared with successful VBAC is associated with an increased risk of uterine rupture, uterine dehiscence, hysterectomy, transfusion, and endometritis.

- **ERCS may increase the risk of serious complications in future pregnancies.**
- The following risks significantly increase with increasing number of repeated CS deliveries:
  * Placenta accreta.   * Injury to bladder, bowel or ureter.
  * Ileus.
  * ICU admission.   * Hysterectomy.
  * The need for postoperative ventilation.
  * Blood transfusion requiring four or more units.
  * The duration of operative time and hospital stay.
- Thus, knowledge of the woman's intended number of future pregnancies is an important factor to consider during the decision-making process for either planned VBAC or ERCS.

- **The risk of anaesthetic complications is extremely low for both planned VBAC and ERCS.**
- Reported rate of maternal death (2.7/100000) attributed to failed intubation.

Risks and benefits of VBAC – fetal

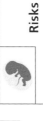

- **Planned VBAC carries a 2–3/10000 additional risk of birth-related perinatal death when compared with ERCS.**
- PNM is significantly greater among women having a planned VBAC than ERCS – 24/10000 vs 9.3/10000.
- The increased risk of PNM is largely due to the statistically significantly increased risk of antepartum SB beyond 37 weeks of gestation in planned VBAC compared with ERCS. Approximately 43% of such SBs in planned VBAC are at or after 39 weeks of gestation.
- Planned VBAC is associated with a 10/10000 risk of antepartum SB beyond 39 weeks of gestation.
- Rates of delivery-related perinatal death are 4/10000 for planned VBAC and 1.4/10000 for ERCS.
- It is likely that these risks can be reduced by ERCS at the start of the 39th week but direct evidence is lacking.
- **The absolute risk of such birth-related perinatal loss is comparable to the risk for women having their first birth.**

- **Planned VBAC carries an 8/10000 risk of the infant developing HIE. The effect on the long-term outcome of the infant upon experiencing HIE is unknown.**
- The incidence of intrapartum HIE at term is significantly greater in planned VBAC (7.8/10000) compared with ERCS (zero rate).
- Approximately 50% of the increased risk in planned VBAC arises from the additional risk of HIE caused by uterine rupture (4.6/10000).
- Severe neonatal metabolic acidosis (pH <7.00) occurs in 33% of term uterine ruptures.
- There is no information comparing long-term outcome, such as cerebral palsy, associated with VBAC and ERCS.

- **Attempting VBAC probably reduces the risk of respiratory problems in the baby after birth: rates are 2–3% with planned VBAC and 3–4% with ERCS.**
- There is a beneficial effect on reducing respiratory morbidity by delaying elective CS to at least 39 weeks.
- Delaying birth by 1 week from 38 to 39 weeks of gestation enables around a 5% reduction in the incidence of respiratory morbidity, although this delay may be associated with a 5/10000 increase in the risk of antepartum SB.
- An approximate 50% reduction in respiratory morbidity (both TTN and RDS) has been reported with prophylactic betamethasone to women having elective CS beyond 37 weeks and this treatment effect remains apparent at 39 weeks. However, it has been suggested that even a single course of antenatal steroids may have long-term consequences for the baby and therefore it may be safer to delay ERCS until 39 weeks of gestation rather than give steroids and deliver at 38 weeks of gestation.

Intrapartum support and intervention

Place of birth

- **At a suitably staffed and equipped delivery suite, with continuous intrapartum care and monitoring and available resources for immediate CS and advanced neonatal resuscitation.** Planned VBAC in low-volume hospitals (<3000 births/year) is not associated with an increased risk of uterine rupture but is associated with an increased risk of uterine rupture that leads to perinatal death. It is likely that the availability of resources for immediate delivery and neonatal resuscitation may reduce the risk of infant morbidity and mortality due to uterine rupture.

Anaesthesia

- Planned VBAC success rates are higher among women receiving epidural analgesia.
- Concerns that epidural analgesia might mask the signs and symptoms associated with uterine rupture are based on a single case report and VBAC is not a contraindication for epidural analgesia.

Continuous intrapartum care

- Provide continuous care to enable prompt identification and management of uterine scar rupture.
- Early diagnosis of uterine scar rupture followed by expeditious laparotomy and resuscitation is essential to reduce associated morbidity and mortality.
- There is no single pathognomonic clinical feature that is indicative of uterine rupture but watch out for: abnormal CTG; severe abdominal pain, especially if persisting between contractions; chest pain or shoulder tip pain; sudden onset of shortness of breath; acute onset scar tenderness; abnormal vaginal bleeding or haematuria; cessation of previously efficient uterine activity; maternal tachycardia, hypotension or shock; loss of station of the presenting part.
- The diagnosis is confirmed at emergency CS or postpartum laparotomy.

Continuous EFM

- Monitor with continuous EFM following the onset of uterine contractions.
- An abnormal CTG is the most consistent finding in uterine rupture and is present in 55–87% of these events.
- The relative and absolute risks of severe adverse events in the absence of continuous EFM are unknown.

Intrauterine pressure catheters

- Do not use intrauterine pressure catheters for early detection of uterine scar rupture.
- Intrauterine pressure catheters may not always be reliable and are unlikely to add significant additional ability to predict uterine rupture over clinical and CTG surveillance. Intrauterine catheter insertion may also be associated with risk.

Induction and augmentation

Risks

- **2- to 3-fold increased risk of uterine rupture and 1.5-fold increased risk of CS in induced and/or augmented labours compared with spontaneous labours.**
- Risk of uterine rupture/10 000 planned VBAC deliveries is 102, 87, and 36 for induced, augmented, and spontaneous labour, respectively. The risk of uterine rupture is 2/10 000 in women with unscarred uteri (risks of induction, augmentation, and spontaneous labour). Rates of CS in women undergoing VBAC are 33%, 26%, and 19% for induced, augmented, and spontaneous labour, respectively.

Prostaglandin induction

- Prostaglandin induction compared with non-prostaglandin induction is associated with a statistically significantly higher uterine rupture risk (87 vs 29/10 000) and a higher risk of perinatal death from uterine rupture (11 vs 4.5/10 000). Risk of perinatal death in women with an unscarred uterus induced by prostaglandin is 6/10 000.
- Given these risks and the absence of direct robust evidence, restrict the dose and keep a lower threshold of total prostaglandin dose. The decision to induce and the method chosen (prostaglandin or non-prostaglandin methods) should be consultant-led.

Cervicometric progress

- There is no evidence to recommend what is acceptable or unacceptable cervicometric progress in women being augmented with a previous CS.
- Among women with unscarred uteri, it is suggested that there is unlikely to be a higher vaginal birth rate if augmentation continues beyond 6–8 hours. The increased risk of uterine rupture in scarred uteri justifies adopting a more conservative threshold to the upper limit of augmentation in women with prior CS.
- Early recognition and intervention for labour dystocia (no cervicometric progress in 2 hours) may prevent a proportion of uterine ruptures among women attempting VBAC.
- Assess cervical progress **for both augmented and non-augmented labours, to ensure that there is adequate cervicometric progress, thereby allowing the planned VBAC to continue.**

Augmentation

- **Consultant obstetrician-led care – the decision to induce, the method chosen, augmentation with oxytocin, the time intervals for serial vaginal examination, and the selected parameters of progress that would necessitate and advise on discontinuing VBAC.**
- The additional risks in augmented VBAC mean that: although augmentation is not contraindicated, undertake a careful obstetric assessment and maternal counselling.
- Oxytocin augmentation – do not exceed the maximum rate of contractions of 4 in 10 minutes; the ideal contraction frequency would be 3–4 in 10 minutes.

Planned VBAC in special circumstances

Preterm birth

- **Planned preterm VBAC has similar success rates to planned term VBAC but with a lower risk of uterine rupture.**
- Women with preterm (24–36 weeks of gestation) VBAC when compared with women at term VBAC –
  - * Similar or higher success rates – (82% vs 74%).
  - * Lower risk of uterine rupture and dehiscence.
  - * Higher risk of VTE, coagulopathy, and transfusion, although overall combined absolute risks are <3% in the preterm VBAC.
- Perinatal outcomes are similar with preterm VBAC and preterm ERCS.
- Therefore, following appropriate counselling and in a carefully selected population, offer planned VBAC as an option to women undergoing preterm birth with a history of prior CS.
- **Twin gestation, fetal macrosomia, short inter-delivery interval** – be cautious when considering planned VBAC, as there is uncertainty in the safety and efficacy of planned VBAC in such situations.
- **Twins** – success rates with VBAC are conflicting. A study reported a lower VBAC success rate (45%) but a comparable risk of uterine rupture (90/10000).
- **Fetal macrosomia** – a review reported a significantly decreased likelihood of successful trial of VBAC for pregnancies with infants weighing 4000 g or more (55–67%) compared with smaller infants (75–83%).
- It is reported that in women with previous CS for dystocia, greater birth weight in the subsequent planned VBAC relative to the first birth weight decreases the likelihood of VBAC success. However, birth weight cannot be accurately predicted by antenatal USS which limits the clinical usefulness of this information.
- **Short interdelivery interval** – a 2 to 3-fold increased risk of uterine scar rupture for women with a short inter-delivery interval (<12–24 months) from their previous CS is reported.

Limitations of evidence

- There are no RCTs comparing planned VBAC with planned elective repeat CS.
- Many studies have limitations in terms of definition of exposures and outcomes, ascertainment, and selection bias.
- Many of the main outcomes of interest are relatively uncommon.

What not to do

- Routine use of intrauterine pressure catheters for early detection of uterine scar rupture.
- Be cautious with prostaglandin IOL.

Birth After Previous Caesarean Birth. RCOG Green-top Guideline No. 45; 2007.

CHAPTER 52 Management of third- and fourth-degree perineal tears

Background and prevalence

- Obstetric anal sphincter injury occurs in 1% of all vaginal deliveries.
- With increasing awareness and training, there appears to be an increase in detection of anal sphincter injury.
- Perineal tears involving the anal sphincter complex and/or the anal epithelium (obstetric anal sphincter injury) occur in 0.6–9.0% of vaginal deliveries where mediolateral episiotomy is performed. With the introduction of endoanal ultrasound, sonographic abnormalities of the anal sphincter anatomy are identified in up to 36% of women after vaginal delivery.

Identification of obstetric anal sphincter injuries

- Examine systematically all women with evidence of genital tract trauma following vaginal delivery to assess the severity of damage prior to suturing.
- The detection rate of anal sphincter injury with the use of endoanal USS immediately following delivery is not significantly increased compared to clinical examination alone.
- As there are clear difficulties with availability, access to staff trained in endoanal USS on the labour ward, image quality, and patient acceptability, the use of endoanal USS in detecting anal sphincter injury immediately after delivery is viewed as a research tool at present.

Classification and terminology

- **First degree**   Injury to perineal skin only.
- **Second degree** Injury to perineum involving perineal muscles but not involving the anal sphincter.
- **Third degree**   Injury to perineum involving the anal sphincter complex:
  3a: less than 50% of external anal sphincter (EAS) thickness torn.
  3b: more than 50% of EAS thickness torn.
  3c: both EAS and internal anal sphincter (IAS) torn.
- **Fourth degree** Injury to perineum involving the anal sphincter complex (EAS and IAS) and anal epithelium.
- **If there is any doubt about the grade of third-degree tear, classify it to the higher degree rather than lower degree.**

Prediction and prevention of obstetric anal sphincter injury

- Be aware of the risk factors for obstetric anal sphincter injury even though known risk factors do not readily allow its prediction or prevention.
- Perform mediolateral episiotomy with careful attention to the angle cut away from the midline where indicated.
- The factors associated with an increased risk of a third degree tear:
  * birth weight > 4 kg (up to 2%);
  * nulliparity (up to 4%);
  * epidural analgesia (up to 2%);
  * shoulder dystocia (up to 4%);
  * forceps delivery (up to 7%).
  * persistent occipito-posterior position (up to 3%);
  * IOL (up to 2%);
  * second stage longer than 1 hour (up to 4%);
  * midline episiotomy (up to 3%);
- A larger angle of episiotomy is associated with a lower risk of third-degree tear with a 50% relative reduction in risk of third-degree tear for every 6 degrees away from the perineal midline.

Risks or complications

Risks – anal incontinence. Defined as any involuntary loss of faeces, flatus or urge incontinence that is adversely affecting a woman's QOL.

- The IAS plays a role in the maintenance of continence. The incidence of anal incontinence is increased in women who had both IAS and EAS damage compared with those who had EAS damage alone.
- In acute obstetric trauma, identification of the IAS may not be possible.
- Assess for any tear that involves only anal mucosa with intact anal sphincter complex (buttonhole tear). If not recognized and repaired this type of tear may cause anovaginal fistula.

Surgical techniques

Method of repair

- For repair of the EAS, use either an overlapping or end-to-end method as both have equivalent outcomes. Where the IAS can be identified, repair it separately with interrupted sutures.
- A systematic review shows that at 12 months there is no significant difference in perineal pain, dyspareunia, flatus incontinence, and faecal incontinence between the two repair techniques. However, there is a significantly lower incidence of faecal urgency and lower anal incontinence score in the overlap group. Overlap technique is also associated with a significantly lower risk of deterioration of anal incontinence symptoms over 12 months. As the experience of the surgeon is not addressed in the studies reviewed, it is inappropriate to recommend one type of repair over another.
- **By whom** – by appropriately trained practitioners since inexperienced attempts at anal sphincter repair may contribute to maternal morbidity, especially subsequent anal incontinence.

Undertake repair in operating theatre, under regional or general anaesthesia.

- Operating theatres will provide aseptic conditions, appropriate instruments, adequate light, and an assistant.
- Regional or general anaesthesia will allow the anal sphincter to relax, which is essential to retrieve the retracted torn ends of the anal sphincter. This also allows the ends of the sphincter to be brought together without any tension.

Suture materials

- EAS muscle – monofilament sutures such as polydiaxanone (PDS) or modern braided sutures such as polyglactin (Vicryl).
- IAS muscle – fine suture such as 3-0 PDS and 2-0 Vicryl may cause less irritation and discomfort.
- Bury the surgical knots beneath the superficial perineal muscles to prevent knot migration to the skin. Warn women of the possibility of knot migration to the perineal surface, with long-acting and non-absorbable suture materials.

Postoperative management

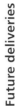

- Intraoperative and postoperative broad-spectrum antibiotics are important to prevent infection. There is a high risk of anal incontinence and fistula formation in the event of infective breakdown of the anal sphincter repair. Prescribe broad-spectrum antibiotics to reduce the incidence of postoperative infections and wound dehiscence. Include metronidazole to cover the possible anaerobic contamination from faecal matter.
- Passage of a hard stool can disrupt the repair. Prescribe stool softener such as Lactulose and a bulking agent such as Fybogelis for about 10 days after the repair to reduce the incidence of postoperative wound dehiscence.

Follow-up

- Commence physiotherapy and pelvic-floor exercises for 6–12 weeks after repair.
- **Review at 6–12 weeks postpartum (by consultant gynaecologist)** to discuss injury sustained, assess for symptoms and offer advice on how to seek help if symptoms develop, offer treatment, and/or refer if indicated and advise on future mode of delivery.
- Provide a patient information leaflet.
- If a woman is experiencing incontinence or pain at follow-up – refer to a specialist gynaecologist or colorectal surgeon for endoanal USS and anorectal manometry. A small number of women may require referral to a colorectal surgeon for consideration of secondary sphincter repair.
- Follow-up – if possible, it should be in a dedicated perineal clinic with access to endoanal USS and anal manometry, as this can aid decision on future delivery.
- Prognosis following EAS repair is good, with 60–80% asymptomatic at 12 months. Most women who remain symptomatic describe incontinence of flatus or faecal urgency.
- Recent RCTs comparing overlap and end-to-end techniques of EAS repair have reported low incidences of anal incontinence symptoms in both arms, with 60–80% of women described as asymptomatic at 12 months.
- Studies using endoanal USS as part of follow-up demonstrate persistent defects in 54–88% of women after primary repair of recognized third-degree tears. More recently, the published RCTs have reported fewer residual defects, about 19–36% overall. The clinical relevance of asymptomatic defects demonstrated by USS is currently unclear.

Future deliveries

- **Counsel about the risks of developing anal incontinence or worsening symptoms with subsequent vaginal delivery.** Subsequent vaginal delivery after third-degree tear can worsen the faecal symptoms in 17% to 24% of women. This seems to occur particularly if there is transient incontinence after the index delivery.
- There is no evidence to support the role of prophylactic episiotomy in subsequent pregnancies.
- Offer an option of elective CS to all women who are symptomatic or have abnormal endoanal USS and/or manometry.

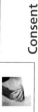

Consent – repair of third- or fourth-degree perineal tears following childbirth

Discuss

- **Inform:**
  * Why the procedure is being carried out.
  * The full extent of the injury sustained and the structures involved.
  * That a systematic examination of the vagina, perineum, and rectum will be carried out.
  * Actual extent of damage might not be identified until she is assessed under anaesthesia.

- **Explain** the repair procedure and the effect the damage that has already occurred might cause if left unrepaired.

- **Intended benefits** – to attempt to restore anorectal and perineal anatomy, facilitate wound healing, and reduce the risk of anal incontinence.

- **What the procedure is likely to involve, the benefits and risks of any available alternative treatments, including no treatment**
  * Repair of a third- or fourth-degree tear involves suturing the disrupted structures of the anorectal complex with a slow absorbing synthetic suture material. Antibiotics and laxatives are prescribed for 7–10 days.
  * Leaving a third- or fourth-degree tear unsutured is not recommended, as this is likely to be associated with increased risk of complications.

- Form of anaesthesia planned.

Risks

- Clarify that the planned procedure is to repair damage that has already happened and that the quoted risks might be linked to sphincter damage rather than the repair.

- **Serious risks:** some of these complications are a result of the tear and not necessarily the repair. However, these complications will be more significant if the repair is not performed.
  * **Common:** incontinence of stools and/or flatus.
  * **Uncommon:** delivery by CS in future pregnancies may be recommended if symptoms of incontinence persist or investigations suggest abnormal anal sphincter structure or function.
  * **Rare:** haematoma; consequences of failure of the repair requiring the need for further interventions in the future such as secondary repair or sacral nerve stimulation.
  * **Very rare:** rectovaginal fistula.

- **Frequent risks:**
  * Fear, difficulty, and discomfort in passing stools in the immediate postnatal period.
  * Migration of suture material requiring removal.
  * Granulation tissue formation.
  * Faecal urgency – 26/100.
  * Perineal pain and dyspareunia – 9/100.
  * Wound infection – 8/100.
  * Urinary infection.

- Surgical and anaesthetic risks are increased with obesity, those who have significant pathology, those who have had previous surgery or those who have pre-existing medical conditions.

Extra procedures

- Any extra procedures which may become necessary:
  * Blood transfusion.
  * Rarely, a vaginal pack is required if haemostasis cannot be achieved.

Risks

Very common	1/1 to 1/10
Common	1/10 to 1/100
Uncommon	1/100 to 1/1000
Rare	1/1000 to 1/10000
Very rare	Less than 1/10000

The Management of Third- and Fourth-Degree Perineal Tears. RCOG Green-top Guideline No. 29; March 2007.
   Please refer to updated guidelines from June 2015.
Repair of Third- and Fourth-Degree Perineal Tears Following Childbirth. RCOG Consent Advice No. 9; June 2010.

CHAPTER 53 Shoulder dystocia

Prevalence and background

- Delivery that requires additional obstetric manoeuvres to release the shoulders after gentle downward traction has failed.
- It occurs when either the anterior or, less commonly, the posterior fetal shoulder impacts on the maternal symphysis or sacral promontory.
- Incidence – 0.6% of deliveries.

Risk factors

- **Prelabour** – previous shoulder dystocia; macrosomia: DM; BMI > 30; IOL.
- **Intrapartum** – prolonged first stage of labour, secondary arrest; OVD; prolonged second stage of labour; oxytocin augmentation.
- Fetal size is not a good predictor. Majority of infants with a birth weight of ≥ 4500 g do not develop shoulder dystocia whereas 48% of shoulder dystocia occur in infants with a birth weight < 4000 g. Moreover, clinical fetal weight estimation is unreliable and third-trimester USS has at least a 10% margin for error for actual birth weight with a sensitivity of just 60% for macrosomia (> 4500 g).

Risks

- High perinatal mortality and morbidity.
- Brachial plexus injuries – 4–16% of such deliveries with < 10% resulting in permanent brachial plexus dysfunction. In the UK, the incidence of brachial plexus injuries is 1/2300 live births. Not all injuries are due to excess traction and there is evidence that maternal propulsive force may contribute to some of these injuries. Moreover, a substantial minority of brachial plexus injuries are not associated with clinically evident shoulder dystocia. In one series, 4% of injuries occurred after a CS.
- Erb's palsy – determine whether the affected shoulder was anterior or posterior at the time of delivery, because damage to the plexus of the posterior shoulder is not due to action by the accoucheur.
- Maternal morbidity – PPH (11%) and fourth-degree perineal tears (4%).

Prediction

- These clinical characteristics have a low PPV both singly and in combination.
- Conventional risk factors predict only 16% of shoulder dystocia that result in infant morbidity. Majority of cases occur in the women with no risk factors.
- Shoulder dystocia is therefore a largely unpredictable and unpreventable event. Be aware of existing risk factors but be alert to the possibility of shoulder dystocia with any delivery.

Prevention

IOL

Suspected non-diabetic macrosomia – early IOL does not improve either maternal or fetal outcome. Do not offer IOL in women without diabetes at term where the fetus is thought to be macrosomic.

Suspected diabetic macrosomia – Cochrane Review reported that IOL in women with DM treated with insulin reduces the risk of macrosomia.

There is a small decrease in the number of deliveries complicated by shoulder dystocia in the IOL group but the risk of maternal or neonatal morbidity is not altered. IOL in women with DM does not reduce the maternal or neonatal morbidity of shoulder dystocia.

Elective CS

Previous shoulder dystocia – recurrence rate of shoulder dystocia is 1–16%.

- Either CS or vaginal delivery is appropriate after a previous shoulder dystocia. There is no requirement to advise elective CS routinely but consider factors such as the severity of any previous neonatal or maternal injury, fetal size, and maternal choice when offering recommendations for the next delivery.

Suspected non-diabetic macrosomia

- Do not offer elective CS to reduce the potential morbidity with suspected fetal macrosomia (EFW > 4.5 kg) without DM. An additional 2345 caesarean deliveries are required at a cost of US$4.9 million to prevent one permanent injury from shoulder dystocia.
- Consider elective CS for an EFW of > 5 kg (ACOG). There are no data that directly support this recommendation. However, there is evidence to suggest that larger infants are more likely to suffer a permanent, rather than transient, brachial plexus injury after shoulder dystocia.

Suspected diabetic macrosomia

- Consider elective CS to reduce the potential morbidity for pregnancies complicated by suspected fetal macrosomia associated with maternal DM.
- Consider elective CS for women with DM suspected of fetal macrosomia (EFW > 4.5 kg). (ACOG)

Diagnosis

- Timely management of shoulder dystocia requires prompt recognition. Observe for: * difficulty with delivery of the face and chin; * the head remaining tightly applied to the vulva or even retracting; * failure of restitution of the fetal head; * failure of the shoulders to descend.
- Employ routine traction in an axial direction to diagnose shoulder dystocia. Avoid lateral and downward traction as it is more likely to cause nerve avulsion.
- Use of the McRoberts' manoeuvre routinely compared with the lithotomy position before clinical diagnosis of shoulder dystocia does not reduce the traction force on the fetal head during vaginal delivery in multiparous women. Do not attempt it to prevent shoulder dystocia.

- **Pre-emptive preparation** – if shoulder dystocia is anticipated, get an experienced obstetrician for the second stage of labour.
- 47% of the babies die within 5 minutes of the head being delivered. Therefore manage the problem efficiently and carefully to avoid hypoxia, acidosis and unnecessary trauma.

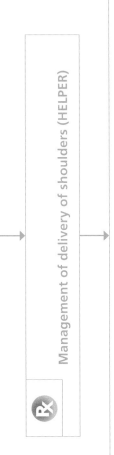

Management of delivery of shoulders (HELPER)

1. Call for extra help immediately – (extra midwives, obstetrician, paediatric resuscitation team, and anaesthetist).
2. Discourage maternal pushing as this may lead to a further impaction of the shoulders, exacerbating the situation.
3. Do not use fundal pressure – it is associated with high neonatal complication rate and may result in uterine rupture.
4. Position – bring the woman's buttocks to the edge of the bed.
5. Episiotomy is not necessary for all cases. The Managing Obstetric Emergencies and Trauma (MOET) Group suggests a selective approach, reserving episiotomy to facilitate manoeuvres such as delivery of the posterior arm or internal rotation of the shoulders. Consider an episiotomy but it is not mandatory.

First-line manoeuvres

- **The McRoberts' manoeuvre** – flexion and abduction of the maternal hips, positioning the maternal thighs on her abdomen. It straightens the lumbo-sacral angle, rotates the maternal pelvis cephalad, and is associated with an increase in uterine pressure and amplitude of contractions.
- The McRoberts' manoeuvre is the single most effective intervention, with reported success rates as high as 90%. It has a low rate of complication and therefore employ it first.
- **Suprapubic pressure** is useful. It can be employed together with McRoberts' manoeuvre to improve success rates. It reduces the bisacromial diameter and rotates the anterior shoulder into the oblique pelvic diameter. The shoulder is then free to slip underneath the symphysis pubis with the aid of routine traction. External suprapubic pressure is applied in a downward and lateral direction to push the posterior aspect of the anterior shoulder towards the fetal chest. Apply for 30 seconds. There is no clear difference in efficacy between continuous pressure and 'rocking' movement.

Fail

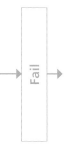

Second-line manoeuvres

Internal manipulation (delivery of the posterior arm and internal rotation manoeuvres) or the all-fours position

- Internal rotation – rotation of shoulders into an oblique diameter or by a full 180-degree rotation of the fetal trunk.
- Delivery of the posterior arm – the fetal trunk will either follow directly or the arm can be used to rotate the fetal trunk to facilitate delivery. Delivery of the posterior arm has a high complication rate: (12% humeral fractures), but the neonatal trauma may be a reflection of the refractory nature of the case, rather than the procedure itself.
- There is no advantage between delivery of the posterior arm and internal rotation manoeuvres. Therefore use clinical judgement and experience to decide their order.
- The all-fours position has been reported with 83% success rate in one case series. For a slim mobile woman without epidural anaesthesia and with a single midwifery attendant, the all-fours position is probably the most appropriate. For a less mobile woman with epidural anaesthesia in place internal manoeuvres are more appropriate.

Fail

Third-line manoeuvres

- Consider carefully to avoid unnecessary maternal morbidity and mortality. These include cleidotomy (bending the clavicle with a finger or surgical division), symphysiotomy (dividing the symphyseal ligament), and the Zavanelli manoeuvre.
- The Zavanelli manoeuvre – cephalic replacement of the head, and delivery by CS. It may be most appropriate for rare bilateral shoulder dystocia, where both the shoulders impact on the pelvic inlet, anteriorly above the pubic symphysis and posteriorly on the sacral promontory. The maternal safety of this procedure is unknown; however, consider that a high proportion of fetuses have irreversible hypoxia–acidosis by this stage.
- Symphysiotomy – there is a high incidence of serious maternal morbidity and poor neonatal outcome.
- It is difficult to recommend a time limit for the management of shoulder dystocia, as there are no conclusive data available.

After delivery be aware of PPH and third- and fourth-degree perineal tears.

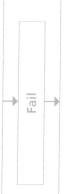

What not to do

- IOL in women without diabetes at term where the fetus is thought to be macrosomic.
- IOL in women with diabetes mellitus does not reduce the maternal or neonatal morbidity of shoulder dystocia.
- Elective CS routinely for previous shoulder dystocia.
- Elective CS for suspected fetal macrosomia (EFW > 4.5 kg) without diabetes.
- The use of the McRoberts' manoeuvre compared with the lithotomy position before clinical diagnosis of shoulder dystocia for prevention of shoulder dystocia.
- Fundal pressure once shoulder dystocia is diagnosed.

Risk management

- Not all cases can be anticipated and therefore all birth attendants should be conversant with the techniques required to facilitate delivery complicated by shoulder dystocia.
- Training – annual 'skill drills'.
- Accurately document a difficult and potentially traumatic delivery.

Shoulder Dystocia. RCOG Guideline No. 42; December 2005.
Shoulder Dystocia. ACOG Practice Bulletin Number 40; November 2002 (replaces Practice Pattern Number 7, October 1997).
Sokol RJ, Blackwell SC. American College of Obstetricians and Gynecologists. Committee on Practice Bulletins – Gynecology. International Journal of Gynaecology and Obstetrics 2003 Jan;80(1):87–92.
www.aps-web.com

CHAPTER 54 Prevention and management of postpartum haemorrhage (PPH)

Background

- One of the major causes of maternal death.
- In the UK CMED (2003–2005), haemorrhage is the third highest direct cause of maternal death (6.6 deaths/million maternities). There is evidence of substandard care in the majority of fatal cases (58%), therefore maternal death was preventable.
- In Scotland, the rate of life-threatening haemorrhage (EBL ≥2.5 litres or women who received >5 units of BT or women who received treatment for coagulopathy after an acute event) is 3.7/1000 maternities.

Causes of PPH – 'the four Ts':

- **Tone** (abnormalities of uterine contraction)
- **Tissue** (retained products of conception)
- **Trauma** (of the genital tract)
- **Thrombin** (abnormalities of coagulation)

Definition

- **Primary PPH** – loss of ≥500 ml of blood from the genital tract within 24 hours of the birth of a baby.
- **Secondary PPH** – excessive bleeding from the birth canal between 24 hours and 12 weeks postnatally.
- **Minor PPH** – EBL of 500–1000 ml (and the absence of clinical signs of shock).
- **Major PPH** – EBL of ≥1000 ml (continuing to bleed or clinical signs of shock associated with a smaller EBL). Major could be moderate (1000–2000 ml) or severe (>2000 ml).
- Most women can readily cope with an EBL of 500 ml. EBL of >1000 ml has been suggested as an appropriate cut-off point for major PPH which should prompt the initiation of a protocol of emergency measures.
- Blood volume depends on the body weight (approximate blood volume equals weight in kilograms divided by 12, expressed as litres). In estimating percentage of blood loss, consider the body weight and the original haemoglobin.
- Allowing for the physiological increase in pregnancy, total blood volume at term is approximately 100ml/kg (an average 70 kg woman – total blood volume of 7000 ml). A blood loss of >40% of total blood volume (approximately 2800ml) is regarded as 'life-threatening'. Initiate PPH protocols at an EBL well below this figure, as the aim of management is to prevent haemorrhage escalating to the point where it is life-threatening.

Risk factors – prediction

- Present antenatally and associated with a substantial increase in the incidence of PPH – suspected or proven placental abruption, placenta praevia, multiple pregnancy, PET/gestational HT. Advise these women to deliver in a consultant-led maternity unit with a blood bank on site.
- Present antenatally and associated with a significant (though smaller) increase in the incidence of PPH – previous PPH, Asian ethnicity, obesity (BMI >35), anaemia (<9 g/dl).
- Become apparent during labour and delivery – emergency or elective CS, IOL, retained placenta, mediolateral episiotomy, OVD, prolonged labour (>12 hours), big baby (>4 kg), pyrexia in labour, age >40 years. Maintain extra vigilance.
- Women who had a previous CS – check the placental site by USS.
- Women with placenta accreta/percreta – See Chapter 30 Antepartum haemorrhage (APH).
- Most cases of PPH have no identifiable risk factors.

Prevention – prophylaxis in the third stage of labour

- Active vs expectant management – active management is associated with lower maternal blood loss and reduced risks of PPH but is associated with an increased incidence of nausea, vomiting, and raised BP. Practise active management of third stage of labour.
- Prophylactic oxytocin versus no uterotonic – oxytocin reduced the risk of PPH by about 60% and the need for therapeutic oxytocics by about 50%. Offer routine prophylactic oxytocics to all women.
- Prophylactic ergometrine–oxytocin (Syntometrine) vs oxytocin – Syntometrine, oxytocin 5 IU, and oxytocin 10 IU have similar efficacy in prevention of PPH >1000 ml. In cases of PPH of at least 500 ml, there is a small reduction in the risk of PPH with Syntometrine. Syntometrine has a 5-fold increased risk in the unpleasant side effects of nausea, vomiting, and elevation of BP. Thus, balance the adverse effects associated with the use of Syntometrine. For women without risk factors for PPH loss against the adverse effects associated with the use of Syntometrine. Syntometrine may be used in the absence of HT as it reduces the risk of minor PPH but increases vomiting.
- For women delivering by CS use oxytocin (5 IU by slow IV) to decrease blood loss (NICE).
- Bolus dose of oxytocin is inappropriate in women with cardiovascular disorders – low-dose infusion is safer.
- Prostaglandins – injectable uterotonics are preferable to prostaglandins for routine prophylaxis.
- Misoprostol is not as effective when compared with oxytocin (10 IU IV) in preventing PPH; it also carries increased adverse effects, which are dose related. However, it may be used in a home-birth setting.
- Carbetocin – a longer-acting oxytocin derivative, is licensed in the UK specifically for the indication of prevention of PPH in the context of CS. A single dose (100 μg) of carbetocin is as effective as oxytocin by infusion. Do not use it routinely because of the paucity of data and its high price.

Management

Four components, all of which must be undertaken simultaneously: communication with relevant professionals; resuscitation; monitoring and investigation; measures to arrest the bleeding.

1. Communication

- **Minor PPH** – basic measures: alert the midwife-in-charge; first-line obstetric and anaesthetic staff.
- **Major PPH (major obstetric haemorrhage [MOH])** – full protocol: call experienced midwife (in addition to midwife in charge), obstetric middle grade and alert consultant, anaesthetic middle grade and alert consultant, porters for delivery of specimens/blood, alert consultant clinical haematologist on call, alert BT laboratory, one member of the team to record events, fluids, drugs, and vital signs.
- Use of the term 'controlled MOH' or 'ongoing MOH' to define the urgency.
- Communicate with the patient and her birthing partner.

3. Monitoring and investigation

Minor PPH – basic measures:
- Group and screen; FBC; coagulation screen including fibrinogen.
- Pulse and BP every 15 minutes.

Major PPH/MOH – full protocol:
- Crossmatch (4 units minimum); FBC; coagulation screen including fibrinogen; renal and liver function for baseline.
- Monitor continuous pulse, BP and respiratory rate; temperature every 15 minutes. Record on a flow chart such as the MOEWS charts or ICU-style charts.
- Foley catheter to monitor urine output.
- Monitor and document fluid balance, blood, blood products, and procedures.
- Replace blood lost aided by the results of FBC and clotting screen, under the guidance of a haematologist and/or consultant in transfusion medicine.
- Central venous and direct arterial pressure monitoring if the cardiovascular system is compromised. The presence of a central line not only provides a means of accurate CVP monitoring but also a route for rapid fluid replacement.
- Transfer to ITU/HDU on delivery suite, once the bleeding is controlled, depending on the severity of the blood loss.

2. Resuscitation

- 'ABC' with a process of simultaneous evaluation and resuscitation.
- **A and B – assess airway and breathing.**
- **Oxygen (10–15 l/minute) via a facemask.** If the airway is compromised owing to impaired conscious level, get anaesthetic assistance urgently. Usually level of consciousness and airway control improve rapidly once the circulating volume is restored.
- **C – evaluate circulation**
- **Two 14-gauge IV lines;** take 20 ml blood sample for diagnostic tests – FBC, coagulation screen, urea and electrolytes, and crossmatch (4 units).
- **Minor PPH – basic measures** – IV access (14-gauge cannula × 1); commence crystalloid infusion.
- **Major PPH/MOH – full protocol:**
  * Position flat; keep the woman warm.
  * Transfuse blood ASAP.
  * Fluid therapy and blood product transfusion
    > Crystalloid up to 2 litres Hartmann's solution.
    > Colloid up to 1–2 litres until blood arrives.
    > Blood – crossmatched; if not available uncrossmatched group-specific blood OR 'O RhD negative' blood.
    > Fresh frozen plasma – 4 units for every 6 units of red cells or prothrombin time/activated partial thromboplastin time > 1.5 × normal (12–15 ml/kg or total 1 litres).
    > Platelet concentrates if PLT count < 50 × 10⁹.
    > Cryoprecipitate if fibrinogen < 1 g/l.
  * Use the best equipment available to achieve rapid warmed infusion of fluids.
  * Do not use special blood filters as they slow infusions.
    > Use of recombinant factor VIIa therapy is based on the results of coagulation.

5. Anaesthetic management

- To assess the woman quickly, to initiate or continue resuscitation to restore intravascular volume and provide adequate anaesthesia.
- The presence of cardiovascular instability is a relative contraindication to regional anaesthesia. Blockage of the sympathetic system can potentially lead to worsening hypotension due to haemorrhage.
- If cardiovascular stability has been achieved and there is no evidence of coagulation failure, regional anaesthesia can be used.
- Continuous epidural block is preferred over spinal, as it allows better BP control and for prolonged surgery.
- When there is continuing bleeding and the cardiovascular stability is compromised, general anaesthesia is more appropriate. Rapid sequence induction is the gold standard to reduce the risk of aspiration.

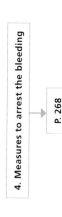

4. Measures to arrest the bleeding

P. 268

Fluids for volume resuscitation

The therapeutic goals of management of massive blood loss are to maintain: haemoglobin > 8g/dl; platelet count >75 × 10⁹/l; prothrombin <1.5 × mean control; activated prothrombin times <1.5 × mean control; fibrinogen >1.0g/l.

Fluid replacement

- Total volume of 3.5 litres of clear fluids (up to 2 litres of warmed Hartmann's solution as rapidly as possible, followed by up to a further 1.5 litres of warmed colloid if blood still not available) is the maximum to be infused while awaiting compatible blood.
- The nature of fluid infused is of less importance than rapid administration and warming of the infusion.

Blood transfusion

- If fully crossmatched blood is unavailable by the time that 3.5 litres of clear fluid have been infused:
  * **Group O RhD-negative blood** is the safest way to avoid a mismatched transfusion. In an extreme situation and when the blood group is unknown, give O RhD-negative red cells (these may be incompatible for patients with irregular antibodies).
  * For most women, the ABO and rhesus groups will have been determined on a current admission sample; if not, testing on a new sample takes 10 minutes; then **ABO & D group-compatible, uncrossmatched** blood can be issued.
- If irregular antibodies are found, or are known to have been present on a previous occasion, then **blood must be crossmatched**. Antibodies may delay crossmatch greatly.

Blood components

- When the blood loss reaches > 4.5 litres (80% of blood volume) and large volumes of replacement fluids have been given, there will be clotting factor defects.
- Follow results of coagulation studies and the advice of a haematologist to guide transfusion of coagulation factors.
- Up to 1 litre of FFP and 10 units of cryoprecipitate (two packs) may be given empirically in the face of relentless bleeding, while awaiting the results of coagulation studies.
- Order these blood products as soon as a need is anticipated, as there is a short delay in supply because of the need for thawing.

Antifibrinolytic drugs

- Fibrinolytic inhibitors such as tranexamic acid may have a place in the management of MOH.

Recombinant factor VIIa (rFVIIa)

- **In the face of life-threatening PPH, and in consultation with a haematologist, rFVIIa may be used as an adjuvant to standard pharmacological and surgical treatments.**
- There have been case reports of thrombosis with its use in cardiac surgery.
- Women with severe PPH are particularly susceptible to defibrination (severe hypofibrinogenaemia); rFVIIa will not work if there is no fibrinogen and effectiveness may also be suboptimal with severe thrombocytopenia (< 20 × 10⁹/l). Therefore, fibrinogen should be above 1g/l and platelets > 20 × 10⁹/l before rFVIIa is given. If there is a suboptimal clinical response to rFVIIa, these should be checked and acted on (cryoprecipitate, fibrinogen concentrate or platelet transfusion) before a second dose is given.
- **Do not use rFVIIa for prophylaxis to reduce blood loss for CS.**
- **The availability of rFVIIa is limited, owing to its financial cost.**
- **The efficacy and safety of the use of rFVIIa for cases of MOH remains to be established.**

4. Measures to arrest the bleeding

The most common cause of primary PPH is uterine atony. However, examine to exclude other or additional causes: retained products (placenta, membranes, clots); vaginal/cervical lacerations or haematoma; ruptured uterus; broad ligament haematoma; extragenital bleeding; uterine inversion.

Uterine atony

Mechanical and pharmacological strategies

1. Bimanual uterine compression.
2. Ensure bladder is empty (Foley catheter, leave in place).
3. **Syntocinon 5 units by slow IV (may have repeat dose).**
4. **Ergometrine 0.5 mg by slow IV/IM (contraindicated in HT).**
5. **Syntocinon infusion (40 units in 500 ml Hartmann's solution at 125 ml/hour)**
   Oxytocin is to be preferred initially especially in women with prior HT or PET. Due to the risk of profound hypotension associated with oxytocin injection when given as an IV bolus, it should be given slowly in a dose of not more than 5 units.
6. **Carboprost 0.25 mg by IM repeated at intervals of not less than 15 min to a maximum of 8 doses (contraindicated in women with asthma).** Carboprost – successful in controlling haemorrhage, without resort to surgical means in 85–95% of cases.
7. **Direct intramyometrial injection of carboprost 0.5 mg** (responsibility of the administering clinician as it is not recommended for intramyometrial use). Use intramyometrial injection of carboprost if bleeding occurs at the time of CS and if laparotomy is undertaken following failure of pharmacological management once the uterus is exposed. It is also possible to inject intramyometrial carboprost through the abdominal wall in the absence of laparotomy.
8. **Misoprostol 1000 µg rectally** – where parenteral prostaglandins are not available or where there are contraindications (usually asthma) to prostaglandin F2α, misoprostol (prostaglandin E1) may be an appropriate alternative. There is no evidence on the use of misoprostol with breastfeeding, therefore consider a washout period of usually 24 hours.

Failure to control the haemorrhage

Intrauterine balloon tamponade

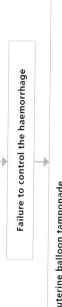

- **Balloon tamponade can avoid hysterectomy in up to 78% of women.**
- Tamponade using various types of hydrostatic balloon catheter (Foley catheter, Bakri balloon, Sengstaken–Blakemore oesophageal catheter, and a condom catheter) has superseded uterine packing for control of atonic PPH. The urological Rusch balloon is preferable by virtue of larger capacity, ease of use, and low cost.
- **Tamponade test** – a 'positive test' (control of PPH following inflation of the balloon) indicates that laparotomy is not required, whereas a 'negative test' (continued PPH following inflation of the balloon) is an indication to proceed to laparotomy.
- There is no clear evidence on how long the balloon tamponade should be left in place. In most cases, 4–6 hours of tamponade is adequate to achieve haemostasis.

Compression of the aorta is a temporary but effective measure to allow time for resuscitation to catch up with the volume replacement and for the appropriate surgical support to arrive.

Failure to control the haemorrhage

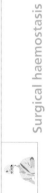

Surgical haemostasis

Haemostatic suturing

- **Haemostatic suture techniques are effective in controlling severe PPH and in reducing the need for hysterectomy in up to 81% of women.**
- Various versions – in the absence of comparative data to demonstrate that any one variant is superior to another, familiarize with one technique.
- B-Lynch (1997) – requires hysterotomy for its insertion therefore particularly suitable when the uterus has already been opened at CS. Reported success in 31/32 cases.
- Hayman (2002) – a modified compression suture which does not require hysterotomy; reported success in 10/11 women.
- Hwu – success in 14/14 women using a simplified technique of vertical compression sutures.
- Kafali – success in 3/3 women using a variant designed to control bleeding of cervical origin.
- Experience with these techniques is limited and few complications have been reported, such as a case of pyometra and partial uterine necrosis.

Internal iliac artery ligation

- Balloon tamponade and haemostatic suturing may be more effective than internal iliac artery ligation and they are easier to perform.
- Internal iliac artery ligation does not impair subsequent fertility and pregnancy outcomes.

Selective arterial occlusion/embolization

- Hysterectomy can be averted in up to 71% of women. The logistics of performing arterial occlusion/embolization where the equipment or an interventional radiologist may not be available mean that uterine balloon tamponade (which has similar efficacy) is a more appropriate first-line treatment.
- Consider it in cases of placenta praevia with accreta if intra-arterial balloons can be placed in the radiology department before the woman goes to theatre for CS.
- It does not impair subsequent menstruation and fertility.

Failure to control the haemorrhage

Hysterectomy

- The decision should be made by an experienced consultant clinician (preferably after discussion with a second experienced consultant clinician) and the procedure should be carried out by a surgeon who is experienced in carrying out hysterectomy.
- Do not delay hysterectomy until the woman is in extremis or while less definitive procedures with which the surgeon has little experience are attempted. Resort to hysterectomy sooner rather than later (especially in cases of placenta accreta or uterine rupture).
- Subtotal hysterectomy is the operation of choice in many instances of PPH requiring hysterectomy unless there is trauma to the cervix or lower segment.

Postoperative care

- Thromboprophylaxis – once the bleeding is arrested and any coagulopathy is corrected, provide thromboprophylaxis as there is a high risk of thrombosis. Use pneumatic compression devices if thromboprophylaxis is contraindicated in cases of thrombocytopenia.
- Continuous physiological monitoring – record parameters over time on a flowchart that will give the reader good visual cues on the clinical progress of the patient. Continually re-evaluate the woman's physiological condition even when bleeding appears to have stopped, to recognize continuing bleeding.
- Proper follow-up and investigations as necessary, such as screening for coagulopathies if there are other indicators and screening for the rare complication of panhypopituitarism (Sheehan syndrome) secondary to hypotension.

Indications for using interventional radiology in PPH

- Access to the anterior division of the internal iliac arteries via a femoral artery approach and subsequent embolization with a suitable embolic material under image guidance.
- Access to imaging is essential.

Emergency intervention

- PPH secondary to:
  * Atonic uterus with or without CS.
  * Surgical complications or uterine tears at the time of CS.
  * Bleeding following hysterectomy.

Elective and prophylactic intervention

- As a prophylactic measure where there is a known or suspected case of placenta accreta, such as placenta praevia on previous CS scar, or placenta accreta diagnosed by scan/colour Doppler or MRI. Balloons are placed in the internal iliac or uterine arteries before delivery. The balloons can be inflated to occlude the vessels in the event of PPH. Embolization can be performed via the balloon catheters if bleeding continues despite inflation. Even if hysterectomy is still required, blood loss, BT, and numbers of admissions to ICU can be reduced.

Secondary PPH

Investigations

- High and low vaginal swabs, blood cultures if pyrexial, FBC, CRP.
- A pelvic USS may help to exclude the presence of retained products of conception, although the appearance of the immediate postpartum uterus may be unreliable.
- Secondary PPH is often associated with infection (endometritis). Treatment involves:
  * Uterotonics – in continuing haemorrhage, insertion of balloon catheter may be effective.
  * Antibiotics – combination of ampicillin (clindamycin if penicillin allergic) and metronidazole. In cases of endomyometritis (tender uterus) or overt sepsis, add gentamicin. This antibiotic therapy does not contraindicate breastfeeding.
  * Surgical measures if there is excessive or continuing bleeding, irrespective of USS findings. Be cautious as any evacuation of retained products of conception carries a high risk for uterine perforation.

Risk management

- Training – annual 'skill drills'.
- Arrange a formal follow-up meeting which analyses the case and addresses what could be done better in the future for every significant PPH.
- Accurate documentation is essential.
- Debrief – MOH can be traumatic to the woman, her family, and the birth attendants, therefore debrief at the earliest opportunity.

Prevention and Management of Postpartum Haemorrhage. RCOG Green-top Guideline No. 52; May 2009; Minor revisions November 2009 and April 2011.

Currie J, Hogg M, Patel N, Madgwick K, Yoong W. Management of women who decline blood and blood products in pregnancy. The Obstetrician & Gynaecologist 2010;12:13–20.

The Role of Emergency and Elective Interventional Radiology in Postpartum Haemorrhage. RCOG Good Practice No. 6; 2007.

Background and prevalence

- Obstetric haemorrhage remains a major cause of maternal mortality in the UK, with substandard management identified as a contributor in 80% of cases.
- There are > 4000 cases of severe haemorrhage each year in the UK. The majority of these need BT.
- **Massive blood loss –**
  * loss of 1 litre blood volume within a 24-hour period. (Normal blood volume in the adult is approximately 7% of ideal body weight.); OR
  * loss of 50% blood volume within 3 hours or a rate of loss of 150 ml/min.

Risks

- BT may be a life-saving procedure but can result in morbidity and mortality if not managed correctly. Adverse events associated with transfusion:
  * Potential infection and potential transmission of prions.
  * Immunological sequelae such as red cell alloimmunization.
  * Transfusion-related acute lung injury.
  * Rising costs and the possible future problems of availability.
- The major risk is of a patient receiving an 'incorrect blood component'.
- In 2006 there were 4 deaths attributable to BT in the UK: 2 from incorrect prescribing, 1 from transfusion of platelets contaminated with *Klebsiella pneumoniae*, and 1 from transfusion-related acute lung injury.
- There is a potential for unrecognized transmission of pathogens. Until 2007, there were 4 reports of variant Creutzfeldt–Jakob disease in recipients of BT in the UK.

Prevention – reduce the chances of transfusion/strategies to minimize the use of banked blood

Identify and treat anaemia – if haemoglobin level is < 10.5 g/dl in the antenatal period, exclude haemoglobinopathies and consider haematinic deficiency.

- Oral iron is the preferred first-line treatment for iron deficiency.
- Parenteral iron when oral iron is not tolerated, or absorbed or patient is not compliant or is a late booker. It offers a shorter duration of treatment and a quicker response than oral therapy but is more invasive and expensive.
- Recombinant human erythropoietin (rHuEPO) is mostly used in the anaemia of end-stage renal disease. It has been used antenatally and postnatally in women without end-stage renal disease without any adverse maternal, fetal or neonatal effects. rHuEPO for non-end-stage renal anaemia should only be used in the context of a controlled clinical trial.
- Blood transfusion – for anaemia not due to haematinic deficiency (haemoglobinopathies and bone marrow failure syndromes) in close conjunction with a haematologist.
- Optimal management of women on anticoagulants, such as LMWH, will minimize blood loss.

Intrapartum and postpartum anaemia – if the Hb is < 7 g/dl in labour or in the immediate postpartum period, where there is no continuing or threat of bleeding, decide to transfuse based on medical history, age, and symptoms. In fit, healthy, asymptomatic patients there is little evidence for the benefit of BT.

- If unexpected severe bleeding is encountered, investigate postnatally for possible bleeding diatheses on a non-urgent basis at least 3–6 months after delivery.

Pre-autologous blood deposit – blood can be pre-deposited and kept for up to 5 weeks. In pregnancy, there are concerns on placental insufficiency, whether the woman will make up her Hb before delivery, and whether the collected units will be sufficient in the event of major obstetric haemorrhage (MOH). It does not prevent the most common error in BT, which is 'incorrect blood component transfusion', nor does it alter the risk of bacterial contamination. Do not offer pre-autologous deposit in pregnancy.

Intraoperative cell salvage (IOCS)

- Blood shed within the surgical field is retrieved by an anticoagulated suction apparatus and collected in a reservoir from where it is centrifuged, washed, and pumped into an infusion bag. This salvaged blood can then be returned to the patient. This process is effective in reducing the need for allogenic red cell transfusion and has been widely used in adult orthopaedic and cardiac surgery without complication. The financial cost of cell salvage may be offset by savings accrued from reducing the amount of allogenic blood transfused.
- Safety concerns – amniotic fluid embolism and fetomaternal isoimmunization in future pregnancies. To minimize fetal contamination of the maternal circulation, a leucocyte depletion filter is used, with separate suction being used for amniotic fluid. However, it will not remove fetal blood cells and therefore adequate anti-D immunization is required to prevent rhesus immunization in RhD-negative women. A standard dose of anti-D is given and a Kleihauer test taken 1 hour after cell salvage has finished to determine whether further anti-D is required.
- Cell salvage is recommended for women in whom an intraoperative blood loss of > 1500 ml is anticipated. IOCS would not, therefore, be required for most CS.
- The total number of obstetric patients who have received salvaged blood in the published studies has been small and without any reported complications; however, the possibility of rare catastrophic events has not been ruled out.
- **The use of IOCS in obstetric practice has been limited.** IOCS has a role in the management of patients who refuse allogenic BT, and for those patients who are at risk of significant intraoperative haemorrhage (placenta percreta or accreta).

Management of major blood loss (MBL)

All delivery units, especially small units without a blood bank on site, should maintain a supply of O RhD-negative blood, as this might offer the only means of restoring oxygen-carrying capacity within an acceptable timescale.

service setup and strategies; red cells transfusion; recombinant factor VIIa (rFVIIa), see Chapter 54: Prevention and management of postpartum haemorrhage (PPH).

Blood components

Fresh frozen plasma (FFP) and cryoprecipitate

- Clinically significant fibrinogen deficiency develops after a loss of about 150% of blood volume – earlier than any other haemostatic abnormality when packed red cell concentrates are used in replacing MBL. Consider FFP before 1 blood volume is lost.
- **DIC** – dilution of coagulation factors is the primary cause of coagulopathy in MBL following volume replacement with crystalloid or colloid and transfusion of red cell components. During DIC, all coagulation factors, especially fibrinogen, factor V, factor VIII, and factor XIII are depleted. Obstetric conditions predisposing to DIC include amniotic fluid embolism, placental abruption, and PET. Suspect DIC when there is profuse bleeding from the site of trauma and oozing from the sites of venepuncture and IV line insertions. If DIC is strongly suspected and clotting studies take a long time, consider transfusion of FFP before results are available if haemorrhage is otherwise difficult to control.
- Once the FFP has been ordered, it takes at least 30 minutes to thaw and issue.
- Administer FFP 12–15 ml/kg to keep the activated partial thromboplastin time (APTT) and prothrombin time ratio < 1:5. Maintain fibrinogen levels above 1.0 g/l by the use of FFP or two pools of cryoprecipitate.
- In the UK most units of FFP (as is the case with red cells, platelets, and cryoprecipitate) are not virally inactivated, so transfusion with these products poses a small risk of transfusion transmitted infection.
- The FFP and cryoprecipitate should ideally be of the same group as the recipient. If unavailable, FFP of a different ABO group is acceptable, provided that it does not have a high titre anti-A or anti-B activity.
- No anti-D prophylaxis is required if an RhD-negative woman receives RhD-positive FFP or cryoprecipitate.

Postpartum anaemia

- Do not offer BT unless the haemoglobin level is < 7 g/dl.
- Healthy women can tolerate an acute drop in haemoglobin to 5 g/dl.
- Anaemia can be treated with iron.

Platelets

- The platelet count should not be allowed to fall < 50 × 10⁹/l in the acutely bleeding patient. A platelet transfusion trigger of 75 × 10⁹/l is recommended to provide a margin of safety.
- A platelet count of 50 × 10⁹/l is anticipated when approximately 2 blood volumes have been replaced by fluid or red cell components.
- Platelets may not be on-site in many units, so anticipate their need and communicate with the transfusion laboratory.
- Give RhD-negative platelets to RhD-negative women. The platelets should ideally also be group compatible. Give anti-RhD immunoglobulin (250 IU) if the platelets are RhD-positive and the recipient RhD-negative. This is not necessary if a caesarean hysterectomy has been performed.
- Anti-D immunoglobulin at a dose of 250 IU will be sufficient to cover five adult therapeutic doses of platelets given within a 6-week period. Doses may be given subcutaneously to minimize bruising and haematomata in women with thrombocytopenia.
- Do not transfuse platelets through a giving set previously used for red cells.

General principles of blood transfusion (BT)

- For all women check blood group and antibodies at booking and at 28 weeks.
- Group and screen or crossmatch samples according to local protocol. If any blood component therapy is contemplated, send a sample for group and screen to the BT laboratory.
- Patient blood samples used for crossmatching red cells should not be > 7 days old. Red cell alloimmunization is most likely to occur in the last trimester, therefore pre-transfusion sample should not be > 7 days old and ideally should be fresh.
- Anti-K in pregnancy is more likely to have been induced by previous transfusion which can be prevented with the use of Kell-negative blood for transfusion in women of childbearing age (high risk of alloimmunization and subsequent HDN, unless a woman is known to be Kell positive).
- Use CMV seronegative red cells and platelets for CMV seronegative pregnant women and where the CMV status is unknown to avoid transmission of CMV to the fetus, although the UK policy of universal leucocyte depletion substantially reduces if not eliminates the risk of CMV transmission. Do not delay urgent transfusion if CMV seronegative components are not immediately available.
- For women with placenta praevia, some obstetric centres make 2 units of crossmatched red cells available in the issue fridge. Replace these units every week.

Women who refuse blood transfusion

Background

- Women attending antenatal clinics – 8% did not want a BT.
- **Reasons** – religion and safety concerns.
- **Safety concerns** – as in previous pages.
- **Religious reasons** – Jehovah's Witnesses (members of a Christian group) – base their refusal of blood on the literal interpretation of certain biblical verses; and administration of blood or blood products to a Jehovah's Witness against their wishes is a gross physical violation.
- Although Jehovah's Witnesses do not accept the use of whole blood or primary blood components (red cells, platelets or plasma), the decision as to whether to accept clotting factors, autologous transfusion or immunoglobulin products such as anti-D is an individual one.
- Autologous pre-deposit is never acceptable to Jehovah's Witnesses, but cell salvage may be acceptable.
- Maternal mortality of women who decline blood is 100 times higher than that of the general population.

Blood conservation techniques

- Intraoperative cell salvage – as in previous pages. In Jehovah's Witness patients the system is set up as a continuous 'loop' which is pre-primed and run without disconnection until the end of the procedure.
- Acute normovolaemic haemodilution – this involves the removal of whole blood immediately preoperatively whilst simultaneously infusing colloid and/or crystalloids. This maintains the circulatory volume but reduces the haematocrit, thus resulting in a smaller red cell mass loss during surgery. There is some concern that this could precipitate cardiac failure or cause placental insufficiency and is probably not adequate in MOH. Currently there is insufficient evidence to recommend a firm conclusion on the efficacy or safety of acute normovolaemic haemodilution, particularly in an obstetric setting.
- Perioperative autologous donation – This has no role in emergency obstetric haemorrhage and is not acceptable to Jehovah's Witnesses. This may have a limited use in women having elective CS who are at a high risk of bleeding and in whom there are exceptional cross-matching difficulties.

Antenatal management

Preconceptual care – optimize haemoglobin levels.

Booking:

- Ask women whether they would accept a BT. If they are unsure, or state that they would decline, explore the reasons and explain the implications.
- Classify as high risk and manage as consultant-led care.
- Routine booking bloods for FBC and group and screen. Discuss about anti-D in rhesus-negative women, including the fact that it is obtained from human blood products.

Advance directives – encourage women to complete an advance directive, which is a legally binding document and is carried in the hand-held notes. A woman can always change her mind about the use of blood products. Establish which blood products (immunoglobulin or clotting factors) or blood sparing techniques (if any) are acceptable.

- Discuss available blood conservation techniques in advance and record their acceptability in the advance directive.

Optimize iron stores – as in previous pages. IV iron sucrose complex increases the rate of rise in haemoglobin in pregnant women more rapidly than oral ferrous sulphate, with no documented serious adverse effects.

Identifying risk factors for haemorrhage:

- Assess placental site; presence of fibroids.
- Clotting disorders; review use of anticoagulant or antiplatelet drugs.

- **Legal issues** – In the UK, a woman may decline any treatment even if this would lead to her demise as long as she is competent and does so voluntarily, no matter how unusual her decision may appear. Advance directives are legally valid and to administer blood to a woman carrying a 'no blood' advance directive would constitute battery. In an emergency, if there is no objective evidence of the woman's beliefs, the doctor must act in the best interests of the woman following discussion with her relatives to gain further information regarding her beliefs.

Intrapartum management

- **Place of delivery** – At a regional centre with intensive care, cell salvage facilities, recombinant factor VII, interventional radiology, and staff who are familiar with the management of women who decline blood products.
- Confirm with the woman that the wishes she has expressed in an advance directive are still strongly held.
- Inform senior obstetric, anaesthetic, midwifery, and haematology staff once the woman is in labour. A consultant obstetrician either performs or directly supervises the CS if the procedure is indicated.
- IV access and FBC.
- If the woman has consented to cell salvage, set up the machine and inform the staff trained in its use.
- In women with an additional risk of bleeding, such as placenta praevia or complicated CS, consider elective interventional radiological techniques.

Active management of the third stage

- Repair perineal damage promptly.
- **Treat PPH aggressively.**
- Anticipate and treat MOH aggressively.
- In addition to standard pharmacological treatment for uterine atony, consider insertion of intrauterine compression balloons and the use of uterine compression sutures.
- Uterine or iliac artery embolization or ligation may be attempted before proceeding to caesarean hysterectomy.
- Maintain a lower threshold for medical and surgical management, including hysterectomy.
- Recombinant factor VIIa – consider or plan in advance with the haematologist.

Currie J, Hogg M, Patel N, Madgwick K, Yoong W. Management of women who decline blood and blood products in pregnancy. The Obstetrician & Gynaecologist 2010;12:13–20.

Prevention and Management of Postpartum Haemorrhage. RCOG Green-top Guideline No. 52; May 2009. Minor revisions November 2009 and April 2011.

Blood Transfusion in Obstetrics. RCOG Green-top Guideline No. 47; December 2007. Minor revisions July 2008. Please refer to updated guidelines from May 2015.

Background and prevalence

- An acute event involving the cardiorespiratory systems and/or brain, resulting in a reduced or absent conscious level (and potentially death), at any stage in pregnancy and up to 6 weeks after delivery.
- UK – the maternal mortality rate is 14/100 000 births, but not all maternal deaths are preceded by maternal collapse. The true rate of maternal collapse lies somewhere between 0.14 and 6/1000 births.

Causes of maternal collapse

4 H's

- Hypovolaemia — Bleeding (may be concealed) (obstetric/other) or relative hypovolaemia of dense spinal block, septic or neurogenic shock
- Hypoxia — Pregnant patients can become hypoxic more quickly Cardiac events: peripartum cardiomyopathy, myocardial infarction, aortic dissection, large-vessel aneurysms
- Hypo/hyperkalaemia and other electrolyte disturbances — No more likely than non-pregnant
- Hypothermia — No more likely than non-pregnant

4 T's

- Thromboembolism — Amniotic fluid embolus, PE, air embolus, myocardial infarction
- Toxicity — Local anaesthetic, magnesium, other
- Tension pneumothorax
- Tamponade (cardiac)
- Eclampsia and pre-eclampsia — Includes intracranial haemorrhage

Prevention

- Maternal collapse occurs with no prior warning in some, although there may be existing risk factors. Often there are clinical signs that precede collapse.
- The first early warning scoring (EWS) systems were introduced on the basis that a deterioration in simple physiological vital signs will precede significant clinical deterioration, and that early intervention will reduce morbidity. EWS systems have not been demonstrated to be highly effective.
- The physiological changes of pregnancy may render the existing EWS systems inappropriate, and no validated system for use in the pregnant woman currently exists. There is continuing work to develop a national obstetrics EWS system.
- Use an obstetric early warning score chart routinely for all women, to allow early recognition of the woman who is becoming critically ill.

Outcomes for mother and baby

- In a review on maternal and fetal outcomes for perimortem CS over an 18-year period from 1986 to 2004, there were 38 procedures, 30 of which resulted in surviving babies (25–42 weeks of gestation) most often with a collapse to delivery interval of ≤ 5 minutes.
  In 18 cases, the cause of the collapse was felt to be irreversible. Of the 20 cases in which the cause of collapse was known and felt to be reversible, 13 women survived, giving a survival rate of 65%. This review also demonstrated the positive effect of the delivery on the maternal circulation, supporting the advice of achieving delivery within 5 minutes of collapse if CPR is ineffective.
- CEMACH reported the neonatal outcomes of the 52 perimortem or postmortem CS that were performed in which the mothers did not survive. 54% babies were liveborn, although 8 out of these 28 babies died in the early neonatal period.
- Neonatal survival is associated with advanced gestation and delivery within a delivery suite or critical care setting, and not the emergency department.

Causes of maternal collapse

- May be pregnancy related or result from conditions pre-existing before pregnancy.
- Common reversible causes of collapse – 4 H's and 4 T's added with eclampsia and intracranial haemorrhage.

Haemorrhage is the most common cause. In most cases of MOH leading to collapse, the cause is obvious, but also consider concealed haemorrhage such as ruptured ectopic, splenic artery rupture, and hepatic rupture.

Sepsis – bacteraemia, which can be present in the absence of pyrexia or a raised white cell count, can progress rapidly to severe sepsis and septic shock leading to collapse. The most common organisms implicated in obstetrics are the streptococcal groups A, B, and D, pneumococcus, and *E. coli*.

Cardiac disease

- Most common overall cause of maternal death in CEMACH report 2003–2005 (48 maternal deaths).
- The majority of women have no previous history. The main causes of death are myocardial infarction, aortic dissection, and cardiomyopathy.
- The incidence of primary cardiac arrest in pregnancy is around 1/30 000 maternities, and most cardiac events have preceding signs and symptoms.
- Aortic root dissection can present in otherwise healthy women, with signs and symptoms such as central chest or interscapular pain, a wide pulse pressure, mainly secondary to systolic HT, and a new cardiac murmur – refer to a cardiologist for appropriate imaging.
- The incidence of congenital and rheumatic heart disease in pregnancy is increasing due to increased survival rates owing to improved management of congenital heart disease and increased immigration – MDT care in regional centres.
- Other cardiac causes include dissection of the coronary artery, acute left ventricular failure, infective endocarditis, and pulmonary oedema.

Thromboembolism (33 PE and 8 cerebral vein thrombosis) is the most common cause of direct maternal death. (CEMACH 2003–2005)

Amniotic fluid embolism (AFE)

- The estimated frequency is 2/100 000 maternities. Survival rates have improved over time, from 14% in 1979 to around 30% in 2005 and 80% in 2010, although neurological morbidity in survivors is well recognized. The perinatal mortality rate is 135/1000 total births.
- AFE presents as collapse during labour or delivery or within 30 minutes of delivery in the form of acute hypotension, respiratory distress, and acute hypoxia. Seizures and cardiac arrest may occur. There are different phases to disease progression, which clearly impacts on maternal survival. Initially, pulmonary hypertension may develop secondary to vascular occlusion either by debris or by vasoconstriction. This often resolves and left ventricular dysfunction or failure develops. Coagulopathy often develops if the mother survives long enough, often giving rise to massive PPH.

Drug toxicity/overdose

- Therapeutic drug toxicity – magnesium sulphate in the presence of renal impairment and local anaesthetic agents injected intravenously by accident.
- Local anaesthetic toxicity resulting from systemic absorption of the local anaesthetic may occur some time after the initial injection. Effects include: a feeling of inebriation and light headedness followed by sedation, circumoral paraesthesia and twitching, convulsions with severe toxicity. On IV injection, convulsions and cardiovascular collapse may occur very rapidly. Signs of severe toxicity include sudden loss of consciousness, with or without tonic–clonic convulsions, and cardiovascular collapse with sinus bradycardia, conduction blocks, asystole, and ventricular tachyarrhythmias.
- Total spinal block or high spinal/epidural block are rarer and usually easily recognized causes of collapse.

Eclampsia

- Eclampsia is usually obvious in the inpatient setting, as often the diagnosis of PET has already been made and the seizure witnessed.
- Consider epilepsy in cases of maternal collapse associated with seizure activity.

Intracranial haemorrhage

- Intracranial haemorrhage is a complication of uncontrolled, particularly systolic HT but can also result from ruptured aneurysms and arteriovenous malformations.
- Initial presentation may be maternal collapse, but often severe headache precedes.

Other causes

- Hypoglycaemia and other metabolic/electrolyte disturbances, other causes of hypoxia such as airway obstruction secondary to aspiration/foreign body, air embolism, tension pneumothorax, cardiac tamponade secondary to trauma, and hypothermia.

Anaphylaxis

- Anaphylaxis is a severe, life-threatening generalized or systemic hypersensitivity reaction resulting in respiratory, cutaneous, and circulatory changes and, possibly, gastrointestinal disturbance and collapse. There is significant intravascular volume redistribution, which can lead to decreased cardiac output. Acute ventricular failure and MI may occur.
- Upper airway occlusion secondary to angioedema, bronchospasm, and mucous plugging of smaller airways all contribute to significant hypoxia and difficulties with ventilation. Common triggers are a variety of drugs, latex, animal allergens, and foods.
- The incidence is 3–10/1000, with a mortality rate of around 1%.
- Anaphylaxis is likely when all of the following 3 criteria are met:
  * Sudden onset and rapid progression of symptoms.
  * Life-threatening airway and/or breathing and/or circulation problems.
  * Skin and/or mucosal changes (flushing, urticaria, angioedema).
- Exposure to a known allergen supports the diagnosis, but many cases occur with no previous history. Mast cell tryptase levels can be useful.

Optimal initial management

Ɍ **Standard A, B, C approach, with some modification**

Help

- Call the obstetric resuscitation team; senior midwife; consultant obstetrician and anaesthetist; neonatal team if > 22 weeks of gestation.
- If the woman survives, involve a consultant intensivist ASAP.

Tilt – from 20 weeks of gestation onwards, relieve the pressure of the gravid uterus from the inferior vena cava and aorta. A left lateral tilt of 15° on a firm surface will relieve aortocaval compression and still allow effective chest compressions.

In the pregnant woman of 20 weeks or more gestation – physiological and anatomical changes of pregnancy.

- Aortocaval compression significantly reduces cardiac output from 20 weeks of gestation onwards.
- Aortocaval compression significantly reduces the efficacy of chest compressions during resuscitation.
- Changes in lung function, diaphragmatic splinting, and increased oxygen consumption make the pregnant woman become hypoxic more readily and make ventilation more difficult.
- Pregnant women are at an increased risk of aspiration.
- Difficult intubation is more likely in pregnancy.
- Increased cardiac output and hyperdynamic circulation of pregnancy mean that large volumes of blood can be lost rapidly, especially from the uterus, which receives 10% of the cardiac output at term.

Airway

- Clear and protect the airway as early as possible followed by intubation **with a cuffed endotracheal tube.** This will protect the airway, ensure good oxygen delivery, and facilitate more efficient ventilation.
- Pregnant women are more likely to regurgitate and aspirate in the absence of a secured airway (tracheal tube) than the non-pregnant patient.

Breathing

- Because of the increased oxygen requirements and rapid onset of hypoxia in pregnancy, ensure optimal oxygen delivery by high-flow 100% oxygen ASAP.
- Undertake bag and mask ventilation until intubation can be achieved.
- Ventilation, by facemask, by a supraglottic airway device and self-inflating bag, or by a cuffed endotracheal tube may be more difficult because of the physiological changes of pregnancy.

- Hand position over the centre of the chest, with the direction of compression perpendicular to the chest wall, thus the angle of tilt must be taken into account.
- **Compressions at a ratio of 30:2.**
- Ventilations unless the woman is intubated, in which case chest compressions and ventilations should be desynchronized, with compressions being performed at a rate of 100/minute and ventilations at a rate of 10/minute.

Circulation

- **In the absence of breathing despite a clear airway, commence chest compressions immediately** and continue until the cardiac rhythm can be checked and cardiac output confirmed.
- Compressions may be difficult because of obesity and the tilted position.
- Insert 2 wide-bore cannulae ASAP with an aggressive approach to volume.
- Abdominal USS can assist in the diagnosis of concealed haemorrhage.

- Because chest compressions are not as effective after 20 weeks of gestation take early recourse to delivery of the fetus and placenta if CPR is not effective. **If no response to CPR after 4 minutes, proceed to delivery/perimortem CS.**

Defibrillation

- Use the same defibrillation energy levels as in the non-pregnant patient as there is no change in thoracic impedance.
- Adhesive defibrillator pads are preferable to defibrillator paddles; apply the left defibrillation pad lateral to the left breast. The energy from the defibrillation shock is directed across the heart and there is no evidence that shocks from a direct current defibrillator have an adverse effect on the fetus.

Drugs

- There is no alteration in algorithm drugs or doses.
- Consider common, reversible causes of maternal cardiopulmonary arrest throughout the resuscitation process.
- Continue resuscitation efforts until a decision is taken by the consultant obstetrician and consultant anaesthetist in consensus with the cardiac arrest team.

Assess rhythm

Non-shockable (PEA/asystole)

Immediately resume CPR for 2 minutes; minimize interruptions

Reversible causes:

- Hypoxia
- Hypovolaemia
- Hypo-/hyperkalaemia/metabolic
- Hypothermia
- Thrombosis – coronary or pulmonary
- Tamponade – cardiac
- Toxins
- Tension pneumothorax

Return of spontaneous circulation

Immediate postcardiac arrest treatment

- Use ABCDE approach
- Controlled oxygenation and ventilation
- 12-lead ECG
- Treat precipitating cause
- Temperature control/therapeutic hypothermia

Shockable (VF/pulseless VT)

1 shock – 150–360 J biphasic or 360 J monophasic

Immediately resume CPR for 2 minutes; minimize interruptions

During CPR:

- Ensure high-quality CPR: rate, depth, recoil
- Plan actions before interrupting CPR
- Give oxygen
- Consider advanced airway and capnography
- Continuous chest compressions when advanced airway in place
- Vascular access (intravenous, intraosseus)
- Give adrenaline every 3–5 minutes
- Correct reversible causes

Perimortem caesarean section

When

- The pregnant woman becomes hypoxic more quickly than the non-pregnant woman, and irreversible brain damage can ensue within 4–6 minutes. The gravid uterus impairs venous return and reduces cardiac output secondary to aortocaval compression. Delivery of the fetus and placenta reduces oxygen consumption, improves venous return and cardiac output, facilitates chest compressions, and makes ventilation easier.
- Before 20 weeks of gestation there is no proven benefit from delivery of the fetus and placenta.
- Perimortem CS is a resuscitative procedure, performed primarily in the interests of maternal, not fetal, survival. Delivery within 5 minutes of maternal collapse improves the chances of survival for the baby, but this is not the reason for delivery. Therefore it is indicated even if the fetus is already dead. There is a possibility of a severely damaged surviving child, but the interests of the mother must come first.
- If there is no response to correctly performed CPR within 4 minutes of maternal collapse or if resuscitation is continued beyond this in women beyond 20 weeks of gestation, deliver to assist maternal resuscitation within 5 minutes of the collapse.

Where

- Do not delay perimortem CS by moving the woman; perform where resuscitation is taking place.
- A scalpel is the only essential equipment required.
- With no circulation, blood loss is minimal and no anaesthetic is required.
- If resuscitation is successful following delivery, transfer to an appropriate environment at that point, as well as anaesthesia and sedation, to control ensuing haemorrhage and complete the operation.
- The doctrine of 'the best interests of the patient' would apply to conduct of this procedure being carried out without consent.

How

- Use the incision that will facilitate the most rapid access.
- A midline abdominal incision and a classic uterine incision will give the most rapid access, but many will be unfamiliar with this approach and, as delivery can be achieved rapidly with a transverse approach, use the approach you are most comfortable with. If resuscitation is successful, close the uterus and abdomen in the usual way to control blood loss and minimize the risk of infection.
- A perimortem CS tray should be available on the resuscitation trolley in all areas where maternal collapse may occur, including the accident and emergency department.

Continuing management – depends on the underlying cause

- Involve senior staff with appropriate experience at an early stage.
- Transfer to a high-dependency/critical care area with appropriate staff and monitoring facilities.

Haemorrhage See Chapter 30 Antepartum haemorrhage (APH) and Chapter 54 Prevention and management of postpartum haemorrhage (PPH).

Thromboembolism See Chapter 43 Prevention and treatment of thrombosis and embolism during pregnancy and the puerperium.

Sepsis See Chapter 60 Bacterial sepsis following pregnancy. The speed and appropriateness of therapy in the initial hours after severe sepsis develops are likely to influence outcome.

Cardiac disease

- Care by cardiology team, which is similar to that in the non-pregnant state, although delivery will be necessary to facilitate this.
- Thrombolysis can be associated with significant bleeding from the placental site; however, it is indicated in women with acute coronary insufficiency, although caution is necessary.
- Percutaneous angioplasty for accurate diagnosis and definitive therapy.

Amniotic fluid embolism (AFE)

- Supportive management, as there is no proven effective therapy.
- Early involvement of senior experienced staff – obstetrician, anaesthetist, haematologist, and intensivist to optimize outcome.
- Arrhythmias may develop and will require standard treatment.
- Inotropic support and measurement of cardiac output may help direct therapy and avoid fluid overload, as this will exacerbate pulmonary oedema and increases the risk of acute respiratory distress syndrome.
- High filling pressures are indicative of a failing left ventricle.
- Coagulopathy – early, aggressive treatment, including use of fresh frozen plasma. The incidence of uterine atony and PPH is increased.
- Various other therapies have been tried, e.g., steroids, heparin, plasmapheresis, and haemofiltration. There is no robust evidence to support their use.

Eclampsia See Chapter 27 Pre-eclampsia (PET) and eclampsia.

Intracranial haemorrhage

- Involve expert neuroradiologist to establish an accurate diagnosis.
- Management as in the non-pregnant state.

Other causes – direct management towards correction of specific causes.

Drug toxicity/overdose

- Many drug overdoses have specific therapy dependent on the drug in question; seek appropriate help.
- *Magnesium sulphate* – the antidote is 10 ml 10% calcium gluconate by slow IV injection.
- *Local anaesthetic agents* – if suspected, stop injecting immediately. Lipid rescue with Intralipid 20% in cases of collapse secondary to local anaesthetic toxicity. Continue CPR throughout this process until an adequate circulation is restored which may take over an hour.
- Manage arrhythmias as usual – they may be very refractory to treatment.
- Prolonged resuscitation may be necessary.
- Some may consider the use of cardiopulmonary bypass.

Anaphylaxis

- Remove all potential causative agents.
- 500 µg (0.5 ml) of 1:1000 adrenaline IM. It can be repeated after 5 minutes if there is no effect. It can be given IV as a 50 µg bolus (0.5 ml of 1:10000 solution).
- Adjuvant therapy – chlorpheniramine 10 mg and hydrocortisone 200 mg given IM or by slow IV injection.

Maternal Collapse in Pregnancy and the Puerperium. RCOG Green-top Guideline No. 56; January 2011.

Background and prevalence

- **Cord prolapse** – the descent of the umbilical cord through the cervix alongside (occult) or past the presenting part (overt) in the presence of ruptured membranes.
- **Cord presentation** – the presence of the umbilical cord between the fetal presenting part and the cervix, with or without membrane rupture.
- **Incidence** – 0.1%–0.6%.
- Higher incidence in breech presentation (the incidence is slightly higher than 1%), male fetuses, multiple gestation, prematurity and congenital malformations.

Antenatal diagnosis

- Routine USS is not sufficiently sensitive or specific for identification of cord presentation antenatally therefore do not perform to predict increased probability of cord prolapse outside a research setting.

Prevention of cord prolapse or its effects

- With transverse, oblique or unstable lie, inpatient care minimizes delays in diagnosis and management of cord prolapse. Consider elective admission to hospital after 37+6 weeks of gestation and advise women to present quickly if there are signs of labour or suspicion of membrane rupture.
- Offer admission to women with non-cephalic presentations and PPROM.
- Avoid ARM whenever possible if the presenting part is mobile. If it is necessary to rupture the membranes, perform it with arrangements in place for immediate CS.
- Vaginal examination and obstetric intervention in the context of ruptured membranes and a high presenting part carry the risk of upward displacement and cord prolapse. Keep upward pressure on the presenting part to a minimum in such women.
- Avoid rupture of membranes if, on vaginal examination, the cord is felt below the presenting part. Perform CS if cord presentation is diagnosed in established labour.

Risks or complications

- Birth asphyxia – hypoxic ischaemic encephalopathy and cerebral palsy. The principal causes of asphyxia are cord compression and umbilical arterial vasospasm preventing venous and arterial blood flow to and from the fetus.
- Perinatal mortality rate is 91/1000.

Risk factors for cord prolapse

- **General** – factors predispose to cord prolapse by preventing close application of the presenting part to the lower part of the uterus and/or pelvic brim.
  - * Multiparity. * Polyhydramnios. * Low-lying placenta.
  - * Other abnormal placentation. * Low birth weight, <2.5 kg. * Prematurity <37 weeks.
  - * Fetal congenital anomalies. * Second twin. * Breech presentation.
  - * Transverse, oblique, and unstable lie. * Unengaged presenting part.
- **Procedure related** – 50% of cases are preceded by obstetric manipulation. The manipulation of the fetus with or without prior membrane rupture and planned artificial rupture of membranes, particularly with an unengaged presenting part, are the interventions that most frequently precede cord prolapse.
  - * Artificial rupture of membranes. * Insertion of uterine pressure transducer.
  - * Vaginal manipulation of the fetus with ruptured membranes. * Stabilizing IOL.
  - * External cephalic version. * Internal podalic version.

DDx

Diagnosis or suspicion of cord prolapse/presentation

- Cord presentation/prolapse may occur without any physical signs and with a normal FHR pattern.
- With spontaneous rupture of membranes in the presence of normal FHR patterns and the absence of risk factors for cord prolapse, routine vaginal examination is not necessary if the liquor is clear.
- Suspect cord prolapse if there is an abnormal FHR pattern (bradycardia or variable fetal heart rate decelerations), particularly if such changes commence soon after membrane rupture. Prompt vaginal examination is the most important aspect of diagnosis.
- Examine for cord at every vaginal examination in labour and after spontaneous rupture of membranes if risk factors are present or if CTG abnormalities commence soon thereafter.
- Perform speculum and/or digital vaginal examination in preterm gestations if cord prolapse is suspected.

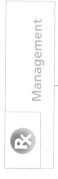

Management

Optimal initial management in hospital settings

- Cord prolapse before full dilatation – deliver immediately.
- Minimal handling of loops of cord prevents vasospasm.
- Elevate the presenting part to prevent cord compression by either:
  * Pushing the presenting part upwards manually.
  * Filling the urinary bladder.
  * Adopting the knee–chest position or head-down tilt (preferably in left-lateral position).
- Consider tocolysis while preparing for CS if there are persistent FHR abnormalities after attempts to prevent compression mechanically and when the delivery is likely to be delayed.
- Although the measures described above are potentially useful during preparation for delivery, they must not result in unnecessary delay.
- There are insufficient data to evaluate manual replacement of the prolapsed cord above the presenting part to allow continuation of labour. This practice is not recommended.

Optimal management in community settings

- Perinatal mortality is increased by more than 10-fold when cord prolapse occurs outside hospital compared with prolapse occurring inside hospital. Neonatal morbidity is also increased.
- Advise women to assume the knee–chest face-down position while waiting for hospital transfer.
- Transfer to the nearest consultant-led unit for delivery, unless an immediate vaginal examination by a competent professional reveals that a spontaneous vaginal delivery is imminent. Still prepare for transfer. During emergency ambulance transfer:
  * Use left-lateral position.
  * Elevate the presenting part by either manual or bladder filling. Community midwives should carry a Foley catheter for this purpose and equipment for fluid infusion. Minimal handling of loops of cord lying outside the vagina prevents vasospasm.

Optimal mode of delivery

- CS is associated with a lower PNM and reduced risk of Apgar score < 3 at 5 minutes compared with spontaneous vaginal delivery when delivery is not imminent. However, when vaginal birth is imminent, outcomes are similar or better when compared with CS.
- **CS** – when vaginal delivery is not imminent, to prevent hypoxia–acidosis.
  * **Category 1 CS** with the aim of delivering within 30 minutes or less if a suspicious or pathological FHR pattern is present.
  * **Category 2 CS** – for women in whom the FHR pattern is normal.
  * Regional anaesthesia may be considered in consultation with an experienced anaesthetist.
- **Operative vaginal birth** can be attempted at full dilatation if it is anticipated that delivery would be accomplished quickly and safely. Attempt vaginal birth only for those women with very favourable characteristics. Choose the instrument most appropriate to the clinical circumstances and level of skill.
- **Breech extraction** after internal podalic version for the second twin may be considered.
- A practitioner competent in the resuscitation of the newborn should be present.
- Take a paired cord blood sample for pH and base excess since a normal paired cord blood gas has a strong predictive value for the exclusion of intrapartum-related hypoxic ischaemic brain damage.

Optimal management of cord prolapse before viability

- Discuss expectant management if gestational age is at the limits of viability.
- Consider uterine cord replacement.
- At extreme preterm gestation (< 24 weeks) – can prolong pregnancy for up to 3 weeks. Prolongation of pregnancy at such gestational ages creates a chance of survival but morbidity from prematurity remains a serious problem.
- Counsel women on both continuation and termination of pregnancy.
- Some women may prefer to choose TOP.
- Consider delivery if there are signs of severe fetal compromise once viability has been reached or a gestational age associated with a reasonable neonatal outcome is achieved.

What not to do

- Routine USS for identification of cord presentation antenatally.
- Routine vaginal examination with spontaneous rupture of membranes in the presence of a normal FHR pattern and the absence of risk factors for cord prolapse.
- Manual replacement of the prolapsed cord above the presenting part to allow continuation of labour.

Clinical governance

- **Debriefing** – after severe obstetric emergencies, women might be psychologically affected with postnatal depression, post-traumatic stress disorder or fear of further childbirth. Offer postnatal debriefing by a professional competent in counselling.
- **Training** – ensure at least annual training in the management of obstetric emergencies including the management of cord prolapse. Annual training seems adequate for those already proficient but more frequent rehearsal is advisable for those initially lacking competency until skill acquisition is achieved.
- **Clinical incident reporting** – submit clinical incident forms.

Umbilical Cord Prolapse. RCOG Green-top Guideline; No. 50; April 2008.
Please refer to – Umbilical Cord Prolapse. RCOG Green-top Guideline No. 50; Nov. 2014.

CHAPTER 58 Neonatal resuscitation

- Most babies born at term need no resuscitation. For uncompromised babies, a delay in cord clamping of at least 1 minute or until the cord stops pulsating from the delivery is recommended as it improves iron status through early infancy. Data are limited on the risks or benefits of delayed cord clamping in the non-vigorous infant.

- HR is the key – the first sign of any improvement will be an increase in HR. Check HR by listening with a stethoscope. It can also be felt by palpating the umbilical cord but a slow rate at the cord is not always indicative of a truly slow HR. Feeling for peripheral pulses is not helpful.
- A healthy baby – will be born blue but with good tone, will cry within a few seconds and will have a good HR within a few minutes of birth (120–150 min).
- A less healthy baby – will be blue but will have less good tone, may have a slow heart rate (< 100 min), and may not establish adequate breathing by 90–120 s.
- An ill baby – will be pale and floppy, not breathing and with a slow or very slow or undetectable HR.
- A pulse oximeter is the best way of assessing HR and oxygenation which gives readings within 90 s of delivery. Use pulse oximetry for all deliveries where it is anticipated that the infant may have problems with transition or need resuscitation. In healthy babies, oxygen saturation increases gradually from approximately 60% soon after birth to over 90% at 10 min.
- Colour – using colour as a proxy for oxygen saturation is usually inaccurate. However, noting whether a baby is initially very pale and therefore either acidotic or anaemic may be an indicator for later therapeutic intervention.

- Most newborn babies have a relatively prominent occiput, which will tend to flex the neck if the baby is placed on his or her back on a flat surface; avoid it by placing some support under the shoulders of the baby, but be careful not to overextend the neck. If the baby is very floppy it may be necessary to apply chin lift or jaw thrust.
- Reserve airway suction only for babies who have obvious airway obstruction that cannot be rectified by appropriate positioning. Rarely, material may be blocking the oropharynx or trachea. In these situations, perform direct visualization and suction of the oropharynx. For tracheal obstruction, intubation and suction on withdrawal of the endotracheal tube may be effective.
- Laryngeal mask airways (LMAs) can be used effectively at birth to ventilate the lungs of babies. Consider if facemask ventilation is unsuccessful and tracheal intubation is unsuccessful or not feasible.

- Most babies have a good HR after birth and establish breathing by about 90 s.
- Until birth the baby's lungs will have been filled with fluid. Aeration of the lungs in these circumstances is likely to require sustained application of pressures of about 30 cm H_2O for 2–3 s.

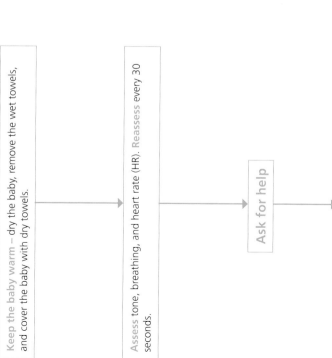

Keep the baby warm – dry the baby, remove the wet towels, and cover the baby with dry towels.

↓

Assess tone, breathing, and heart rate (HR). Reassess every 30 seconds.

↓

Ask for help

↓

Airway

The airway must be open – place the baby on his/her back with the head in the neutral position, i.e., with the neck neither flexed nor extended.

↓

Breathing

If the baby is not breathing adequately give 5 inflation breaths, preferably using air.

↓

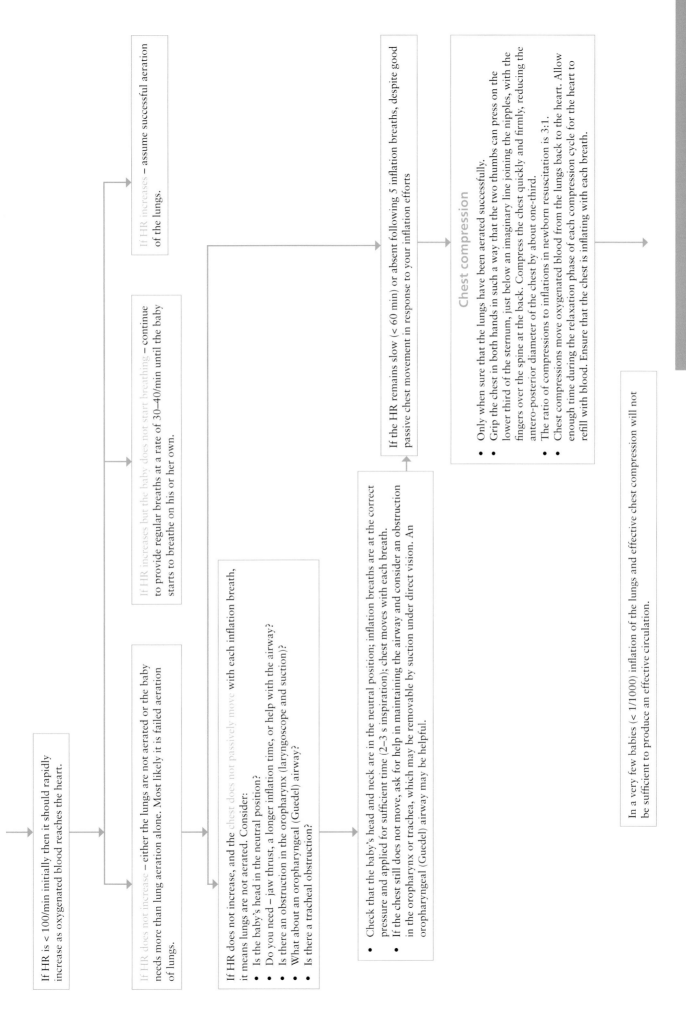

If HR is < 100/min initially then it should rapidly increase as oxygenated blood reaches the heart.

If HR does not increase – either the lungs are not aerated or the baby needs more than lung aeration alone. Most likely it is failed aeration of lungs.

If HR increases but the baby does not start breathing – continue to provide regular breaths at a rate of 30–40/min until the baby starts to breathe on his or her own.

If HR increases – assume successful aeration of the lungs.

If HR does nor increase, and the chest does not passively move with each inflation breath, it means lungs are not aerated. Consider:
• Is the baby's head in the neutral position?
• Do you need – jaw thrust, a longer inflation time, or help with the airway?
• Is there an obstruction in the oropharynx (laryngoscope and suction)?
• What about an oropharyngeal (Guedel) airway?
• Is there a tracheal obstruction?

• Check that the baby's head and neck are in the neutral position; inflation breaths are at the correct pressure and applied for sufficient time (2–3 s inspiration); chest moves with each breath.
• If the chest still does not move, ask for help in maintaining the airway and consider an obstruction in the oropharynx or trachea, which may be removable by suction under direct vision. An oropharyngeal (Guedel) airway may be helpful.

If the HR remains slow (< 60 min) or absent following 5 inflation breaths, despite good passive chest movement in response to your inflation efforts

Chest compression

• Only when sure that the lungs have been aerated successfully.
• Grip the chest in both hands in such a way that the two thumbs can press on the lower third of the sternum, just below an imaginary line joining the nipples, with the fingers over the spine at the back. Compress the chest quickly and firmly, reducing the antero-posterior diameter of the chest by about one-third.
• The ratio of compressions to inflations in newborn resuscitation is 3:1.
• Chest compressions move oxygenated blood from the lungs back to the heart. Allow enough time during the relaxation phase of each compression cycle for the heart to refill with blood. Ensure that the chest is inflating with each breath.

In a very few babies (< 1/1000) inflation of the lungs and effective chest compression will not be sufficient to produce an effective circulation.

Drugs

- Only if there is no significant cardiac output despite effective lung inflation and chest compression.
- Adrenaline (1:10 000), occasionally sodium bicarbonate (ideally 4.2%), and dextrose (10%).
- They are best delivered via an umbilical venous catheter.
- The recommended IV dose for adrenaline is 10 µg/kg (0.1 ml/kg of 1:10000 solution). If this is not effective, a dose of up to 30 µg/kg (0.3 ml/kg of 1:10000 solution) may be tried. The tracheal dose is 50–100 µg/kg.
- The dose for sodium bicarbonate is 1–2 mmol of bicarbonate/kg (2–4 ml of 4.2% bicarbonate solution).
- The dose of dextrose recommended is 250 mg/kg (2.5 ml/kg of 10% dextrose).
- Very rarely, HR cannot increase because the baby has lost significant blood volume. There is often a history of blood loss from the baby, but not always. Use of isotonic crystalloid rather than albumin is preferred for emergency volume replacement. In the presence of hypovolaemia, a bolus of 10 ml/kg of 0.9% sodium chloride or similar given over 10–20 s will often produce a rapid response and can be repeated safely if needed.

Therapeutic hypothermia

- Treat term or near-term infants with evolving moderate to severe hypoxic ischaemic encephalopathy with therapeutic hypothermia.
- Whole body cooling and selective head cooling are both appropriate strategies.

When to stop

- In a newly born baby with no detectable cardiac activity, and with cardiac activity that remains undetectable for 10 min, it is appropriate to consider stopping resuscitation.
- The decision to continue resuscitation efforts beyond 10 min with no cardiac activity is often complex and may be influenced by issues such as the presumed aetiology of the arrest, the gestation of the baby, the presence or absence of complications, and the parents' previously expressed feelings about acceptable risk of morbidity.

Airway suctioning with or without meconium

- Routine elective intubation and suctioning of vigorous infants at birth does not reduce meconium aspiration syndrome (MAS).
- Suctioning the nose and mouth of such babies on the perineum and before delivery of the shoulders (intrapartum suctioning) is also ineffective.
- Whilst non-vigorous infants born through meconium-stained amniotic fluid are at increased risk of MAS, tracheal suctioning has not been shown to improve the outcome.
- Routine intrapartum oropharyngeal and nasopharyngeal suctioning for infants born with clear and/or meconium-stained amniotic fluid is not recommended.
- There is insufficient evidence to recommend a change in the current practice of performing direct oropharyngeal and tracheal suctioning of non-vigorous babies after birth with meconium-stained amniotic fluid if feasible. However, if attempted intubation is prolonged or unsuccessful, mask ventilation should be implemented, particularly if there is persistent bradycardia.

Resuscitation Council (UK). Newborn Life Support Guidelines 2010.

CHAPTER 59 Postnatal care

The essential care for woman and her baby in the first 6–8 weeks after birth.

Service setup

- Postnatal services with local protocols regarding the transfer of care between clinical sectors for efficient and effective service.
- An individualized postnatal care plan including
  * Relevant factors from the antenatal, intrapartum, and immediate postnatal period.
  * Plans for the postnatal period.
- Give all mothers – DOH booklet 'Birth to five' (guide to parenthood for the first 5 years of a child's life) within 3 days of birth and child health record ASAP.

- **At each postnatal contact:**
  * Ask and assess the woman about her and baby's health and wellbeing.
  * Advise women of the signs and symptoms of potentially life-threatening conditions and to contact immediately or call for emergency help if any signs and symptoms occur.
  * Provide information and reassurance on the physiological process of recovery after birth, normal patterns of emotional changes in the postnatal period and that these usually resolve within 10–14 days of giving birth (within 3 days); common health concerns as appropriate (weeks 2–8).

Maternal health – life-threatening conditions

Pre-eclampsia/eclampsia

- Record minimum of one BP measurement within 6 hours of the birth.
- Do not assess for proteinuria routinely.
- Consider and evaluate for PET in women with severe or persistent headache (emergency).
- If DBP is > 90 mmHg, and there are no other signs and symptoms of PET, repeat BP within 4 hours. Evaluate for PET if DBP is > 90mm Hg and does not fall below 90 mmHg within 4 hours (emergency).
- Evaluate further if DBP is > 90 mmHg and accompanied by other signs or symptoms of PET (emergency).

Genital tract sepsis

- Assess temperature if infection is suspected. If the temperature is > 38°C, repeat it in 4–6 hours. Evaluate further if the temperature remains > 38°C on the second reading or there are other symptoms and signs of sepsis (emergency).
- In the absence of any signs and symptoms of infection, routine assessment of temperature is unnecessary.

Postpartum haemorrhage

- Assess vaginal loss and uterine involution and position in women with excessive or offensive vaginal loss, abdominal tenderness or fever. Evaluate any abnormalities in the size, tone, and position of the uterus. If no uterine abnormality is found, consider other causes of symptoms (urgent).
- Evaluate sudden or profuse blood loss, or blood loss accompanied by any of the signs and symptoms of shock (emergency).
- In the absence of abnormal vaginal loss, assessment of the uterus by abdominal palpation or measurement as a routine observation is unnecessary.

Mental health and wellbeing

- Ask women about their emotional wellbeing, family and social support, and their usual coping strategies. Encourage women and their families/partners to discuss any changes in mood, emotional state, and behaviour that are outside of the woman's normal pattern.
- Do not provide formal debriefing of the birth experience.
- Be aware of signs and symptoms of maternal mental health problems that may be experienced in the weeks and months after the birth.
- At 10–14 days after birth – ask women about resolution of symptoms of baby blues (for example, tearfulness, feelings of anxiety and low mood). If symptoms have not resolved, assess for postnatal depression, and evaluate further if symptoms persist (urgent).

Thromboembolism

- Encourage women to mobilize as soon as appropriate following birth.
- Obese women are at higher risk of VTE – provide individualized care.
- Evaluate for DVT in women with unilateral calf pain, redness or swelling (emergency).
- Evaluate for PE in women with shortness of breath or chest pain (emergency).
- Do not routinely use Homan's sign as a tool for evaluation of thromboembolism.

Postnatal – general physical health and wellbeing

- **Perineal care** – Ask for symptoms of perineal pain, discomfort or stinging, offensive odour or dyspareunia.
  * Assess the perineum if pain or discomfort.
  * Topical cold therapy, for example crushed ice or gel pads are effective methods of pain relief.
  * Analgesia if required – paracetamol; oral or rectal non-steroidal anti-inflammatory (NSAID).
  * Evaluate any signs and symptoms of infection, inadequate repair, wound breakdown or non-healing (urgent).
- **Dyspareunia** – Ask about resumption of sexual intercourse and possible dyspareunia 2–6 weeks after birth. If a woman expresses anxiety about resuming intercourse, explore the reasons.
  * Assess the perineum in women with perineal trauma with dyspareunia.
  * Advise a water-based lubricant gel to help ease discomfort during intercourse, particularly if a woman is breastfeeding.
  * Evaluate women who continue to express anxiety about sexual health problems.

- **Headache** – Ask about headache at each contact.
  * For severe headache – consider PET.
  * Women who had epidural or spinal anaesthesia – advise to report any severe headache, particularly one which occurs while sitting or standing.
  * Management of mild headache is based on differential diagnosis of headache type.
  * Women with tension or migraine headaches – advise on relaxation and how to avoid factors associated with the onset of headaches.
- **Fatigue** – Women who report persistent fatigue – ask about their general wellbeing, and offer advice on diet, exercise, and planning activities.
  * If persistent postnatal fatigue impacts on the woman's care of herself or baby, evaluate underlying physical, psychological or social causes.
  * Evaluate haemoglobin level if a woman had a PPH, or is experiencing persistent fatigue and treat it if low.
  * **Backache** – manage as in the general population.

- **Immunization**
  * Provide anti-D immunoglobulin injection to non-sensitized RhD-negative woman within 72 hours following the delivery of an RhD-positive baby.
  * Women found to be sero-negative on antenatal screening for rubella – provide MMR vaccination following birth. Advise to avoid pregnancy for 1 month after receiving MMR; breastfeeding may continue.
  * MMR vaccine may be given with anti-D immunoglobulin injection provided that separate syringes are used and the products are administered into different limbs.
  * If not given simultaneously, give MMR 3 months after anti-D immunoglobulin.

- **Constipation** – Assess diet and fluid intake and offer advice. Prescribe a gentle laxative if dietary measures are not effective.
- **Haemorrhoids** – Advise to take dietary measures to avoid constipation and offer management if necessary. Evaluate women with a severe, swollen or prolapsed haemorrhoid or any rectal bleeding (urgent).
- **Faecal incontinence** – Assess for severity, duration, and frequency of symptoms. If symptoms do not resolve, evaluate further (urgent).
- **Urinary retention** – If urine has not been passed within 6 hours after the birth, advise on efforts to assist urination such as taking a warm bath or shower; if not immediately successful, assess bladder volume and consider catheterization (urgent).
- **Urinary incontinence** – Refer for pelvic floor exercises women with involuntary leakage of a small volume of urine. Evaluate further the women with involuntary leakage of urine which does not resolve or becomes worse.

- **Contraception** – discuss and provide methods and timing of resumption of contraception within the first week of the birth.
- **Domestic abuse** – be aware of the risks, signs, and symptoms of domestic abuse and know who to contact for advice and management.
- **6- to 8-week check** – at the end of the postnatal period, review the woman's physical, emotional, and social wellbeing.

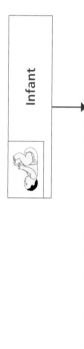

Infant

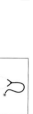

Physical examination and screening

- A complete examination of the baby within 72 hours of birth.
- Review medical history: family, maternal, antenatal, and perinatal history; fetal, neonatal, and infant history including any previously plotted birth weight and head circumference; whether the baby has passed meconium and urine (urine stream in a boy).
- Physical examination:
  * Appearance – colour, breathing, behaviour, activity, and posture.
  * Head (including fontanelles), face, nose, mouth including palate, ears, neck, and general symmetry of head and facial features. Measure and plot head circumference.
  * Eyes – opacities and red reflex.
  * Neck and clavicles, limbs, hands, feet, and digits. assess proportions and symmetry.
  * Heart – position, heart rate, rhythm and sounds, murmurs and femoral pulse volume.
  * Lungs – effort, rate, and lung sounds.
  * Abdomen – shape and palpation to identify any organomegaly; condition of umbilical cord.
  * Genitalia and anus – completeness and patency and undescended testes in males.
  * Spine – inspect and palpate bony structures and check integrity of the skin.
  * Skin – colour and texture as well as any birthmarks or rashes.
  * Central nervous system – tone, behaviour, movements, and posture. Elicit newborn reflexes only if concerned.
  * Hips, symmetry of the limbs and skin folds (Barlow and Ortolani's manoeuvres).
  * Cry; note sound; weight; measure and plot.
- Newborn blood spot test when baby is 5–8 days old.
- At 6–8 weeks – an examination and assessment of social smiling and visual fixing.
- A hearing screen before discharge from hospital or by week 4 in the hospital programme or by week 5 in the community programme.
- Routine immunizations for the baby according to the DOH recommendations.

Preventing, identifying, and treating breastfeeding concerns

- Provide breastfeeding support, discuss the benefits of breastfeeding, colostrum, and the timing of the first breastfeed.
- Do not give formula milk to breastfed babies unless medically indicated.
- Encourage unrestricted breastfeeding frequency and duration.
- **Nipple pain** – if their nipples are painful or cracked, it is probably due to incorrect attachment. If nipple pain persists after repositioning and re-attachment, assess for thrush.
- **Engorgement** – treat breast engorgement with: frequent unlimited breastfeeding including prolonged feeding from the affected breast; breast massage; and, if necessary, hand expression and analgesia.
- **Mastitis** – advise women to report any signs and symptoms of mastitis including flu-like symptoms, red, tender and painful breasts. Offer assistance with positioning and attachment and advise to:
  * Continue breastfeeding and/or hand expression to ensure effective milk removal; if necessary, with gentle massaging of the breast to overcome any blockage; take analgesia, for example paracetamol; increase fluid intake.
  * If the signs and symptoms of mastitis have not eased, evaluate for need for antibiotics (urgent).
- **Inverted nipples** – provide extra support and care to ensure successful breastfeeding.
- **Ankyloglossia (tongue tie)** – evaluate for ankyloglossia if breastfeeding concerns persist after a review of positioning and attachment. Evaluate further babies who appear to have ankyloglossia (non-urgent).

What not to do

- In the absence of abnormal vaginal loss, a routine assessment of the uterus by abdominal palpation or measurement.
- In the absence of any signs and symptoms of infection, routine assessment of temperature.
- Routine assessment of proteinuria.
- Formal debriefing of the birth experience.
- Routine use of Homan's sign as a tool for evaluation of thromboembolism.
- Dicycloverine (dicyclomine) in the treatment of colic.

Newborn – physical health and wellbeing

- **Jaundice** – Advise parents to contact HCP if the baby is jaundiced, jaundice is worsening, or baby is passing pale stools.
  * Evaluate babies who develop jaundice within the first 24 hours after birth (emergency).
  * If jaundice develops in babies aged 24 hours and older, monitor its intensity and record it along with the baby's overall wellbeing, hydration, and alertness. Encourage the mother of a breastfed baby who has signs of jaundice to breastfeed frequently. Do not routinely supplement with formula milk, water or dextrose water. Evaluate for serum bilirubin level if a baby is significantly jaundiced or appears unwell.
  * Evaluate if jaundice first develops after 7 days or jaundice remains after 14 days in an otherwise healthy baby and a cause has not already been identified (urgent).

- **Fever** – The temperature of a baby does not need to be taken, unless there are specific risk factors, for example maternal pyrexia during labour.
  * Evaluate a temperature of 38°C or more (emergency) – full assessment, including physical examination.

- **Vitamin K** – Offer vitamin K prophylaxis for their babies to prevent disorder of vitamin K deficiency bleeding.
  * A single dose of 1 mg IM (most cost-effective).
  * If parents decline IM vitamin K, offer oral vitamin K in multiple doses.

- **Constipation** – * If a baby has not passed meconium within 24 hours, evaluate to determine the cause, which may be related to feeding patterns or underlying pathology (emergency).
  * If a baby is constipated and is formula fed, evaluate: feed preparation technique, quantity of fluid taken, frequency of feeding; composition of feed (urgent).

- **Diarrhoea** – * Evaluate if a baby who is experiencing increased frequency and/or looser stools than usual (urgent).

- **Colic** – * A baby who is crying excessively and inconsolable, most often during the evening, either drawing its knees up to its abdomen or arching its back – assess for an underlying cause, including infant colic (urgent).
  * Assess: general health, antenatal and perinatal history, onset and length of crying, nature of the stools, feeding, woman's diet if breastfeeding, family history of allergy, any factors which lessen or worsen crying. Reassure that colic is usually a phase that will pass, holding the baby through the crying episode may be helpful.
  * Consider use of hypoallergenic formula in bottle-fed babies for treating colic under medical guidance.
  * Do not offer dicycloverine (dicyclomine) for the treatment of colic due to side effects such as breathing difficulties and coma.

- **Skin** – * Advise not to add cleansing agents to a baby's bath water, nor to use lotions or medicated wipes. The only cleansing agent suggested, where it is needed, is a mild non-perfumed soap.
  * Advise how to keep the umbilical cord clean and dry and not to use antiseptics routinely.

- **Thrush** – * treat with an antifungal medication if the symptoms are causing pain to the woman or the baby or feeding concerns to either.
  * If thrush is non-symptomatic, antifungal treatment is not required.

- **Nappy rash** – * Consider: hygiene and skin care, sensitivity to detergents, fabric softeners or external products that have contact with the skin, infection.
  * If painful nappy rash persists it is usually caused by thrush; consider antifungal treatment.
  * If after a course of treatment the rash does not resolve, evaluate it further (non-urgent).

- **Safety** – Use all home visits as an opportunity to assess relevant safety issues.
  * Give information on sudden infant death syndrome (SIDS) and co-sleeping.
  * If parents choose to share a bed with their baby, advice that there is an increased risk of SIDS, especially when the baby is < 11 weeks old, if either parent: is a smoker, has recently drunk any alcohol, has taken medication or drugs that make them sleep more heavily, is very tired.
  * If a baby has become accustomed to using a pacifier (dummy) while sleeping, do not stop suddenly during the first 26 weeks.

- **Child abuse** – Be aware of risk factors and signs and symptoms of child abuse.

Routine Postnatal Care of Women and their Babies. NICE CGN 37; 2006.

CHAPTER 60 Bacterial sepsis following pregnancy

Background and prevalence

- Sepsis in the puerperium remains an important cause of maternal death, accounting for around 10 deaths per year in the UK. Severe sepsis with acute organ dysfunction has a mortality rate of 20–40%, rising to around 60% if septicaemic shock develops.
- Most common site of sepsis in the puerperium is the genital tract. The uterus is particularly susceptible, resulting in endometritis.
- **Common organisms** – GAS (*Streptococcus pyogenes*); *E. coli*; *Staphylococcus aureus*; *Streptococcus pneumoniae*; MRSA; *Clostridium septicum*; and *Morganella morganii*. GAS was directly responsible for 13 of the 29 maternal deaths from infection in the UK during 2006–2008.

Risk factors for severe sepsis

- Risk factors – obesity; impaired glucose tolerance/diabetes; impaired immunity: HIV/immunosuppressive drugs; anaemia; vaginal discharge; history of pelvic infection amniocentesis and other invasive procedures; cervical cerclage; prolonged spontaneous rupture of membranes; vaginal trauma, CS, wound haematoma; retained products of conception; GAS infection in close contacts/family members; black or minority ethnic group origin. Acquisition or carriage of invasive organisms, especially GAS.

Pneumonia

- Haemoptysis may be a feature of pneumococcal pneumonia.
- Severe haemoptysis and low peripheral white cell count suggest Panton–Valentine leucocidin (PVL)-associated staphylococcal necrotizing pneumonia, which has a mortality rate of > 70%.
- Diagnosis – sputum for culture; a urinary sample may be tested for pneumococcal antigen when sputum is not easily available.
- Manage severe pneumonia in consultation with a respiratory physician and a medical microbiologist.
- Treat with a beta-lactam antibiotic together with a macrolide to cover typical and atypical organisms.

Mastitis

- It may lead to breast abscesses, necrotizing fasciitis, and toxic shock syndrome.
- Refer to hospital if the woman with mastitis is clinically unwell, if there is no response to oral antibiotics within 48 hours, if mastitis recurs or if there are severe or unusual symptoms.

UTI

- Gram-negative bacteria.
- Admit women with signs of sepsis, those who are unable to remain hydrated, and those who are vomiting.
- Diagnosis – primarily clinical; presence of leucocytes, protein, and blood in urinalysis; send a specimen for culture.
- Treat acute pyelonephritis aggressively.
- Extended-spectrum beta-lactamases (ESBL)-producing coliforms are resistant to commonly used antimicrobials such as cephalosporins and co-amoxiclav and may need carbapenems or more unusual IV antimicrobials such as colistin.

Gastroenteritis

- *Salmonella* and *Campylobacter* rarely cause severe systemic infection.
- Manage supportively unless features of bacteraemia are present.
- *C. difficile* is rare but increasingly found in obstetric patients.

Pharyngitis

- Most are viral, but approximately 10% are attributable to GAS.
- Treat with antibiotics if 3 of the 4 Centor criteria (fever, tonsillar exudate, no cough, tender anterior cervical lymphadenopathy) are present.

Infection related to regional anaesthesia

- Spinal abscess is a very rare complication after regional anaesthesia.
- The usual organisms responsible are S. *aureus*, streptococci, and gram-negative rods.
- Consider the diagnosis, investigate, and treat in a timely manner as permanent spinal cord or cauda equina damage may result if neural compression is prolonged.

Skin and soft-tissue infection

- These are particularly associated with toxic shock syndromes.
- Check IV cannulae or injection sites and caesarean or episiotomy wounds.
- Swabs for culture if any discharge.
- If drains, vascular access devices or other indwelling devices are suspected as the source of infection, remove them as soon as practicable.
- Recurrent abscess formation is a feature of PVL-producing staphylococci.
- Septicaemic seeding of streptococci from a uterine focus may give rise to a secondary focus in a limb, simulating a venous thrombosis.
- Early necrotizing fasciitis occurs deep in the tissues; therefore, in early necrotizing fasciitis there may be no visible skin changes. As the necrotizing process ascends to the skin, late infection produces blisters and obvious necrosis. The cardinal feature of necrotizing fasciitis is agonising pain, necessitating increasing amounts of strong analgesia. Examine carefully all women with suspected thrombosis who are systemically unwell with any features of sepsis.

Symptoms

Fever, rigors (persistent swinging temperature suggests abscess). Normal temperature may be attributable to antipyretics or NSAIDs.
Diarrhoea or vomiting – may indicate exotoxin production (early toxic shock).
Breast engorgement/redness.
Rash (generalized maculopapular rash); abdominal/pelvic pain and tenderness.
Wound infection – spreading cellulitis or discharge.
Offensive vaginal discharge (smelly; suggestive of anaerobes; serosanguineous: suggestive of streptococcal infection); delay in uterine involution, heavy lochia.
Productive cough; urinary symptoms.
General – non-specific signs such as lethargy, reduced appetite.

Signs – pyrexia, hypothermia, tachycardia, tachypnoea, hypoxia, hypotension, oliguria, impaired consciousness, and failure to respond to treatment. These signs may not always be present and are not necessarily related to the severity of sepsis. Some cases may present only with severe abdominal pain, in the absence of fever and tachycardia.
Any widespread rash suggests early toxic shock syndrome, especially if conjunctival hyperaemia or suffusion is present. Conjunctival suffusion is a classic sign of toxic shock syndrome.
A generalized macular rash is present in most cases of staphylococcal toxic shock syndrome but in only 10% of cases of streptococcal toxic shock syndrome.

Hospitalization – suspicion of significant sepsis ('red flag' signs and symptoms) – refer urgently to secondary care:

* Pyrexia > 38°C.
* Sustained tachycardia > 90 beats/minute.
* Breathlessness (respiratory rate > 20 breaths/minute; a serious symptom).
* Abdominal or chest pain.
* Diarrhoea and/or vomiting.
* Uterine or renal angle pain and tenderness.
* Woman is generally unwell or seems unduly anxious or distressed.

* Early presentation of sepsis (< 12 hours postbirth) is more likely to be caused by streptococcal infection, particularly GAS.
* Rule out sepsis if persistent vaginal bleeding and abdominal pain.
* Abdominal pain, fever (> 38°C), and tachycardia (> 90 beats/minute) are indications for urgent broad-spectrum IV antibiotics (within an hour of suspected sepsis).

* Discuss with a clinical microbiologist or infectious diseases physician.
* Women with previously documented carriage of or infection with multiresistant organisms (e.g., ESBL-producing organisms, MRSA, GAS or PVL-producing staphylococci) – notify the infection control team.
* Suspicion of necrotizing fasciitis – involve intensive care physicians and refer for surgical opinion, ideally from plastic and reconstructive surgeons if available.

Diagnostic criteria for sepsis – See Chapter 24

Bacterial sepsis in pregnancy

History and examination

* Symptoms of sepsis may be less distinctive than in the non-pregnant population and may not necessarily present in all cases; therefore, maintain a high index of suspicion.
* Consider sepsis in all recently delivered women who feel unwell and have pyrexia or hypothermia.
* Genital tract sepsis – constant, severe abdominal pain and tenderness unrelieved by usual analgesia.
* Take a history to identify the source of sepsis. A history of recent sore throat or prolonged (household) contact with family members with known streptococcal infections (pharyngitis, impetigo, cellulitis) is implicated in cases of GAS sepsis.
* IV drug misuse carries a high risk of staphylococcal and streptococcal sepsis as well as generalized immunosuppression of chronic disease, endocarditis, and blood-borne viruses.
* Recent febrile illnesses, especially if associated with chills and rigors, suggest bacteraemia.
* Gastrointestinal symptoms such as diarrhoea and vomiting may be attributable to food-borne pathogens, *C. difficile*, infection or early toxic shock.
* Ingestion of unpasteurized milk products raises the possibility of infection with *Salmonella, Campylobacter* or *Listeria*.
* *Chlamydophila psittaci* is acquired by contact with aborting sheep or infected birds or by crossinfection from washing contaminated clothing.
* Q fever is caused by *Coxiella burnetii* after inhalation of infectious particles from birthing animals or contaminated dust.
* Recent foreign travel or hospitalization abroad is associated with a high carriage rate of multiresistant organisms.
* Any intercurrent illness warranting antimicrobials should be noted on admission.
* Prior carriage of or infection with multiresistant organisms such as ESBL-producing gram-negative bacteria, vancomycin-resistant enterococci, and MRSA will affect the empirical antimicrobial choice.

Investigations

* Blood cultures prior to antibiotic administration.
* Measure serum lactate within 6 hours of suspicion of severe sepsis. Serum lactate ≥ 4 mmol/l is indicative of tissue hypoperfusion.
* Relevant imaging studies – chest X-ray, pelvic USS or CT scan if pelvic abscess is suspected.
* Other samples – MSU, HVS, throat swab, placental swabs, sputum, cerebrospinal fluid, epidural site swab, CS or episiotomy site wound swabs, and expressed breast milk.
* Routine blood tests – FBC, urea, electrolytes, and CRP.
* Woman with symptoms of tonsillitis/pharyngitis – throat swab for culture.
* If the MRSA status is unknown – send a premoistened nose swab for rapid MRSA screening.
* If diarrhoea is particularly offensive following antimicrobial therapy – stool sample for *C. difficile* toxin.
* A history of diarrhoea – routine culture (e.g. *Salmonella, Campylobacter*).
* Inform the laboratory if suspicion of unusual pathogens such as *Listeria monocytogenes* (consumption of soft cheese or cured meats) or if there is a history of foreign travel (parasites, typhoid or cholera).
* Gram staining can guide empirical prescribing. A paucity of leucocytes and presence of gram-positive cocci in chains indicate streptococcal infection. 'Mixed organisms' would suggest the possibility of gut organisms, including anaerobes, as part of a synergistic infection.
* Thrombocytosis with a rising CRP and a swinging pyrexia indicates a collection of pus or an infected haematoma.

Management – maternal

- Place of care – in a hospital where diagnostic services are easy to access and intensive care facilities are readily available.
- Regular observations of all vital signs (including temperature, pulse rate, BP, and respiratory rate) and record on a modified early obstetric warning score (MEOWS) chart. Abnormal scores should trigger an appropriate response.
- Avoid NSAIDs as they impede the ability of polymorphs to fight GAS infection.
- Find and treat the source of sepsis – this may be by uterine evacuation or by drainage of a breast, wound or pelvic abscess.

Antibiotics –

- If genital tract sepsis suspected – combination of high-dose broad-spectrum IV antibiotics. A combination of either piperacillin/tazobactam or a carbapenem plus clindamycin. Clindamycin is not nephrotoxic and switches off the production of superantigens and other exotoxins. Therefore, together with either piperacillin/tazobactam or a carbapenem, it provides broad cover in severe sepsis.
- MRSA may be resistant to clindamycin, hence if the woman is or is highly likely to be MRSA-positive – a glycopeptide such as vancomycin or teicoplanin may be added until sensitivity is known.
- Breastfeeding – seek advice of a consultant microbiologist.
- Cefuroxime and metronidazole – cefuroxime is associated with C. difficile. Neither agent provides any protection against MRSA, Pseudomonas or ESBL.
- In ESBL infection, piperacillin/tazobactam is likely to be ineffective.

Adverse effects of antibiotics –

- Allergic reactions, including skin rashes. However, in toxic shock, a maculopapular or blanching erythema may be exotoxin related and not an allergy to the therapy.
- C. difficile infection – does not infect neonates but can cause up to 30% mortality in mothers if untreated. Send stool for culture and commence oral metronidazole or oral vancomycin empirically.
- Appropriate infection control precautions.

Tasks to be performed within the first 6 hours of the identification of severe sepsis

- Obtain blood cultures prior to antibiotic administration.
- Broad-spectrum antibiotic within 1 hour of recognition of severe sepsis.
- Measure serum lactate.
- Hypotension and/or a serum lactate >4mmol/l – give an initial minimum 20 ml/kg of crystalloid or an equivalent. If hypotension is not responding, give vasopressors to maintain mean arterial pressure (MAP) > 65 mmHg.
- Persistent hypotension despite fluid resuscitation (septic shock) and/or lactate >4 mmol/l:
  a. Achieve a CVP of ≥ 8 mmHg.
  b. Achieve a central venous oxygen saturation (ScvO₂) ≥ 70% or mixed venous oxygen saturation (SvO₂) ≥ 65%.

Transfer to ICU

- Liaise with critical care team, obstetric consultant, and the consultant obstetric anaesthetist.
- **Indications for transfer to ICU** – the presence of shock or other organ dysfunction.
  * Persistent cardiovascular hypotension or raised serum lactate persisting despite fluid resuscitation, suggests the need for inotrope support.
  * Respiratory – pulmonary oedema, mechanical ventilation, airway protection.
  * Renal dialysis.
  * Significantly decreased conscious level.
  * Multiorgan failure; uncorrected acidosis, hypothermia.
  * Fluid replacement – postpartum women may be more susceptible to the development of pulmonary oedema than non-pregnant patients after circulatory fluid overload. To achieve the correct balance central venous pressure monitoring and vasopressor treatment are likely to be required on the ICU.
- Give IVIG for severe invasive streptococcal or staphylococcal infection if other therapies have failed. IVIG has an immunomodulatory effect, neutralizing the superantigen effect of exotoxins, and inhibits production of tumour necrosis factor (TNF) and interleukins.

It is effective in exotoxic shock (i.e., toxic shock due to streptococci and staphylococci) but with little evidence of benefit in gram-negative (endotoxin related) sepsis.
Congenital deficiency of immunoglobulin A is the main contraindication.

Infection control issues

Mothers or neonates infected or colonized with high-risk organisms such as GAS, MRSA or PVL-producing staphylococci may generate outbreaks within the healthcare setting, especially for other babies in nursery units and staff. Inform the local infection control team of any such cases and follow appropriate isolation precautions.

- Isolate the woman in a single room with en suite facilities.
- Healthcare workers should wear personal protective equipment including disposable gloves and aprons when in contact with the woman, equipment, and their immediate surroundings.
- Breaks in the skin of the woman or carer must be covered with a waterproof dressing.
- Fluid-repellent surgical masks with visors must be used at operative debridement/change of dressings of GAS necrotizing fasciitis and for other procedures where droplet spread is possible.
- Offer visitors suitable information and relevant personal protective equipment.
- Liaise with a microbiologist to ensure isolation procedures and diagnostic tests are appropriate.
- If GAS is isolated in non-maternity patients, such as in health care workers, notify the infection control team and occupational health department.

Women who use illicit drugs

- Monitor under MDT care. Liaise with the local drugs advisory specialist team.
- Swab any injection-site lesions and screen for MRSA.
- Sepsis of unknown site – search for bacterial endocarditis or abscesses spread via the bloodstream.
- Current or former intravenous drug users usually have very difficult vascular access. Alternative access devices such as a central venous catheter or peripherally inserted central catheter may be required, therefore refer early to a vascular access team.

Indications for prophylaxis to family/staff

- Warn close household contacts about the symptoms of GAS infection and to seek medical attention if any symptoms develop; provide antibiotic prophylaxis if needed.
- Asymptomatic contacts may warrant prophylaxis. Liaise with the local health protection unit or consultant for communicable disease control.
- Only the meningococcus (*Neisseria meningitidis*) and GAS merit consideration of prophylaxis for family or staff.
- MRSA and PVL-producing *S. aureus* are transmitted during breastfeeding and close contact. Although routine prophylaxis is not indicated, observe the neonate closely and liaise with the infection control team.
- Generally, prophylaxis for GAS organisms would be administered in the event of close contact (kissing or household contacts) and for healthcare workers with exposure to respiratory secretions (e.g., suctioning).

Newborn

- The baby is at risk of streptococcal and staphylococcal infection during birth and during breastfeeding.
- Examine the umbilical area and liaise with paediatrician.
- If either the mother or the baby is infected with invasive GAS in the postpartum period, treat both with antibiotics. GAS and PVL-producing *S. aureus* infections have been transmitted to babies during breastfeeding, causing severe infection. GAS poses the highest risk of sepsis in the neonate; hence, provide antimicrobial prophylaxis routinely to neonates of mothers with GAS infection.
- GBS – See Chapter 14: Group B streptococcal disease in pregnancy.

Bacterial sepsis following pregnancy. RCOG Green-top Guideline No. 64b; 1st edition April 2012.

CHAPTER 61 Obesity in pregnancy

- Defined as body mass index (BMI) of ≥ 30 kg/m^2 at the first antenatal consultation.
- BMI = weight in kilograms divided by the square of height in metres (kg/m^2).
- There are 3 different classes of obesity: which recognize the continuous relationship between BMI and morbidity and mortality.
  - * BMI 30.0–34.9 (Class 1).
  - * BMI 35.0–39.9 (Class 2).
  - * BMI ≥ 40 (Class 3/morbid obesity).
- In the UK 32% of women aged 35–64 years are overweight (BMI 25–30) and 21% are obese (BMI > 30).
- The prevalence of obesity in pregnancy has increased, rising from 9–10% in the early 1990s to 16–19% in the 2000s.

Service provision

For pregnant women with a booking BMI > 30 – all maternity units should have:

- MDT guidelines.
- A documented environmental risk assessment regarding the availability of facilities.
- A central list of all facilities and equipment required to provide safe care.
- All HCPs involved in the care of pregnant women should receive:
  - * Education about maternal nutrition and its impact on maternal, fetal, and child health.
  - * Training in manual handling techniques and the use of specialist equipment which may be required for pregnant and postnatal women with obesity.

Risks or complications

Maternal

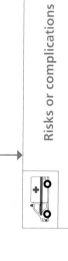

- **Prepregnancy** – menstrual disorders, infertility.
- **Early pregnancy** – increased risk of miscarriage, fetal anomalies, difficult and less accurate USS resulting in difficulties in fetal surveillance and screening for anomalies.
- **Pregnancy** – VTE, GDM, PIH, PET.
- **Labour and delivery** – IOL, failed IOL, dysfunctional labour (slow progress of labour), CS, operative vaginal delivery (OVD), shoulder dystocia, third and fourth degree tear, PPH, difficulty in surveillance in labour, technical difficulty with OVD and CS.
- **Anaesthetic complications** – failed epidurals, increased aspiration during GA, and difficulty with intubation.
- **Postpartum** – wound infections and dehiscence, endometritis, prolonged hospitalization, and lower breastfeeding rate.
- Obesity may be a risk factor for maternal death: the CEMACE report (2006–2008) – 27% of mothers who died were obese. 49% of all women who died from direct or indirect causes were either overweight or obese.

Fetal – neonatal

- Increased risk of congenital anomalies/birth defects, prematurity, macrosomia, stillbirth, neonatal death, and admission to NICU.
- Up to a 2-fold increase in risk for neural tube defects where there is prepregnancy maternal obesity. The greater the maternal BMI the higher the risk of congenital malformation.
- Macrosomia – prepregnancy BMI is a strong positive predictor of birth weight. The OR for an obese mother delivering a large-for-dates infant is 1.4–18.
- Almost a 3-fold increased risk of SB (OR 2.8) and neonatal death (OR 2.6). No single cause of death explains the higher mortality in children of obese women but more stillbirths are either unexplained intrauterine deaths or associated with fetoplacental dysfunction among obese compared with normal weight women.
- Up to 1.5 times more likely to be admitted to an NICU. The odds of admission increases with each increasing BMI category.
- Intrauterine exposure to maternal obesity is also associated with an increased risk of developing obesity, metabolic disorders in childhood, and coronary heart disease.

Pre-pregnancy care

Women of childbearing age with obesity

Care in the primary care setting

Index pregnancy

- Women of childbearing age with a BMI > 30 – provide information and advice about the risks of obesity during pregnancy and childbirth and support to lose weight before conception.
- Ensure that all women of childbearing age have the opportunity to optimize their weight before pregnancy. Advise on weight and lifestyle during family planning consultations, and monitor weight, BMI, and waist circumference regularly.

Interpregnancy weight

- There is an association of increase in BMI between successive pregnancies with adverse outcomes during the second pregnancy. The risks of obesity in pregnancy are linearly related to interpregnancy weight gain. **Interpregnancy weight reduction among women with obesity has been shown to significantly reduce the risks.**
- Women with maternal obesity prior to their first singleton pregnancy – a weight loss of at least 4.5 kg before the second pregnancy reduces the risk of developing GDM by up to 40%.
- Although it has been suggested that some weight loss regimens during the first trimester may increase the risk of fetal neural tube defects (NTD), weight loss prior to pregnancy does not appear to carry this risk.

Nutritional supplements

Folic acid

Periconceptual folic acid supplementation reduces the risk of the first occurrence, as well as the recurrence, of NTDs (RR 0.28) in general population. In women at high risk of fetal NTD (previous pregnancy with NTD), a higher dose of folic acid supplementation (5 mg/day) reduces the risk of a subsequent NTD by 72%.

- Women with a raised BMI are at increased risk of NTD – systematic review – OR of 1.2, 1.7, and 3 for women defined as overweight, obese, and severely obese, respectively.
- Compared to women with a BMI < 27, women with a BMI > 27 have lower serum folate levels even after controlling for folate intake. Advise women with a BMI > 30 wishing to become pregnant to take 5 mg folic acid supplementation daily, starting at least 1 month before conception and continuing during the first trimester of pregnancy.

Vitamin D

- Pre-pregnancy BMI is inversely associated with serum vitamin D concentrations among pregnant women, and women with obesity (BMI ≥ 30) are at increased risk of vitamin D deficiency.
- About a quarter of British women aged 19–24 and a sixth of those aged 25–34 are at risk of vitamin D deficiency. Maternal skin exposure alone may not always be enough to achieve the optimal vitamin D status needed for pregnancy. Advise women with a booking BMI ≥ 30 to take 10 μg Vitamin D supplementation daily during pregnancy and while breastfeeding.

Antenatal care – booking

Measure weight, height, and BMI

- Self-reported height is often overestimated and self-reported weight underestimated, particularly in obese women, which may lead to inaccurate risk assessment during pregnancy.
- Measure weight and height and calculate BMI at the booking visit.
- For women with obesity in pregnancy, re-measure maternal weight during the third trimester to allow appropriate plans to be made for equipment and personnel required during labour and delivery.

Risk assessment for anaesthetic issues

- Obese pregnant women are at higher risk of anaesthesia-related complications and obesity is a significant risk factor for anaesthesia-related maternal mortality. Women with class III obesity will be at highest risk and anaesthetic resources should be focused on this group of women.
- Epidural re-site rates increase with increasing BMI, with a failure rate of epidural as high as 42% in morbid obesity. For these reasons, an early epidural is advisable.
- Obesity may increase the risk of aspiration of gastric contents under GA, difficult endotracheal intubation, and postoperative atelectasis. These women are also more likely to have comorbidities such as HT and ischaemic heart disease.
- Pregnant women with a booking BMI ≥ 40 – arrange an antenatal consultation with an obstetric anaesthetist, so that potential difficulties with venous access, regional or GA can be identified. Discuss and document an anaesthetic management plan for labour and delivery.

Information during pregnancy – women with a booking BMI ≥ 30:

- Provide with accurate and accessible information about the risks associated with obesity in pregnancy and how they may be minimized.
- Advise on the importance of healthy eating and appropriate exercise during pregnancy in order to prevent excessive weight gain and GDM.
- Dietetic advice by trained dietician in early pregnancy.

Service provision – integrate management of women with obesity in pregnancy into all antenatal clinics, with clear policies and guidelines for care.

Manual handling requirements – safe working loads of beds and theatre tables, appropriate lateral transfer equipment, hoists, and appropriately sized thromboembolic deterrent stockings (TEDS). Women with a booking BMI ≥ 40 – assessment in the third trimester to determine manual handling requirements for childbirth and tissue viability issues. Some women with a booking BMI < 40 may also benefit from assessment of manual handling requirements.

Increased risk of pressure sores when a woman may be relatively immobile; regular inspection of potential pressure areas is important. Assess with validated scoring tools, and plan regarding body positions, repositioning schedules, skin care, and support surfaces.

Antenatal care (contd) – maternal surveillance and screening

Anomaly screen – get a detailed anomaly scan and serum screening for congenital abnormality. Adipose tissue can significantly attenuate the ultrasound signal resulting in the reduced sensitivity of ultrasound as a screening test for fetal anomaly. This reduction is most marked when visualizing the fetal heart, umbilical cord, and spine.

BP measurement – the differences in readings are smallest in non-obese subjects and become progressively greater with increasing arm circumference in the obese population. Less error is introduced by using too large a cuff than by too small a cuff. **Use and document an appropriate size of arm cuff.**

Gestational diabetes (GDM) – maternal obesity is known to be a risk factor for GDM with a 3-fold increased risk. Screen all pregnant women with a booking BMI > 30 for GDM. Arrange 2-hour 75 g oral GTT at 24–28 weeks (WHO criteria) for women with a BMI > 30.

Pre-eclampsia (PET) – elevated pre-pregnancy BMI is an independent risk factor for the development of PIH; risk is approximately doubled (OR 1.8). Incidence of PET ranges from 1.4% among women with a BMI 20–26 to 3.5% among those with a booking BMI > 35 for PET. Monitor women with a booking BMI > 35 for PET.

Antenatal prophylaxis for PET

- Among women with a BMI > 35 as the only risk, the incidence of PET is 3%, resulting in 714 women needing treatment to prevent one case of PET.
- When a woman with a BMI > 35 also had other risk factors, such as primigravidity or diabetes, the risk was greatly elevated and the number needed to treat in order to prevent one case of PET is only 37.
- **NICE** – Although moderate risk factors for PET (obesity, first pregnancy, maternal age > 40 years, family history of PET, multiple pregnancy) are poorly defined, women with more than one moderate risk factor may benefit from taking 75 mg aspirin daily from 12 weeks' gestation until birth of the baby.

Thromboprophylaxis

- Maternal obesity is associated with a significant risk of VTE during antenatal and postnatal periods; with BMI ≥ 30, OR of VTE is 5.3 and an OR of 2.7 for antenatal PE.
- Assess women with a booking BMI ≥ 30 at their first antenatal visit and throughout pregnancy for the risk of VTE. Consider antenatal and post-delivery thromboprophylaxis.

Mobilization – both immobility and obesity are independently associated with VTE; in combination, they pose a much greater risk.

- Raised BMI (≥ 25) and immobilization has OR of 62 for antenatal VTE and 40 for postnatal VTE compared with women with a BMI < 25 and no immobilization.
- Women with a BMI ≥ 25 without immobilization have a much lower OR of 1.8 for antenatal VTE and 2.4 for postnatal VTE.
- Encourage women with a BMI ≥ 30 to mobilize as early as practicable following childbirth to reduce the risk of VTE.

LMWH – for women with a booking BMI ≥ 30 requiring pharmacological thromboprophylaxis, prescribe doses appropriate for maternal weight.

- A woman with a BMI ≥ 30 who also has ≥ 2 additional risk factors for VTE – consider prophylactic LMWH antenatally as early in pregnancy as practical.
- Advise all women receiving LMWH antenatally to continue it until 6 weeks postpartum, but undertake a postnatal risk assessment.

Postnatal – Offer all women with a BMI ≥ 40 postnatal thromboprophylaxis regardless of the mode of delivery and continue for a minimum of 1 week.

- Women with a BMI ≥ 30 who have ≥ 1 additional persisting risk factor for VTE – consider for LMWH for 7 days after delivery.
- Women with a booking BMI ≥ 30 who have ≥ 2 additional persisting risk factors – give graduated compression stockings in addition to LMWH.

PRECOG guideline

- Women with a booking BMI > 35 with no additional risk factor can have monitoring at a minimum of 3 weekly intervals between 24 and 32 weeks' gestation, and 2-weekly intervals from 32 weeks to delivery.
- Women with a booking BMI > 35 who also have at least 1 additional risk factor for PET – refer early in pregnancy for specialist input.

Additional risk factors include: first pregnancy, previous PET, >10 years since last baby, > 40 years, family history of PET, booking diastolic BP > 80 mmHg, booking proteinuria >1+ on more than one occasion or > 0.3 g/24 hours, multiple pregnancy, and certain underlying medical conditions such as antiphospholipid antibodies or pre-existing HT, renal disease or diabetes.

Labour and delivery – planning mode of delivery

- CS can be technically difficult with a higher risk of anaesthetic complications; there is also a higher incidence of intrapartum complications in labour – carefully consider the mode of delivery and in conjunction with the full MDT and the woman.
- **NICE –**
  - * Advise women with BMI > 35 to give birth in a consultant-led obstetric unit with appropriate neonatal services to reduce the risk of maternal and fetal adverse outcomes.
  - * Individualize place of birth for women with a booking BMI of 30–34 after risk assessment.

IOL – In the absence of other obstetric or medical indications, do not offer IOL for obesity alone and encourage a normal birth. IOL carries the risk of failed induction and emergency CS, which can be a high risk procedure in women with obesity. Offer IOL for specific obstetric or medical indication.

VBAC – Consider the circumstances of previous CS and the current clinical situation.
- Obesity is a risk factor for unsuccessful VBAC, and morbid obesity carries a greater risk for uterine rupture and neonatal injury during trial of labour.
- Emergency CS in women with obesity is associated with an increased risk of serious maternal morbidity because anaesthetic and operative difficulties are more prevalent in these women.
- Women with a booking BMI > 30 – individualize decision for VBAC following informed discussion and consideration of all relevant clinical factors.

Intrapartum care

- Women with a BMI > 40 – establish venous access early in labour.
- Women with a BMI > 40 in established labour – provide continuous midwifery care.
- FHR monitoring might be difficult; use fetal scalp electrode or USS of the fetal heart if necessary.
- Increased risk of PPH – offer active management of the third stage of labour for all women with a BMI > 30.

- Inform the duty anaesthetist covering the labour ward when a woman with a BMI > 40 is admitted to the labour ward if delivery or operative intervention is anticipated. Early assessment will allow the anaesthetist to review the antenatal anaesthetic consultation, identify potential difficulties with regional and/or GA, and alert senior colleagues if necessary. Appropriately experienced clinicians should be present to perform or supervise delivery.
- Alert operating theatre staff regarding any woman whose weight exceeds 120 kg and who is due to have an operative intervention in theatre. An operating table with the appropriate safe working load and appropriate lateral transfer equipment should be available.
- Give prophylactic antibiotics at the time of surgery for women with a BMI > 30.
- NICE – suture the subcutaneous tissue space in women undergoing CS who have > 2 cm subcutaneous fat to reduce the risk of wound infection and wound separation.

Postnatal care and follow-up

Breastfeeding – obesity is associated with low breastfeeding initiation and maintenance rates. This is likely to be multifactorial in origin: women's perception of breastfeeding; difficulty with correct positioning of the baby; and the possibility of an impaired prolactin response to suckling.
- Women with a booking BMI > 30 – provide specialist advice and support antenatally and postnatally regarding the benefits, initiation, and maintenance of breastfeeding.

Weight reduction – women with a booking BMI > 30 – nutritional advice from an appropriately trained professional, with a view to weight reduction. Modification of dietary and physical activity behaviour are associated with a significant reduction in body weight compared to no lifestyle intervention.

Diabetes
- Women with a booking BMI > 30 who have been diagnosed with GDM:
  - * GTT approximately 6 weeks after giving birth.
  - * Annual screening for cardio-metabolic risk factors.
  - * Offer lifestyle and weight management advice.
- Lifestyle interventions can prevent or delay the development of diabetes in high-risk individuals.
- Women with a booking BMI > 30 and GDM who have a normal GTT following childbirth – provide regular follow-up with GP to screen for the development of type 2 DM.

All women with BMI > 30	Women with BMI > 35 – additional measures	Women with BMI > 40 – additional measures
Prepregnancy		
• Information and advise about risks of obesity in pregnancy. • Support women to lose weight. • Folic acid 5 mg daily, at least 1 month prior to conception.		
Booking visit		
• Measure height, weight, calculate BMI; use appropriate size BP cuff. • Vit D 10 mg daily, throughout pregnancy and breastfeeding. • Consider 75 mg aspirin, if additional moderate risk factors for PET. • Assess VTE risk – thromboprophylaxis if indicated. • Book GTT at 24–28 weeks. • Refer to consultant obstetrician to discuss delivery plan.	Refer to specialist care if one or more additional risk factors for PET.	Arrange antenatal anaesthetic review.
Throughout pregnancy		
• Use appropriate size BP cuff. • Assess VTE risk – thromboprophylaxis if indicated.	Monitor for PET 3-weekly between 24 and 32 weeks and 2-weekly from 32 weeks onwards.	Monitor for PET 3-weekly between 24 and 32 weeks and 2-weekly from 32 weeks onwards.
Third trimester		
• 75 g oral GTT at 24–28 weeks. • Advise and support on initiation and maintenance of breastfeeding		• Re-measure maternal weight and BMI. • Risk assessment for manual handling requirement.
Labour and delivery		
• Individual risk assessment to decide mode and place of birth. • Active management of third stage of labour. • Obesity itself is not an indication for IOL. • Prophylactic antibiotics at CS. • Suture subcutaneous tissue at CS if >2 cm subcutaneous fat.	• Place of birth – consultant-led obstetric unit. • Alert theatre staff if weight >120 kg and needs operative intervention in theatre.	• Continuous midwifery care; inform duty anaesthetist. • Establish early venous access. • Consider early epidural in labour. • Inform senior obstetrician and anaesthetist – review patient on ward round and supervise/attend operative vaginal delivery or CS.
Postpartum		

• Encourage to mobilize as soon as possible.
• Thromboprophylaxis for 7 days if ≥ 1 additional risk factors for VTE.
• Compression stockings if ≥ 2 additional risk factors for VTE.
• Advise and support on initiation and maintenance of breastfeeding.
• Refer for ongoing dietetic and life style advice.
• If GDM:
  ※ GTT 6 weeks later.
  ※ Lifestyle and weight management advice.
  ※ Annual screening for type 2 DM and cardiometabolic risk factors.
		• Thromboprophylaxis for 7 days regardless of delivery mode.

Management of Women with Obesity in Pregnancy. CMACE/RCOG Joint Guideline; March 2010.

Weight Management Before, During and after Pregnancy; NICE July 2010.

Obesity and Reproductive Health – RCOG Study Group Statement; 2007.

Stewart FM, Ramsay JE, Greer IA. Obesity: impact on obstetric practice and outcome. The Obstetrician & Gynaecologist 2009;11:25–31.

CHAPTER 62 Alcohol consumption in pregnancy

Prevalence and background

- A survey of antenatal clinics in UK – 45% consumed no alcohol, 44% consumed < 1 unit per week, 10% consumed up to one unit a day, and 1% consumed > 1 unit a day.
- USA – 9–15% of women drink alcohol at least once a month during their pregnancy.
- Most women who suffer from 'problem drinking' have other behaviours (such as smoking, drug abuse, poor nutrition) which may independently or synergistically contribute to an adverse outcome of pregnancy.

- **Measuring consumption** – in units: the amount of alcohol found in many standard drinks (one small glass of wine, one measure of spirits, half pint of beer/lager) is measured at 7.9 g or 10 ml of ethanol.
- Drinking 5 or more drinks at one session for women is known as 'binge drinking'.

Adverse outcomes of alcohol consumption on the reproductive process

Fertility

- Effect on anovulatory infertility – evidence is controversial. One study reported an OR of 1.3 in women consuming < 100 g of alcohol a week compared to non-drinkers and an OR of 1.6 in those consuming >100 g of alcohol a week.
- Less information on male fertility. Postmortem testicular biopsies – normal spermatogenesis in men consuming < 40 g of alcohol a day. There is a dose-response reduction in spermatogenesis at consumption levels higher than this, with a significant number of aspermic men among a group consuming >80 g of alcohol a day.
- Binge drinking – infrequent binge drinkers are 3 times more likely and frequent binge drinkers 7 times more likely to have STDs and unplanned pregnancy than non-drinkers or women who do not binge drink.

Miscarriage and structural congenital malformations

- Miscarriage – some evidence that there may be an increase in first-trimester and second trimester loss with alcohol consumption of > 5 units a week.
- Major structural malformations are seen about 3 times more commonly in women drinking > 3.5 g a day compared with those consuming less or none at all.

Fetal growth and development

- There is a dose-response relationship between alcohol consumption in the second half of pregnancy and FGR. Women who continue to drink > 2 units/day throughout the third trimester – 45% have an infant with a birth weight < 10th centile for gestational age. Whereas in those who successfully reduce or discontinue their alcohol during the last 3 months of pregnancy, only 8% have infants < 10th centile.
- Binge drinking – there are concerns about the longer-term effects. Children at 7 years of age have learning problems, low academic achievement, and hyperkinetic and impulsive behaviour problems. Alcohol-related neurodevelopmental disorder has been reported in relation to binge drinking in early pregnancy.

Preterm labour

- There may be a relationship between alcohol consumption, both in early pregnancy and in late pregnancy, and PTB at levels of consumption in excess of 10 drinks a week.

Fetal alcohol syndrome and fetal alcohol spectrum disorders

Fetal alcohol syndrome (FAS) and fetal alcohol spectrum disorders (FASD)

- The effects of alcohol consumption in the offspring may not always be recognized.
- **FASD** includes the pattern of disorders which might be associated with lesser degrees of harm from maternal alcohol consumption:
  * **Fetal alcohol syndrome (FAS)**
  * FAS without a confirmed history of alcohol consumption.
  * Partial FAS – where some but not all of the 4 usual features are present.
  * Alcohol-related birth defects:
    > structural defects are seen without the pattern of neurodevelopmental disorder; and
    > alcohol-related neurodevelopmental disorder with no obvious structural defects.
- Estimated incidence of the full-blown FAS is 0.6/1000 live births, and that of FASDs is 9/1000 live births (North America). North American prevalence rates are up to 20 times higher than those seen in Europe and African American background.
- Low socioeconomic status predicts a 10-fold increase in FAS.

Diagnostic criteria for FAS (Stratton et al.) –

- Confirmed maternal alcohol exposure.
- Characteristic pattern of facial anomalies – short palpebral fissures and abnormalities in the premaxillary zone (e.g., flat upper lip, flattened philtrum, and flat midface).
- FGR with one of the following:
  * LBW for gestational age.
  * Decelerating weight over time not due to nutrition.
  * Disproportionally low weight to height.
- CNS neurodevelopmental abnormalities, with one of the following:
  * Decreased cranial size at birth.
  * Structural brain abnormalities (e.g., microcephaly, partial or complete agenesis of the corpus callosum, cerebellar hypoplasia).
  * Neurological hard or soft signs (e.g., impaired fine motor skills, neurosensory hearing loss, poor tandem gait, poor eye–hand coordination).

- **FASD is a diagnosis of exclusion** because 'many genetic and malformation syndromes have some of the clinical characteristics of FAS'. Therefore, do not assign a diagnosis of FASD continuum automatically to a child with disabilities just because his or her mother drank alcohol during the pregnancy.

Do low levels of alcohol consumption harm the fetus?

There is considerable doubt as to whether infrequent and low levels of alcohol consumption during pregnancy convey any long-term risk.

Fetal behavioural studies

- In late pregnancy, spontaneous and provoked fetal activity is reduced and the effects are also seen in infants at 5 months of age; significance of these findings is uncertain.

Neurodevelopmental studies

- Alcohol-related neurodevelopmental disorder may be related to the timing of exposure, levels of consumption, genetic factors affecting maternal or fetal metabolism or individual susceptibility, as well as interaction with other harmful behaviours. It is not clear whether these effects fit a threshold or a dose-response model.
- Follow-up study of children aged 6–7 years whose mothers reported alcohol consumption of at least 15 g of alcohol per day –
  * OR for delinquent behaviour is 3.2; but not significantly higher in the subgroup with low alcohol exposure.
  * Aggressive behaviour is significantly more common in the offspring of mothers even consuming low levels of alcohol compared with children who are not exposed to alcohol.
- A Danish study – maternal alcohol intake up to one drink (12 g alcohol) a day is unlikely to have an impact on child development.

Childhood growth studies

- Even low levels of consumption (0 to <0.2 drinks a day) are associated with a body weight reduction of 1.5 kg at 14 years compared with the offspring of non-drinkers.
- A consistent dose-response relationship is seen with increasing alcohol consumption.
- The effect is related to first- and second-trimester exposures but not third trimester. Height and head circumference are both negatively associated with first but not second- or third-trimester maternal alcohol exposure.

Assessment and management

Maternal alcohol screening

- Universally screen for alcohol consumption in all pregnant women and women of childbearing age. Identify at-risk drinking before pregnancy, allowing for change. Interventions to reduce alcohol consumption in pregnancy are effective. Ideally offer at the stage of preconception counselling.
- **Risk factors associated with maternal drinking** – smoking, illicit drug use, unemployment, low income, age 15 to 24 years, non-white, less educated, single, little social support, history of depression, and physical or sexual abuse.

Management – SOGC

- Brief interventions for women with 'at-risk drinking' are effective.
- If a woman continues to use alcohol during pregnancy, encourage harm reduction/treatment strategies.
- Priority access to pregnant women for withdrawal management and treatment.
- Low-level consumption of alcohol in early pregnancy is not an indication for TOP.

Alcohol interventions with women of child-bearing years

3 As – Assess, Advice, Assist
Inform all women about health risks and FASD.

All women and low risk

- **Discuss low-risk drinking guidelines:**
  - * Pre-conception – avoid at-risk drinking.
  - * Pregnant – safest not to drink (no known safe amount).
- **Brief intervention in all women.**

Moderate to high risk

- Pre-conception – avoid at risk drinking and/or use contraception.
- Pregnant – safest to not drink (no known safe amount), or reduce to lowest possible level and reduce harms associated with drinking.
- **Multiple contact with brief interventions.**
- Referral to services and follow-up as needed.

Alcohol dependent

- Inform on the process of withdrawal, stages of recovery, treatment, and support options.
- **Multiple brief interventions, assistance with goal setting.**
- Referral and support to access treatment.
- Withdrawal management/treatment options.
- Explore need for medication.
- Follow-up visit – continue to support.

The most common type of brief intervention reported in pregnant women and women of childbearing age is motivational interviewing. It motivates individuals to change behaviours through exploring and resolving discrepancy and ambivalence. It is especially effective in helping women who are drinking problematically. It helps to prevent an alcohol-exposed pregnancy and to reduce alcohol intake and participate in alcohol treatment.

Women who are alcohol dependent find it more difficult to stop drinking when they are pregnant. They need more intense and specialized counselling and support. Harm reduction involves assisting women with reducing harms associated with substance use, as well as with establishing realistic and achievable goals to reduce their alcohol use as they work toward abstinence or when abstinence is not possible. Medical support during the process of withdrawal is key. Intense home-visiting advocacy programs are effective in helping alcohol-dependent women of childbearing years get the help they need to effect change in their lives.

RCOG – recommendations

- The most vulnerable period for the fetus is from 4 to 10 weeks of gestation but alcohol-related damage may occur throughout pregnancy. Thus, benefit to the infant can be obtained if alcohol is withdrawn at any stage of gestation.
- Advise women to avoid alcohol during the first trimester and limit their intake to 1–2 units once or twice a week for the remainder of their pregnancy.
- NICE – women should limit alcohol consumption to no more than one standard unit per day.
- Binge drinking in early pregnancy is particularly harmful.
- In antenatal clinics, improve objective history about alcohol intake and other substance abuse, this will identify the high-risk group of women with problem drinking or other behaviour that can be harmful to the fetus.
- Counselling and detoxification programmes should be easily available to women.
- It is quite likely that many cases of FASD are being missed and training in the recognition of this disorder and the availability of tertiary referral for confirmation of the diagnosis should be made more widespread in the UK.

Guideline comparator

- **US Department of Health 2005** – alcoholic beverages should not be consumed by women of childbearing age who may become pregnant, are pregnant or breastfeeding.
- **SOGC** – there is insufficient evidence regarding fetal safety or harm at low levels of alcohol consumption in pregnancy. There is insufficient evidence to define any threshold for low-level drinking in pregnancy. Abstinence is the prudent choice for a woman who is or might become pregnant.
- **While the safest approach may be to avoid any alcohol intake during pregnancy, it remains the case that there is no evidence of harm from low levels of alcohol consumption, defined as no more than one or two units of alcohol once or twice a week. RCOG**
- **The UK DOH (2007)** – pregnant women or women trying to conceive should avoid drinking alcohol. If they do choose to drink, to minimize the risk to the baby, they should not drink more than 1 to 2 units of alcohol once or twice a week and should not get drunk.
- **NICE (2008)** – pregnant women and women planning a pregnancy should be advised to avoid drinking alcohol in the first 3 months of pregnancy if possible because it may be associated with an increased risk of miscarriage. If women choose to drink alcohol during pregnancy they should be advised to drink no more than 1 to 2 units once or twice a week.
- It is suggested that the evidence of harm from low levels of alcohol consumption in pregnancy is such that UK guidelines should be revised to recommend complete abstinence, in line with the US advice.

Alcohol Use and Pregnancy Consensus. RCOG Clinical Guidelines No. 245; August 2010.

Alcohol Consumption and the Outcomes of Pregnancy. RCOG Statement No. 5; March 2006.

Alcohol Use and Pregnancy Consensus Clinical Guidelines. SOGC. Journal of Obstetrics and Gynaecology Canada; Volume 32; Number 8; August 2010; Supplement 3.

International Guidelines On Drinking and Pregnancy. http://www.icap.org/Table/InternationalGuidelinesOnDrinkingAndPregnancy

CHAPTER 63 Smoking in pregnancy

Prevalence and background

- Smoking remains the single largest preventable cause of fetal and infant morbidity in the UK.
- Prevalence among pregnant women:
  - * Nearly a third smoke in the 12-month period before and/or during pregnancy.
  - * 14% of mothers continue to smoke throughout pregnancy.
- 49% of mothers <20 years smoked throughout pregnancy compared with only 9% aged >35 years.
- Socioeconomic status – mothers in managerial and professional occupations are 4 times less likely to smoke throughout pregnancy (7%) than those in routine and manual occupations (29%).
- Smoking in partners and close family is strongly linked with continued smoking.
- Levels of self-esteem and self-confidence have also been shown to be predictors of cessation success.

Risks or complications

Maternal

- Ectopic pregnancy – smoking has an independent dose-related risk for ectopic pregnancy, with an OR of 1.9.
- Increased incidence of miscarriage.
- PROM – OR of 1.8 in smokers compared with controls.
- Placental complications (such as placenta praevia and abruption) – smokers are up to 3 times more likely to experience these than non-smokers.
- GDM – OR 1.5; CS – OR 1.20.
- Reduced duration of breastfeeding.
- Women who stop smoking prior to 15 weeks of gestation are at no greater risk of adverse outcome than non-smokers.

Fetal and neonatal

- FGR – OR 2; birthweight <2500 g – OR 1.7.
- Linear relationship between the number of cigarettes smoked in the third trimester and decreased birth weight. LBW babies are at increased risk of illness in both the neonatal period and later life.
- PTB – incidence is 4% in non-smokers and stopped smokers compared with 10% in the current smokers.
- Incidence of PET is reduced – OR 0.88. The mechanism is unclear; smoking may modulate factors involved in angiogenesis, endothelial function, and the immune response.
- Health in children – an impact on health in both early and adult life.
- Sudden infant death syndrome – increased risk by up to 4-fold. The mechanism is unclear; exposure to a hypoxic state in the womb may diminish the normal physiological response to hypoxia in the neonate. This may also be responsible for increased susceptibility to respiratory conditions.
- A clear relationship between respiratory symptoms in children (including chronic cough, wheeze, and breathlessness) and exposure to parental smoke.
- Developmental/behavioural problems and obesity.

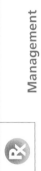

Management

One-to-one and group counselling

- Begin with brief intervention at the initial point of care, moving on to one-to-one counselling and/or group therapy clinics.
- Brief intervention – provide information regarding cessation service availability, the risks of smoking during pregnancy, and the benefits of quitting.
- Brief intervention increases cessation rates between 1 and 3% compared with no intervention.
- Motivational assessment – '5 As' assessment and planning tool:
  * Ask – identify smokers at each clinic visit.
  * Advise – inform on health benefits of smoking cessation.
  * Assess – individual's willingness and motivation to quit.
  * Assist – information & access to smoking cessation services.
  * Arrange – follow-up contact.
- Second-stage intervention involves one-to-one or group counselling sessions Group therapy is typically offered to groups of between 5 and 25 individuals. The effectiveness of one-to-one behavioural counselling improves cessation rates substantially compared with controls, with a relative risk for smoking cessation at long-term follow-up of 1.4.
- The difference in success rates between the group and individual counselling is not shown to be significant.
- Cochrane review examined the efficacy of all the interventions in pregnant women smokers and reported that not only are these interventions effective, but they also lead to a reduction in the incidence of PTB and LBW.

Nicotine replacement therapy (NRT)

- Goal – to reduce nicotine withdrawal cravings by providing nicotine in a controlled dose regimen during smoking cessation attempts. It is available as lozenges, patches, and nasal spray.
- In general population – NRT use increases cessation by 50–70% compared with controls. Evidence for NRT efficacy and safety in pregnancy is limited.
- As nicotine crosses the placenta and has been shown to cause a dose-related rise in maternal BP and heart rate, this may expose the fetus to consequent health risks. It has also been suggested that, as nicotine is metabolized 30% more quickly in pregnancy, this could limit the efficacy of NRT and potentially lead to a compensatory increase in smoking.
- NICE –
  * Discuss the risks and benefits of NRT.
  * Use only if smoking cessation without NRT fails.
  * Use if women express a clear wish to receive NRT.
  * Only prescribe 2 weeks of NRT.
  * Only give subsequent prescriptions to women who have demonstrated on re-assessment that they are still not smoking.
  * Advise women to remove NRT before going to bed.
- Committee on Safety of Medicines on NRT use in pregnancy –
  * Available data are limited; NRT use in pregnancy does not give undue concern. Although NRT efficacy is unproven in pregnant women, its use may be justified in terms of reducing risk of poor health outcomes in the neonate. Smoking exposes the fetus to nicotine as well as other toxins and hypoxia because of increased carbon monoxide concentrations in maternal blood. NRT exposes the fetus to only one of these risks; therefore, weigh the risks of using NRT against the harm potentially caused by continued smoking.
  * Use NRT early in pregnancy with the aim of discontinuing after 2–3 months.
  * NRT can be transmitted to a baby through breastfeeding; any risk is theoretical and not evidence-based, whereas the risk of continued smoking is known.

Pharmacological therapies

- Bupropion and varenicline have proven effective in increasing cessation rates in the general population. But the drug manufacturers and NICE state they are contraindicated in pregnancy.

Management – at booking and subsequent visits (NICE)

- **Enquire –**
  - ✳ If she or anyone else in her household smokes.
  - ✳ Whether she is a light or infrequent smoker.
  - ✳ The time since she last smoked and the number of cigarettes smoked (and when) on the test day.
- **Use of a CO test** – will allow a physical measure of smoking and exposure to other people's smoking to be seen.
- CO levels fall overnight so morning readings may give low results.

- Provide information about the risks to the unborn child of smoking and the hazards of exposure to second-hand smoke for both mother and baby.
- Explain the health benefits of stopping for the woman and her baby.
- **Advise her to stop – not just cut down.**

Refer to NHS Stop Smoking Services
- All women who smoke.
- Women who have stopped smoking within the last 2 weeks.
- Those with a CO reading of 7 ppm or above.
- Light or infrequent smokers, even if they register a lower reading, e.g., 3 ppm.

Next appointment – check whether the woman took up her referral.

- If not, ask if she is interested in stopping smoking and offer another referral to the service.
- If she declines the referral, accept the answer.
- Leave the offer of help open.
- Review at a later appointment.

- If the referral was taken up, provide feedback.
- Review at subsequent appointments, as appropriate

- If a high CO reading (>10ppm) but say they do not smoke, advise them about possible CO poisoning.
- If her partner or others in the household smoke, suggest they contact NHS Stop Smoking Services.
- If no one smokes, give positive feedback.

Recommendation for partners and others in the household who smoke –
- Advise about the danger that other people's tobacco smoke poses to the pregnant woman and to the baby – before and after birth.
- Advise not to smoke around the pregnant woman, mother or baby. This includes not smoking in the house or car.
- Offer partners who smoke help to stop using multicomponent interventions. Choose medication, the one that seems most likely to succeed.

Published Guidance Outlining the Intended Scope and Availability of Smoking Cessation Services in the UK; NICE 2008.
Quitting Smoking in Pregnancy and Following Childbirth. NICE. Issue date: June 2010.
Eastham R, Gosakan R. Smoking and smoking cessation in pregnancy. The Obstetrician & Gynaecologist 2010;12:103–109.

CHAPTER 64 Teenage pregnancy

Background and prevalence

- In 2004 the pregnancy rate in girls aged 15–17 years in England was 42/1000.
- There has been an overall decline of 11% since 1998. UK still has the highest rate of teenage pregnancy in Western Europe under 16 years of age.
- Sociodemographic variables associated with teenage pregnancy increase the risk of adverse outcomes. However, the risks remain significantly elevated for teenage mothers after adjustment for marital status, level of education, and adequacy of prenatal care.
- Socioeconomic deprivation – CEMACE (2006–2008) – 13 deaths in mothers aged < 20 years; 4 girls were aged between 15 and 16. Seven of these girls were either in social care or known to social services.

Risk factors – multiple socioeconomic factors

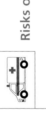

- Teenagers from socially deprived areas are up to 6 times more likely to become pregnant than teenagers from other areas. Rates higher in more deprived areas – 56/1000 girls aged 15–17 years vs 25/1000 in least deprived areas, in 2004.
- Teenagers from unskilled manual backgrounds (social class V) are 10 times more likely to become pregnant than those from professional backgrounds (social class I).
- Low educational achievement – young people scoring below average on educational achievement are at increased risk of becoming teenage parents. 29% of sexually active young women who left school at 16 years of age without any qualifications had a child before the age of 18 years, compared with 14% of those who left at 16 with qualifications and 1% of those who left at age 17 years or over.
- Having had teenage parents – women who were themselves children of teenage mothers are more likely to have a teenage pregnancy compared with those born to older mothers. • Crime.
- Being in the care of social services. • Sexual abuse. • Mental health problems.

Risks or complications

Risks of teenage pregnancy

- Biological risks may have been exaggerated in previous studies. Risks are likely to reflect a complex interplay between sociodemographic variables, gynaecological immaturity, and the growth and nutritional status of the mother.
- Fetal –
  * PTD – especially in the 13–16 years age group.
  * SGA infants. * LBW. * Increased neonatal mortality.
  * Rates of spontaneous miscarriage and of very PTD (< 32 weeks of gestation) are highest in girls aged 13–15 years.
- Maternal – * Anaemia. * PIH. * Postnatal depression. * STIs.
- Offspring – * Poorer cognitive development. * Lower educational attainment. * More frequent criminal activity. * Higher risks of abuse, neglect and behavioural problems during childhood.
- Gynaecological immaturity – high risk of adverse pregnancy outcome in the adolescent has been attributed to gynaecological immaturity and the growth and nutritional status of the mother. Almost 50% of adolescents continue to grow while pregnant. This growth is associated with larger pregnancy weight gains, increased fat stores, and greater postpartum weight retention than in non-growing adolescents and mature women. In spite of the changes typically associated with increased fetal size (larger pregnancy weight gains, increased fat stores), the offspring are smaller in growing than non-growing adolescents. This significant reduction in fetal growth rate is attributed to a competition for nutrients between the maternal body and the gravid uterus.

Other risks associated with teenage pregnancy

- **STIs** – 1 in 8 teenagers attending a family planning clinic in Nottingham had an STI. The incidence of gonorrhoea is increased by 35% between 1997 and 1999 in the UK and those most at risk in the female population were aged 16–19 years.
- **Alcohol and substance misuse and smoking** – UK survey – 36% of those aged 15 and 16 years smoked cigarettes. Girls who have had a teenage pregnancy are more likely to have smoked than those who have not conceived as teenagers. The birth weight for gestational age curves of smoking adolescents show a marked fall off in weight from 36 weeks of gestation. At least 10% of adolescent smokers have pregnancies affected by severe early onset (before 32 weeks of gestation) FGR.
- **Poor diet** – poor eating habits and neglect to take vitamin supplements. Teenagers are less likely than older women to be of adequate prepregnancy weight or to gain an adequate amount of weight during pregnancy. Low weight gain increases the risk of having a low birth weight baby.
- **Postnatal depression and difficulties with breastfeeding** – teenage mothers are more likely to suffer from postnatal depression than older mothers. 37–54% reduction in milk production 6 months after childbirth in adolescents compared with older mothers.

CHAPTER 64 Teenage pregnancy

309

Prevention

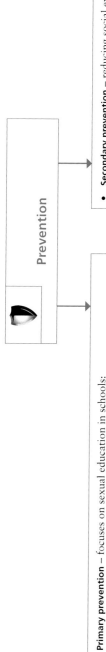

- **Primary prevention** – focuses on sexual education in schools:
  * Sex and relationships education and school-based health services.
  * Encouraging abstinence and delay as approaches to sexual health.
  * Use of effective contraceptive methods.
  * Services in keeping with lifestyle – on-site contraceptive and sexual health advice.

- **Secondary prevention** – reducing social exclusion rates among teenage parents and their children:
  * Supporting pregnant teenagers and teenage mothers.
  * Specially trained midwives and HCPs in maternity services.
  * Access to a dedicated personal adviser providing individualized support.
  * Continued education and training.
  * Advice on contact with housing support services.

Management

General measures

- There is no evidence of medical interventions that can specifically improve pregnancy outcome.
- Supportive care and social support.
- Smoking cessation.
- Effective postnatal counselling regarding contraception can help prevent subsequent pregnancies and STIs.

Termination of pregnancy and adoption

- Approximately 40% of teenagers in the UK terminate their pregnancies.
- Over 25% will become pregnant again during their teenage years, including 18% of those who terminate their first pregnancy.
- Teenagers are more likely to have later terminations, to resort to unskilled practitioners, and dangerous methods and, when complications do arise, they are more likely to present late.
- While termination and adoption are options that are available, most girls choose to continue with their pregnancies and keep their infants.

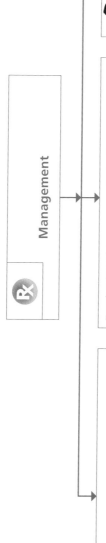

Antenatal care

- Encourage adolescents to attend for antenatal care.
- Confirm gestational age with early USS.
- Advise on nutrition and adverse habits such as smoking and alcohol use.
- Social support – early referral to a specialist midwife or social worker.
- Provide information regarding antenatal care and labour in a format that is accessible and easily understood.

Intrapartum care

- Manage as for other labouring women. However, be aware of increased likelihood of obstructed labour because of a small, immature pelvis in very young adolescents.

Postnatal care

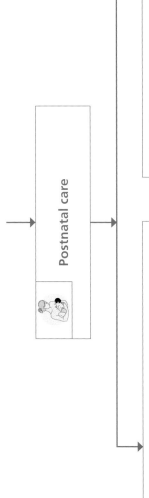

Care and counselling

- Infants at greater risk of inadequate growth, infection, and chemical dependence. Observe infant feeding, growth, and safety.
- Below the age of 20 years, the younger the mother, the greater the risk of her infant dying during the first year of life.
- Women in this group are also less likely to receive child support from the biological fathers, over 50% of children of adolescent mothers never live with their biological father. They are less likely to complete their education and establish their independence and financial security. Therefore, pay special attention to discuss financial issues and returning to school.

Contraception

- Condoms are the most widely used contraceptive in adolescence but teenagers are relatively poor users of both barrier and hormonal contraceptives. The combined use of condoms plus the contraceptive pill ('double Dutch') is the most effective option.
- Use of the combined pill in a vaginal ring or in patch form may improve compliance.
- Long-acting contraception may help to reduce teenage pregnancy but it does not protect against STIs.
- Advise not to use emergency contraception as an alternative for a regular form of contraception.
- Contraceptive services should be easily accessible, confidential, cheap or free, and safe. They also benefit from having close links with STI clinics, smoking cessation programmes, substance abuse clinics, social services, maternity hospitals, and termination services.

Teenage Pregnancy and Reproductive Health. RCOG Summary Review; June 2007.
Horgan RP, Kenny LC. Management of Teenage Pregnancy. The Obstetrician & Gynaecologist 2007;9:153–158.

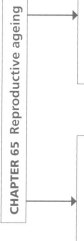

CHAPTER 65 Reproductive ageing

Background

- UK – the mean age of childbearing was 23 years in 1968 and 29 in 2008. Women aged 30–34 have nearly doubled their fecundity overtaking women in the 25–29 age group.
- UK – the proportion of maternities in women aged 35 years or over has increased from 8% (180 000 maternities) in 1985–87 to 20% (460 000 maternities) in 2006–8.
- There are a variety of social, psychological or economic reasons why women may delay starting a family – career concerns (63%), financial reasons (53%), and finding a suitable partner (53%).
- There has been a significant rise in the incidence of dizygotic twins, both from natural conception, caused by an increase in the release of FSH with age, and from assisted conception. Women over 40 are the group with the highest proportion of multiple pregnancies.
- Older women are also more likely to be nulliparous, require ART for conception, and have multiple pregnancies (naturally and after ART), all of which predispose to increased obstetric and neonatal morbidity.

Declining fertility

- Women are born with all the oocytes they will ever have, which are formed within a few weeks of conception in the female fetus. There are up to 7 million primary oocytes in a typical 20-week fetus. This number is more than halved by apoptosis by the time of birth and just 400 000 remain by puberty. On average, 400 oocytes reach maturity and ovulate in a woman's lifetime. This decline in the number of oocytes continues up to the menopause, with older women demonstrating both decreased ovarian reserve and poorer quality in those remaining oocytes.
- Decline in oocyte 'quality' – age-related changes in nuclear and cytoplasmic competence affect fundamental processes of spindle formation and chromosome segregation, mitochondrial function, and the integrity of the cytoskeleton. A poor-quality oocyte is less likely to be fertilized and, if fertilized, will produce an embryo which is generally slow to divide and unlikely to implant.
- The rate of decline in fertility accelerates with age. Ageing results in poorer quality gametes causing increased chances of chromosomal abnormality resulting in miscarriage. The proportion who experience infertility, miscarriage or fetal abnormality increases rapidly after 35 such that only 2 in 5 of those who wish to have a child at 40 years of age will be able to do so.
- At the age of 25 just 5% of women take longer than a year to conceive with regular intercourse, rising to 30% in those aged 35.

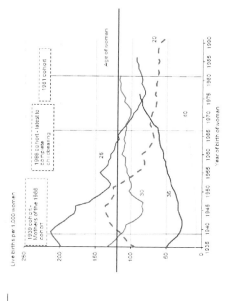

Age-specific fertility rates at selected ages, by year of birth of woman, 1935 to 1991 England and Wales

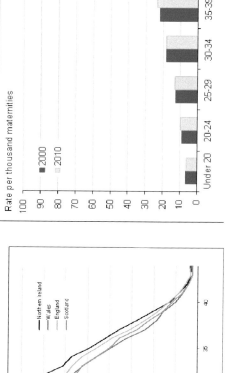

Maternities with multiple births by age of mother, 2000 and 2010, England and Wales

Age-specific fertility rates (ASFRs), constituent countries of the UK, 2010

Fertility

Ovarian reserve testing

- It tests for the quantity of oocytes remaining within the ovaries of a woman at a certain time point.
- **Serum FSH in early follicular phase** – as the size of the oocyte pool diminishes, higher levels of pituitary stimulation are needed to promote development of a dominant follicle. Hence, high concentrations of FSH reflect low ovarian reserve.
- However, no cut-off level predictive of poor outcome has been agreed.
- **Serum anti-müllerian hormone (AMH) and inhibin** – inhibin B is produced by small antral follicles in response to FSH stimulation, while AMH is derived from pre-antral follicles and is non-FSH dependent. AMH has the best predictive value. AMH concentrations are fairly stable throughout the cycle and there is limited cycle-to-cycle variation.
- **Antral follicle count (AFC)** – using high-resolution TVS to count small antral follicles 2–10 mm in diameter.
- AFC correlates with oocyte yield in IVF.
- Drawbacks – test is operator-dependent and requires attendance at the ultrasound facility. Recent studies have not shown evidence of benefit over AMH measurement.

Adverse effects of age on reproduction

- Gynaecological problems increase with age such as premature menopause, STIs, PID, endometriosis, fibroids, cervical surgery.
- Conception – reduced fertility, increased miscarriage and ectopic pregnancy; chromosomal anomaly, birth defects, multiple pregnancy.
- Avoidable factors that adversely affect fertility such as smoking, alcohol, BMI >30, STIs.

Prevention of infertility

- Age is a key factor amenable to action through education and social support for parenting. Provide full, clear fertility facts to women of all ages.
- Reinforce the information in schools, family planning, sexual health clinics, and in the media, to remind young couples of the biological realities of reproductive ageing.
- Provide fertility graphs in general practice surgeries and at family planning clinics to remind patients that the optimal age for childbearing is between 20 and 35 years.
- IVF cannot make up for the delay and physiological decline in the quality of gametes.
- Mixed media messages about fecundity or IVF may also be partially responsible for exacerbating the delay in starting a family, giving women a false sense of security.

Assisted reproductive technology (ART) options

- Fertility success with ART starts to decline from the age of 35.
- There is a 32% chance of live birth from 1 cycle of IVF with fresh eggs in women under 35, falling to 3% in women over 44.
- More than half of the IVF live births in women over the age of 40 have used donor eggs.

Preimplantation genetic screening (PGS)

- Embryo biopsy and testing, to screen IVF embryos for aneuploidy using PGS, with transfer of euploid embryos.
- Despite the scientific and clinical rationale for PGS, meta-analysis failed to show a significant increase in live birth rates following PGS.
- The mitotic error rate in cleavage-stage embryos results in mosaicism; as a consequence, the genome of a single blastomere is not representative of the whole genome of the embryo, which may account for the results of the clinical trials being at odds with the scientific rationale for PGS.

Oocyte storage

- Oocyte vitrification offers young healthy women the possibility of preserving oocytes until the less fertile years of life.
- Chances of healthy pregnancy resulting from a vitrified oocyte are small (4%), so many eggs need to be collected and frozen to give a realistic chance of success later on.
- This exposes the healthy woman to superovulation and oocyte collection with its associated complications.
- The best age for oocyte vitrification is probably under 30 years, resulting in medicalization of relatively young women.
- Unrealistic reliance on their store of vitrified oocytes may lead women to defer pregnancy for many years only to experience disappointment when the stored oocytes later fail to fertilize or implant.
- Anxieties about the effects of prolonged vitrification on the offspring remain.

Oocyte donation

- To use oocytes from a younger, fertile donor.
- Oocyte donors are required to go through superovulation and transvaginal oocyte collection.
- Current UK law does not permit commercial oocyte donation and the number of available oocyte donors is small.
- This has caused an exodus of potential recipients of this technique to countries that permit payment to egg donors, such as Spain, Cyprus, USA. This cross-border reproductive care carries significant disadvantages for both the recipient and the donor.

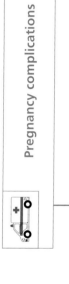

Pregnancy complications

Maternal risks –

- Acquired medical problems: development of age-related medical disorders such as chronic HT, gestational HT, type 2 diabetes, and obesity.
- Cancer of the breast, thyroid, and cervix are the three most common malignancies encountered in pregnancy. The incidence of cancer in pregnant women over 40 is 6 times higher than in those aged 24–29.
- Obstetric complications: malpresentation, prematurity, PET, placenta praevia (OR 2.8), GDM (OR 2.4), abruption (OR 2.3), CS (OR 2.0), DVT, CS, PPH, and maternal death.
- The maternal mortality rate in the UK is highest in the 40 years and over age group, with a rate of 29/100 000 maternities compared with a rate of 11/100 000 for all ages. (CMACE 2006–2008)

Fetal risk –

- Risk of miscarriage in a woman 35–39 years is 24%, doubles to 51% at 40–44 years.
- Higher risk of birth defects or genetic/chromosomal abnormality, such as trisomy 21. The risk of trisomy 21 rises from 1 in 1600 in mothers aged <23 years to 1 in 40 for mothers aged 43 years.
- Increased LBW, PTD, post-term delivery; FGR; stillbirth, birth asphyxia, and neonatal death. Rates of stillbirth have an OR of 2.4 at over 35 years of age, rising to 5.2 at 40 years, with a peak at 41 weeks of gestation.
- Advanced maternal age is independently associated with an increase in antenatal and intrapartum stillbirth and an increase in neonatal mortality.

Risk of stillbirth in older mothers

- Women aged ≥40 years have a similar SB risk at 39 weeks of gestation to 25- to 29-year-olds at 41 weeks of gestation.
- Unexplained SB increase with advancing maternal age and with increasing gestational age in both nulliparous and multiparous women.
- Recent American data – at 41 weeks the risk of stillbirth is 0.75/1000 women under the age of 35 years, and 2.5/1000 women aged ≥40 years. The effect of maternal age persist despite accounting for medical disease, parity, race, and ethnicity.
- Scottish retrospective cohort study: women that are nulliparous and aged ≥ 40 years old and at term have an increased rate of intrapartum SB due to intrapartum anoxia with an adjusted odds ratio (aOR) of 5.3 compared to younger women.

Reason for the excess risk of SB in advanced maternal age

- Remains unknown.
- FGR increases with maternal age. Reported OR for FGR is 1.4 in women aged 35–39 years compared with 3.2 in women who are ≥40 years.
- No association between other clinical markers of uteroplacental insufficiency and older mothers is found suggesting that uteroplacental insufficiency may not be the full explanation for the increase in SB in the 3rd trimester in women that are older.

Risk of neonatal death

- Women ≥ 40 years old are 1.3 times more likely to have a neonatal death compared to women aged 25–29 years old.

Intrapartum complications

- Ageing impairs myometrial function resulting in increased rates of CS for dystocia and instrumental delivery in older mothers in spontaneous or induced labour.
- The incidence of prolonged labour (>12 hours) and surgical intervention because of dystocia is reported to be one-third higher in spontaneously labouring nulliparous women aged ≥ 35 years compared to younger women.
- Women ≥ 35 years of age require oxytocin at higher doses and for a longer duration in order to achieve a successful vaginal delivery.
- Scottish study – spontaneous and induced labour; the OR for a 5-year increase in age was 1.49 for the risk of an instrumental delivery and 1.49 for the risk of intrapartum CS.

Antenatal care

- Routine ANC as per the general population but be aware of higher risk of development of antenatal complications.
- No evidence to support routine assessment of fetal growth or umbilical artery and uterine artery Doppler in older mothers to identify FGR.

Time and mode of delivery

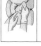

- 37% of obstetricians offer IOL at term to women aged 40–44 years of age and 55% to those ≥45 years old.
- Elective CSs in older women are also rising with a reported lower threshold among patients and providers to perform a CS in older women.
- Reasons for elective CS: anxiety regarding maternal age, the use of ART, medical comorbidities, and concerns to prevent neonatal harm.
- Planned CS result in increased NICU admissions compared to vaginal delivery (RR 2.2) and those performed before 39 weeks of gestation are at risk of neonatal adverse respiratory outcomes.
- Vaginal birth remains more likely than an emergency CS following IOL in women who are older and nulliparous. Data from women of all ages addressing the maternal and neonatal outcomes of IOL at term compared to those expectantly managed shows favourable outcomes for the IOL at term. There remains a paucity of data specifically in older women.
- The maternal and gestational age-specific SB risks suggest that if all women aged ≥ 40 years old, with a singleton pregnancy are induced at 39 weeks of gestation instead of 41 weeks of gestation, 17 SBs could be prevented. This equates to inducing an extra 9350 women to prevent one SB. Inducing at 40 weeks of gestation, instead of 41, would prevent 7 SBs and require an extra 4750 women to be induced.

- The incidence of SB is higher in women of advanced maternal age. This at 39–40 weeks of gestation equates to 2 in 1000 for women ≥40 years of age compared to 1 in 1000 for women < 35 years old.
- IOL at 39–40 weeks of gestation to women ≥40 years of age would reduce late antenatal SBs, especially where there are concurrent medical comorbidities, nulliparity, or Afro-Caribbean ethnicity; all of which are known to have higher SB rates.
- However, at present there are insufficient data available on the effect such a policy would have on surgical deliveries and perinatal mortality specifically in older mothers.
- **Elective CS** – women who are older and nulliparous, may request elective delivery rather than IOL. A discussion of risks and benefits of IOL versus elective CS is appropriate in these circumstances.

Reproductive ageing

Reproductive ageing in males

- Men start producing mature sperm at puberty and this continues throughout life.
- While many men remain fertile into their fifth decade and beyond, the proportion of men with disorders of spermatogenesis increases with advancing age.
- Men over 40 years of age contribute to reduced fertility and fecundity of a couple, especially when the female partner is also of advanced age.
- Increasing paternal age can be associated with decreased serum androgen concentration, decreased sexual activity, alterations of testicular morphology, and deterioration of semen quality.
- Increased paternal age has an influence on the DNA integrity of sperm, and is suggested to have epigenetic effects.
- The reproductive impact of paternal ageing is suggested to be (though less pronounced than that of female ageing) at least in part responsible for the association with reduced fertility and the increase in pregnancy-associated complications and adverse outcome in the offspring.

- While still remaining within WHO guidelines for 'normal' semen analysis, there is a decline in motility, morphology, and volume from the age of 50.
- Time to pregnancy for one group of women all aged under 25 was significantly affected by the male partner's age when adjusted for female variables. For men aged below 25 the average length of time for their partners to get pregnant was 4.6 months, compared with nearly 2 years for those men over 40.
- The rate of miscarriage in pregnancies from men older than 50 also increases when accounted for age-matched women, although there is no change in birth outcomes.
- Paternally inherited diseases caused by missense copy errors or genetic mutations increase with advancing age.

Induction of Labour at Term in Older Mothers. RCOG Scientific Impact Paper No.34; February 2013.
Reproductive Ageing. RCOG Scientific Advisory Committee Opinion Paper 24; January 2011.
Utting D, Bewley S. Family planning and age-related reproductive risk. The Obstetrician & Gynaecologist 2011;13:35–41.
http://www.ons.gov.uk
Delayed Child-Bearing; SOGC Committee Opinion No. 271. Journal of Obstetrics & Gynaecology Canada 2012;34(1):80–93.

CHAPTER 66 Air travel in pregnancy

Physiological and environmental changes associated with commercial air travel

- Cabin altitude is maintained between 4000 and 8000 feet at cruising altitude. The barometric pressure is significantly lower than at sea level with a reduction in the partial pressure of oxygen, which results in a reduction in blood oxygen saturation by around 10%. Such a reduction does not pose a problem for healthy individuals and in pregnancy.

- Owing to the higher count of red blood cells in the fetal circulation and the favourable properties of fetal haemoglobin, there is little change in fetal oxygen pressures.

- However, in significantly anaemic pregnant women, this may be enough to induce symptoms. **Therefore advise women with sickle cell disease who are at risk of sickling crisis against flying** (relative contraindication).

- Radiation exposure from one transatlantic flight is 2.5 times the dose of a single chest X-ray with abdominal shielding. The increased cosmic radiation exposure associated with flying is not significant in terms of risk to the mother or fetus for occasional flights but flight crew are not allowed to fly while pregnant as their exposure would be substantially greater.

- Humidity in aircraft cabins is low at around 15% which leads to an increase in insensible fluid loss; this is insufficient to cause dehydration, although drying of mucous membranes occurs.

  Use of body scanners (back scatter machines and millimetre wave units) utilizing ionizing radiation for security checks prior to flying is safe. With regard to pregnancy, negligible radiation doses are absorbed into the body and therefore the fetal dose is much lower than the dose to a pregnant woman.

Contraindication

- Medical complications which may occur during pregnancy and which contraindicate commercial air travel include:
  * Severe anaemia with a haemoglobin < 7.5 g/dl.
  * Unstable fracture, where significant leg swelling can occur in flight, particularly hazardous if a cast is in place.
  * Recent haemorrhage.
  * Otitis media and sinusitis.
  * Serious respiratory disease, particularly with marked breathlessness.
  * Recent sickling crisis.
  * Recent gastrointestinal surgery where suture lines on the intestine could come under stress due to the reduction in pressure and gaseous expansion.

Risks or complications

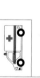

- With increasing altitude and reduction in barometric pressure, gases expand. This leads to problems within the ear, particularly if there is nasal congestion, which is more common because of the vasodilatation of pregnancy.

- Motion sickness may be a problem and this may exacerbate morning sickness.

- In non-pregnant populations, around 4–5% of those at high risk will develop DVT associated with air travel. The risk of new thrombosis associated with air travel is approximately 2- to 4-fold in non-pregnant individuals. There is some evidence to suggest that flights of 8 hours or more increase the risk of DVT in pregnant women with additional risk factors (previous DVT or obesity). Although the absolute risk is small, this risk is likely to be increased by air travel owing to immobility and cramped conditions.

- Prolonged air travel results in a small increase in the absolute incidence of VTE of around 3-fold, with an 18% higher risk of VTE for each 2-hour increase in flight duration. However, the overall absolute incidence of a symptomatic VTE is low, with a rate of 1 in 4600 flights in the month following a flight of 4 hours' duration. The risk will depend on the individual's risk factors such as thrombophilia and combined oral contraceptive use.

- Graduated elastic compression stockings worn during a flight significantly reduce the risk of asymptomatic DVT with a RR of 0.10; i.e., 4.5 fewer in low-risk population and 16.2 fewer symptomatic DVT per 10000 people in a high-risk population. These data relate to the non-pregnant population, although may be reasonable to apply to pregnant women.

Gestation of pregnancy

- The main concern restricting the airlines from accepting pregnant women as passengers relates to the risk of labour, which may disrupt the flight along with the problem of lack of appropriate care providers and facilities to manage labour or any obstetric complication. Many airlines do not allow women to fly after 36 completed weeks because of this risk.

- If there are significant risk factors for PTL, such as multiple pregnancy, advise women against flying after 32 completed weeks.

- Many airlines require a letter from a midwife or doctor confirming that there are no anticipated complications for flights taken after the 28th week of pregnancy and confirmation of the expected date of delivery.

Obstetric emergencies, though rare, could have serious consequences in the absence of appropriate medical facilities (both personnel and equipment).

Practical considerations and advice

General advice

- Women with an uncomplicated pregnancy and no medical or obstetric risk factors that would contraindicate air travel can safely use air travel.
- Advise women at risk of miscarriage or ectopic pregnancy (previous ectopic pregnancy or history of recurrent miscarriage) to confirm the location and/or viability of the pregnancy by ultrasound prior to travel.
- In view of the difficulties associated with labour occurring in flight, it would appear to be prudent to avoid air travel from 37 weeks of gestation in an uncomplicated singleton pregnancy and beyond 34 weeks of gestation in an uncomplicated multiple dichorionic pregnancy.
- Advise women travelling abroad to obtain medical insurance. Travel insurance may be difficult to obtain in the latter stages of pregnancy. Most insurance companies do not cover women beyond 32 weeks of gestation. Prior to this both maternal and neonatal expenses should be covered.
- Issues associated with destination include immunization and antimalarial medication.
- General precautions regarding avoiding contaminated food and water.
- For seat belt use, advise woman to ensure that the strap is reasonably tightly fastened under her abdomen and across the top of her thighs.

Minimizing the risk of DVT

- General advice – to have an aisle seat to facilitate ease of movement; to take regular walks around the cabin every 30 minutes or so on a medium- or long-haul flight; to maintain a good fluid intake and minimize caffeine and alcohol intake to avoid dehydration.
- Undertake a specific individualized risk assessment for thrombosis.
- For short-haul journeys – no specific measures.
- For medium- to long-haul flights lasting >4 hours –
  * All pregnant women – graduated elastic compression stockings.
  * In presence of additional risk factors such as a previous DVT, morbid obesity or medical problems, consider prophylaxis with LMWH in the doses recommended for antenatal prophylaxis for the day of travel and several days thereafter.
- In such cases, the woman is likely to be on antenatal thromboprophylaxis with LMWH which should be continued. She may require a letter to confirm the gestation and also for security purposes if she is carrying a supply of LMWH injections.
- Do not offer aspirin alone as VTE prophylaxis, primarily because more effective methods of prophylaxis are readily available and there is an association with potential haemorrhagic complications.

CEC Kingman, DL Economides. Air travel in pregnancy. The Obstetrician & Gynaecologist 2002;4;188–192. Air Travel and Pregnancy. RCOG Scientific Impact Paper No. 1; May 2013.

CHAPTER 67 Women with breast cancer in pregnancy

Prevalence and background

- Breast cancer is the most common cancer in females (lifetime risk 1 in 9) in the UK, and is the leading cause of death in women aged 35–54 years. The 5-year survival is around 80% for the under 50s age group.
- It affects almost 5000 women of reproductive age in the UK annually. About 10% of women diagnosed with breast cancer subsequently become pregnant.
- 10–20% cases of breast cancer in women aged 30 years or less may be associated with pregnancy or occur within 1 year postpartum.
- Pregnancy does not worsen the prognosis. However, as pregnancy-associated breast cancer occurs in a younger population who may have features that carry a higher risk of metastases, these younger women may be expected to have an inferior prognosis.

- **Refer women presenting with a breast lump during pregnancy to a breast specialist team. MDT care.**
- Prognostic factors – tumour size, grade, nodal status, oestrogen and progesterone receptor, and HER2 status.

Diagnosis and staging

- Diagnosis may be difficult in women who are pregnant or lactating.
- Ultrasound first to assess a discrete lump, but if cancer is confirmed, perform mammography (with fetal shielding) to assess the extent of disease and the contralateral breast.
- Use tissue diagnosis with ultrasound-guided biopsy for histology rather than cytology, as proliferative change during pregnancy renders cytology inconclusive in many women.
- Histological grade, receptor status, and human epidermal growth factor receptor 2 (HER2) will help treatment planning.
- For staging for metastases in non-pregnant women – use X-ray, CT, and isotope bone scan. Bone scanning and pelvic X-ray CT are contraindicated in pregnancy because of the possible effect of irradiation on the fetus. In pregnant women undertake staging for metastases if there is high clinical suspicion – chest X-ray and liver USS. If there is concern about bone involvement, arrange a plain film of the relevant area and/or MRI to minimize radiation exposure to the fetus.

Treatment during pregnancy – breast cancer

Surgical treatment

- Can be undertaken in all trimesters.
- Consider breast conserving surgery or mastectomy based on tumour characteristics and breast size.
- Delay reconstruction to avoid prolonged anaesthesia and to allow optimal symmetrization of the breasts after delivery.
- Sentinel node assessment using radioisotope scintigraphy does not cause significant uterine radiation, but avoid blue dye as the effect upon the fetus is unknown.
- Sentinel node biopsy is indicated in women who have a negative result from a preoperative axillary ultrasound and needle biopsy. If the axilla is positive, axillary clearance is indicated.

Radiotherapy (RT)

- Do not offer RT until delivery unless it is life saving or to preserve organ function (e.g., spinal cord compression).
- If necessary, consider RT with fetal shielding or, depending on gestational age, consider early elective delivery.
- Defer routine breast/chest wall RT until after delivery.

Chemotherapy (ChT)

- Do not offer ChT in the first trimester because of a high rate of fetal abnormality. It can be safely given from the second trimester.
- There is no evidence for an increased rate of second-trimester miscarriage or FGR, organ dysfunction or long-term adverse outcome with the use of ChT.
- Anthracylines are safe. There are fewer data on taxanes; reserve them for high-risk (node-positive) or metastatic disease.
- Neoadjuvant ChT before surgery may allow tumour down staging and facilitate surgery.

Others

- Tamoxifen and trastuzumab are contraindicated in pregnancy. There are no data on other targeted therapies such as vascular endothelial growth factor antagonists, including bevacizumab.
- Standard antiemetics including 5HT3 serotonin antagonists and dexamethasone.
- There are no data on a neurokinin receptor antagonist which has very high efficacy in ChT-induced emesis.
- Haemopoietic growth factors (granulocyte colony stimulating factor) to minimize potential maternal and fetal problems associated with neutropenia.

Management of pregnancy

℞

Termination of pregnancy

- Offer it based on discussion of the cancer prognosis, treatment, and future fertility with the woman and MDT.

Timing of delivery

- Time the birth of the baby after discussion with the woman and the MDT.
- Most women can go to full term of pregnancy and have a normal or induced delivery.
- If early delivery of the baby is necessary, consider corticosteroids for fetal lung maturity.
- Time birth more than 2–3 weeks after the last ChT session to allow maternal bone marrow recovery and to minimize problems with neutropenia.

Breastfeeding

- Ability to breastfeed depends on surgery and whether major ducts have been excised.
- Do not advise breastfeeding while on ChT as the drugs cross into breast milk and may cause neonatal leucopenia. A time interval of 14 days or more from the last ChT session to start of breastfeeding is needed to allow drug clearance from breast milk. If ChT is restarted, breastfeeding must cease.
- Women taking tamoxifen or trastuzumab should not breastfeed.

Contraception

- **Offer non-hormonal contraceptive methods.**
- Do not offer hormonal contraception to women with current or recent breast cancer.
- This advice does not differentiate between hormone-sensitive and hormone-insensitive tumours. Although hormonal contraception may be considered after at least 5 years free of recurrence, there is insufficient evidence to support the use of combined or progestagen-only hormonal contraceptives when alternative non-hormonal methods are suitable and acceptable.
- The LNG-IUS may reduce the risk of endometrial abnormalities during tamoxifen therapy, but further evidence is required on its safety in breast cancer survivors.

Women planning pregnancy following breast cancer

Impact of pregnancy on risk of recurrence

- Refer for MDT discussion – clinical oncologist, breast surgeon, and obstetrician.
- Women with metastatic disease – advise against pregnancy as life expectancy is limited and treatment of metastatic disease would be compromised.
- Women treated for early-stage disease on tamoxifen – advise to:
  * Stop treatment 3 months before trying to conceive.
  * Have any imaging before trying to conceive to avoid the need for imaging during pregnancy.
- Reassure that long-term survival after breast cancer is not adversely affected by pregnancy. Prognosis is good for women with early-stage breast cancer.
- In women with BRCA mutations, the risks associated with subsequent pregnancy are uncertain. BRCA carriers may consider PGD.

Time interval before pregnancy

- Advice on postponement of pregnancy – individualize based on treatment needs and prognosis.
- Weigh up the benefit of postponing conception to complete adjuvant therapy, against the risk of infertility as a result of delay.
- The rate of disease recurrence is highest in the first 3 years and then declines, although late relapses do occur up to 10 years and more. Most women should wait at least 2 years after treatment, which is when the risk of cancer recurrence is highest.
- Women with oestrogen receptor positive disease – the recommended duration of tamoxifen treatment is 5 years. Age is a major determinant of fertility and delay with already poor ovarian function owing to ChT is likely to lead to infertility. Women in their 30s desiring pregnancy may consider discontinuation of tamoxifen after 2–3 years. Resuming treatment with tamoxifen after childbearing has not been studied, but it is a reasonable strategy.

Outcome of pregnancy

- The majority of pregnancies after breast cancer proceed to live birth. There may be an increased miscarriage rate. One reported series – full-term births (51%), spontaneous miscarriages (8%), and TOPs (41%).
- Risk of malformation in children conceived after treatment for breast cancer – data are limited and conflicting. Reassure.

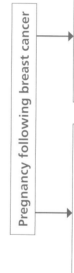

Pregnancy following breast cancer

Women wishing to breastfeed

- Reassure that they can breastfeed from the unaffected breast.
- There is no evidence that breastfeeding increases the risk of recurrence in women who have completed treatment for breast cancer.
- Breast-conserving surgery may not inhibit lactation in the affected breast, but RT causes fibrosis, making lactation unlikely.
- There is no evidence that previous ChT affects the safety of breastfeeding.
- In view of the well-recognized benefits of breastfeeding to the baby, encourage women who wish to breastfeed to do so.

Management of pregnancy

- MDT – obstetrician, oncologist, and breast surgeon.
- During pregnancy, a breast treated by surgery/RT may not undergo hormonal change and the woman may require a temporary prosthesis.
- If breast imaging is needed, ultrasound is preferred.
- Metastatic relapse may be harder to detect and common complaints in pregnancy such as backache can be difficult to assess.
- In women who have received adjuvant ChT with anthracyclines, cumulative dose-dependent left ventricular dysfunction can occur and, rarely, cardiomyopathy. Although cardiac complications during pregnancy are rare in cancer survivors, perform echocardiography in women at risk to detect cardiomyopathy.
- There may be a slightly increased risk of delivery complications and CS.

Non-pregnant women after diagnosis or treatment of breast cancer

- Discuss the effect of treatment on fertility of potential gonadotoxicity before treatment.

- Fertility preservation – refer to a fertility specialist for assisted conception.
- Specialist psychological support and counselling.

GnRH analogues – early studies on use of GnRH analogues during ChT to protect the oocyte pool from depletion are suggestive of benefit with reduced risk of ovarian damage. However, there are concerns that they may lessen tumour response to ChT. Do not offer GnRH analogues for ovarian protection in oestrogen receptor positive breast cancer routinely.

Cryopreservation – egg or embryo freezing.
- Embryo cryopreservation – success rates of 20% per cycle; success rates may be lower when oocytes are retrieved from women with cancer. Time required for ovarian stimulation may postpone ChT, and there is a small risk of procedural complications such as OHSS.
- Due to the concern that elevated oestrogen levels may be deleterious in oestrogen receptor positive breast cancer, stimulation regimens with tamoxifen or letrozole, combined with gonadotrophins are proposed. **Consider modified stimulation regimes for women with oestrogen-sensitive breast cancer.**
- Oocyte storage in women without a partner. There are no long-term safety data.

Cryopreservation of ovarian cortex or the whole ovary – reports of a few pregnancies after regrafting. The need for a surgical procedure is a disadvantage, but this technique does not delay ChT. There are insufficient data to support ovarian tissue storage; offer it only in the context of a research trial.

Adjuvant chemotherapy

- Gonadotoxicity may cause permanent amenorrhoea with complete loss of germ cells, transient amenorrhoea, menstrual irregularity, and subfertility. Degree of gonadotoxicity depends on the specific agents used, the cumulative dose administered, and the woman's age.
- Rate of amenorrhoea – < 5% in women under 30 years of age; up to 50% in women aged 36–40 years; 20–70% in premenopausal women.
- Alkylating agents such as cyclophosphamide cause a higher incidence of amenorrhoea than anthracycline-based regimens. The newer taxanes are less gonadotoxic.

Adjuvant hormonal therapy

- Does not cause long-term effects on fertility.
- Tamoxifen – causes menstrual irregularity with an increased risk of endometrial pathology; avoid pregnancy during tamoxifen therapy because of potential teratogenicity. Advise a 'washout period' of 2–3 months.
- GnRH analogues – are used in hormone-sensitive breast cancer, as they induce profound ovarian suppression and create a low-oestrogen state. They cause amenorrhoea and menopausal symptoms, but the effect is reversible.
- Trastuzumab – no evidence that it impairs fertility, but avoid pregnancy during treatment.

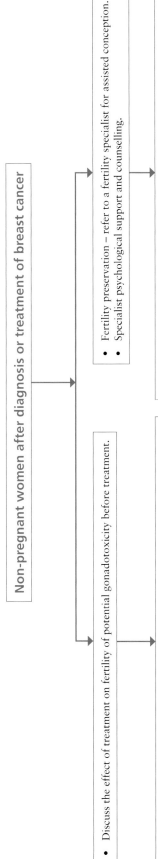

What not to do

- Gadolinium-enhanced MRI; tumour markers such as CA15-3, CEA, and CA125; bone scanning and pelvic X-ray CT.
- RT unless it is life saving or to preserve organ function.
- ChT in the first trimester.
- Tamoxifen and trastuzumab.
- Breastfeeding while on ChT, tamoxifen or trastuzumab.
- Hormonal contraception in women with current or recent breast cancer.
- Routine use of GnRH analogues for ovarian protection.
- Ovarian tissue storage outside the context of a research trial.

Pregnancy and Breast Cancer. RCOG Green-top Guideline No. 12; March 2011.

CHAPTER 68 Complex social issues and pregnancy

Background and definition

- Women whose social situation may impact adversely on the outcomes of pregnancy for them and their baby.
- **Complex social factors** – poverty, homelessness, substance misuse, recent arrival as a migrant, asylum seeker or refugee status, difficulty speaking or understanding English, age under 20, domestic abuse.
- **Domestic abuse** – "an incident of threatening behaviour, violence or abuse (psychological, physical, sexual, financial or emotional) between adults who are or have been partners or family members". It can also include forced marriage, female genital mutilation, and 'honour violence'.
- **Recent migrants** – women who moved to the UK within the previous 12 months.
- **Substance misuse (alcohol and/or drugs)** – regular use of recreational drugs, misuse of over-the-counter medications; prescription medications; alcohol or volatile substances (such as solvents or inhalants) to an extent where physical dependence or harm is a risk.

Risks or complications

- Socially excluded women are at higher risk of death during or after pregnancy. These women are far less likely to seek antenatal care (ANC) early in pregnancy or to stay in regular contact with maternity services. 17% of the women who died from direct or indirect causes booked for maternity care after 22 weeks of gestation or had missed >4 routine antenatal visits compared to 2% of the general population.
- These women are likely to recognize their pregnancy later and delay seeing a HCP.
- Compared to women who booked prior to 20 weeks, women who booked late or missed >4 routine appointments were more likely to be: black African or Caribbean, experiencing domestic abuse, substance misusers, known to social services or child protection services, or unemployed.
- Perinatal mortality – women from non-white ethnic groups and women in the most deprived population quintile had SB and neonatal death rates that were twice those of white women and those living in the least deprived areas.
- Maternal stress in pregnancy has a detrimental effect on subsequent childhood development.

General recommendations for all pregnant women with complex social factors

Some pregnant women with complex social factors are discouraged from using antenatal care services due to language barriers or through lack of knowledge regarding how the health services work. There is a great need to understand barriers to services for these women to enable them to initiate and maintain contact, and to provide services that are flexible to meet their needs.

Provide training for HCP

Improve service organization

Tailor services to meet the needs of the local population

- To guide service provision, record:
  * The number of women presenting with any complex social factor.
  * The number within each complex social factor group identified locally.
- For each complex social factor group, record the number of women who:
  * attend for booking by 10, 12+6, and 20 weeks;
  * attend for the recommended number of antenatal appointments;
  * experience, or have babies who experience, mortality or significant morbidity; and
  * the number of appointments each woman attends;
  * the number of scheduled appointments each woman does not attend.
- **Involve women in their antenatal care** – ask women about their satisfaction with the services provided and record, monitor, and use their responses to guide service development. Involve women and their families in determining local needs and how these might be met.

Enhance care delivery

Give information and offer referral at the first contact – At the first contact with any HCP if the woman does not have a booking appointment arranged – * discuss the need for antenatal care; offer a booking appointment ideally before 10 weeks, or if she is considering TOP offer referral to sexual health services; * ask her to tell her HCP if her address changes and give her a phone number for this purpose.

Reinforce contact at the booking appointment – remind her to tell her HCP if her address changes and make sure she has a phone number for this purpose; give her an out-of-hours phone number, for example the hospital triage contact, the labour ward or the birth centre.

Coordinate care – consider initiating a multiagency needs assessment, including safeguarding issues.

Communicate sensitively – * respect a woman's right to confidentiality and sensitively discuss her fears in a non-judgemental manner; * tell her why and when information may need to be shared with other agencies; * to allow for discussion of sensitive issues, provide each woman with a one-to-one consultation, without partners, family members or legal guardians present, on at least one occasion.

Keep the hand-held maternity notes up to date – make sure the hand-held maternity notes contain a full record of care and the results of all antenatal tests.

A. Pregnant women who misuse substances (alcohol and/or drugs)

Improve service organization

- **Coordinate care with local agencies** – including social care and agencies that provide substance misuse services.
  - * Jointly develop care plans across agencies.
  - * Include information about opiate replacement therapy in care plans.
  - * Offer women information about other services.
- **Track each woman's progress** – Consider ways of ensuring that, for each woman:
  - * Progress is tracked through the agencies involved in her care.
  - * Clinic notes from the different agencies involved in her care are combined into a single document.
  - * There is a coordinated care plan.
- **Offer a named midwife or doctor** and provide a direct phone number.

Enhance care delivery

- **Offer referral to a substance misuse programme** the first time a woman who misuses substances discloses that she is pregnant.
- **Offer information and support** about additional services (such as drug and alcohol misuse support services) and encourage her to use them according to her needs.
  - * Offer information about the potential effects of substance misuse on her unborn baby and what to expect when the baby is born, for example: medical care the baby might need; where the baby will be cared for; any potential involvement of social services.
- **Work with social care professionals to provide supportive and coordinated care** – these women may be anxious about the potential role of social services.
  - * Address women's fears about the involvement of children's services and potential removal of her child by giving her information tailored to her needs.
  - * Address her feelings of guilt about her substance misuse and the potential effects on her baby.

B. Pregnant women who are recent migrants, asylum seekers or refugees, or who have difficulty reading or speaking English

Improve service organization

- These women may not make full use of antenatal care services; because of unfamiliarity with the health service or because they find it hard to communicate with HCPs.
- **Adapt antenatal services to meet local needs** – monitor emergent local needs and plan and adjust services accordingly.
- **Work with other agencies** that provide housing and other services for recent migrants, asylum seekers, and refugees, such as asylum centres, to ensure that antenatal care services have accurate information about a woman's current address and contact details during her pregnancy.
- **Allow enough time for interpretation** – offer flexibility in the number and length of antenatal appointments when interpreting services are used.
- **Provide accessible information about pregnancy and how to find and use antenatal services** in a variety of: * formats, such as posters, leaflets, photographs, drawings/diagrams, online video clips, audio clips, and DVDs; * settings, including pharmacies, community centres, faith groups and centres, GP surgeries, family planning clinics, and children's centres.

Enhance care delivery

- **Offer information and support** on access to healthcare.
  - * At the booking appointment discuss with the woman the importance of keeping her hand-held maternity record with her at all times.
  - * Avoid making assumptions based on a woman's culture, ethnic origin or religious beliefs.
- **Help women who have difficulty reading or speaking English to communicate**
  - * Provide an interpreter (who may be a link worker or advocate and should not be a member of the woman's family, her legal guardian or her partner) who can communicate with the woman in her preferred language.
  - * When giving spoken information, ask the woman about her understanding of what she has been told to ensure she has understood correctly.

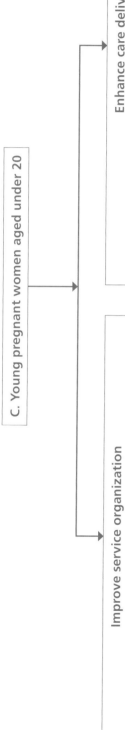

C. Young pregnant women aged under 20

Improve service organization

- These women may feel uncomfortable using antenatal care services in which the majority of service users are in older age groups.
- **Form working partnerships with education authorities and other agencies** to improve access to antenatal services for young women aged under 20.
- **Consider a specialist antenatal service** for these women, using a flexible model of care tailored to the needs of the local population. Components may include:
  - ANC and education in peer groups in a variety of settings, such as GP surgeries, children's centres, and schools.
  - Antenatal education in peer groups offered at the same time and location as antenatal appointments, such as a 'one-stop shop' (where a range of services can be accessed at the same time).
- **Offer a named midwife** who should take responsibility for and provide the majority of the woman's ANC, and provide a direct phone number for the midwife.

Enhance care delivery

- These women may be reluctant to recognize their pregnancy or inhibited by embarrassment and fear of parental reaction. They may also have practical problems such as difficulty getting to and from antenatal appointments.
- **Take into account the young woman's age**
  - Be aware that the young woman may be dealing with other social problems.
  - Offer age-appropriate information in a variety of formats.
  - Include information about:
    - > care services
    - > help with transport to appointments
    - > antenatal peer group education or drop-in sessions
    - > housing benefit and other benefits.
- **Provide opportunities for the baby's father to be involved** – if the young woman agrees, provide opportunities for her baby's father to be involved in her ANC.

Provide training for HCP on

- The social and psychological needs of women who misuse substances and how to communicate sensitively with such women.
- Social, religious, psychological, and health needs of women who are recent migrants, asylum seekers or refugees, such as needs arising from female genital mutilation or HIV. The most recent government policies on access and entitlement to care for women in these groups.
- The safeguarding responsibilities for both the young woman and her unborn baby. The most recent government guidance on consent for examination or treatment in young women.

Domestic violence (DV)

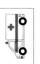

Definition and prevalence

- "Any incident of threatening behaviour, violence or abuse (psychological, physical, sexual, financial or emotional) between adults who are or have been intimate partners or family members, regardless of gender or sexuality".
- In the UK the lifetime prevalence of DV is estimated to be 1 in 3–4 women with an annual prevalence rate of 1 in 9–10 women.
- DV accounts for between 16% and 25% of all recorded violent crime. In any one year, there are 13 million separate incidents of physical violence or threats of violence against women from partners or former partners.
- 26% of women have experienced at least one incident of non-sexual domestic abuse since they were 16. If sexual assault and stalking are included, then 45% of women have experienced at least one incident of inter-personal abuse in their lifetimes.
- The police receives one call about DV every minute in the UK.
- All forms of DV – psychological, economic, emotional, and physical – come from the abuser's desire for power and control over other family members or intimate partners.
- Women experience DV regardless of race, ethnic or religious group, class, disability or lifestyle.
- Factors associated with increased risk of DV include poverty (though not social class) and youth: women < 30 years are at considerably greater risk than those > 40 years.
- The misuse of substances is not the underlying cause of DV.
- Pregnancy can often trigger or exacerbate the DV. In 30% of cases of DV, the abuse first started during pregnancy. The pattern of violence may change with assaults directed to the abdomen, breasts or genitalia.
- Women appear to be at greater risk of DV during the postpartum period and higher rates have been reported in teenage pregnancies.
- 12% of all the women who died of any cause during or immediately after pregnancy had features of DV. (CMACE 2006–2008).
- Higher rates have been associated with increased parity, being divorced or separated, and being better educated than the partner.

Risks or complications

- Serious consequences on physical and mental health.
- Physical health – physical injury due to the assault and sexual injury.
- Mental health – depression, anxiety, post-traumatic stress disorder, suicide.
- Children are involved in up to 36% of cases witnessing or experiencing violence between their parents.
- Adverse effect on pregnancy – obstetric outcome: miscarriage, placental abruption, chorioamnionitis, still birth, LBW babies, and PTL.
- Abdominal trauma may lead to uterine rupture, liver or spleen rupture, fetal fractures, maternal or fetal death in extreme cases.
- An association between risk behaviour and DV has been reported. Smoking, alcohol, and illicit drug use can be an attempt to cope with the trauma and stress of living in an abusive relationship.
- Women experiencing DV appear to be less able to make use of antenatal care, with many booking late and not attending scheduled appointments. More likely to describe pregnancy as unplanned and elect for TOP.

Features of domestic violence

- Various forms of abusive relationship – destructive criticism and verbal abuse; pressure tactics; disrespect; breaking trust; isolation; harassment; threats; sexual violence; physical violence; denial.
- Presence of abuse should be suspected when the women present with – late booking; poor obstetric history; vaginal bleeding; genitourinary infection; injuries to face, head, neck, chest or abdomen; unresolved admissions; repeated presentations with depression, anxiety, self harming, and psychosomatic disorders; substance abuse and alcohol abuse.
- The failure of HCPs to identify DV and offer appropriate intervention has been attributed to a number of factors, including: lack of knowledge and adequate training; lack of time; fear of offending the woman; fear of opening up issues that could get out of control; a belief that domestic violence is not the province of HCPs; feeling powerless to 'fix' the situation.
- In the absence of direct questioning, women do not volunteer information about experiences of DV due to embarrassment and shame.

D. Pregnant women who experience domestic abuse – intervention

- Use of repeat screening and a structured screening questionnaire significantly increases the rate of detection of DV.
- Obstetricians should be alert to DV being the hidden cause of many presenting/recurrent presenting symptoms.

Improve service organization

- **Discuss women's needs with their domestic abuse support agencies** – to provide coordinated care and support during pregnancy.
- **Develop a local protocol** – ensure that an HCP with expertise in the care of women experiencing domestic abuse works with social care providers, the police, and other agencies to jointly develop a local protocol.
- **Provide flexible antenatal services** – provide for flexibility in the length and frequency of antenatal appointments, to allow more time for women to discuss the domestic abuse they are experiencing.
- **Offer a named midwife** who takes responsibility for and provides the majority of her ANC.

Enhance care delivery

- These women may have particular difficulties using antenatal care services. For example, the perpetrator of the abuse may try to prevent her from attending appointments. She may also be afraid that disclosure of the abuse to a HCP will worsen her situation, or be worried about their reaction.
- **Offer confidentiality** – Do not include information which may be used against her in the hand-held antenatal record.
- **Offer information and support** –
  * Offer information about other agencies that provide support for women who experience domestic abuse.
  * Give the woman a credit-card sized information card that includes local and national helpline numbers.

Local protocol for women who experience domestic abuse

- Clear referral pathways that set out the information and care.
- The latest government guidance on responding to domestic abuse.
- Sources of support for women, including addresses and phone numbers, such as social services, the police, support groups, and women's refuges.
- Safety information for women.
- Plan for follow-up care, such as additional appointments or referral to a domestic abuse support worker.
- Obtain a phone number that is safe to contact her.
- Contact details of other people who should be told that the woman is experiencing domestic abuse, including her GP.

Provide training for HCPs

- HCPs need to be alert to features suggesting domestic abuse and offer women the opportunity to disclose it in an environment in which they feel secure.
- **Provide joint training with social care professionals** to:
  * Facilitate greater understanding of each other's roles.
  * Enable HCPs to inform and reassure women who are apprehensive about the involvement of social services.
- **Provide training on domestic abuse** – on the care of women known or suspected to be experiencing domestic abuse that includes:
  * Local protocols; local resources for both the woman and the HCPs.
  * Features suggesting domestic abuse.
  * How to discuss domestic abuse with women experiencing it and how to respond to disclosure of domestic abuse.

Pregnancy and Complex Social Factors: A Model for Service Provision for Pregnant Women with Complex Social Factors; NICE September 2010.
Domestic Violence: Frequently Asked Questions; Factsheet 2009; www.womensaid.org.uk
Statistics: Domestic Violence; www.womensaid.org.uk
Centre for Maternal and Child Enquiries (CMACE). Saving mothers' lives: reviewing maternal deaths to make motherhood safer: 2006–2008. The 8th Report on Confidential Enquiries into maternal deaths in the UK. BJOG 2011; 118 (suppl. 1): 1–203.

INDEX

Printed in the United States
By Bookmasters